Time and
the Inner Future

A TEMPORAL APPROACH TO
PSYCHIATRIC DISORDERS

Time and the Inner Future

A TEMPORAL APPROACH TO PSYCHIATRIC DISORDERS

FREDERICK TOWNE MELGES, M.D.

Professor of Psychiatry
Department of Psychiatry
Duke University School of Medicine

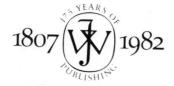

A WILEY-INTERSCIENCE PUBLICATION

JOHN WILEY & SONS

New York · Chichester · Brisbane · Toronto · Singapore

Library of Congress Cataloging in Publication Data

Melges, Frederick Towne, 1935-
  Time and the inner future.

  "A Wiley-Interscience publication."
  Bibliography: p. 325
  Includes index.
  1. Psychology, Pathological. 2. Time perspective.
3. Time perception disorders. 4. Psychotherapy.
I. Title.

RC454.4.M45   616.89   82-6879
ISBN 0-471-86075-1   AACR2

Printed in the United States of America

10 9 8 7 6 5 4 3 2 1

To my mother,
Elizabeth Towne Melges,
who twice gave me life,
first at birth and later by donating her kidney

Foreword

Occasionally there is a new volume in our field which is destined to influence the clinical practice of psychiatry. This book is such a volume. Melges, in a highly creative synthesis, focuses the reader's attention on the importance of time distortions in psychiatric illness. He builds a theory of psychopathology around time and the personal future.

Beginning with an excellent review of research on temporal distortion and psychological time, Melges develops a temporal approach to the psychiatric patient, emphasizing the relevance of time distortions as they cloud the personal future of psychiatric patients. He develops the concept that psychosis is a loss of control of the future, that paranoid thinking is the result of over-futuring, and that depression is a block to the future related to the development of spirals of hopelessness. He relates anxiety and the neuroses to a dread of the future.

The most important components of the book relate to the treatment of psychiatric disorders through an understanding of the temporal distortions they produce. Melges contributes new and highly significant knowledge to the literature on treatment approaches through his excellent chapters on grief-resolution therapy and future-oriented psychotherapy. These chapters outline approaches to the neurotic and psychotic patient that will prove of great utility to our field and impact immeasurably on the overall treatment strategy for mental illness. Melges's principal thesis is that the mentally ill suffer a vicious cycle, or temporal spiral, related to changes induced in their perception of a personal future that may further aggravate their problems with time—with sequence, rate, and temporal perspective.

The treatment of these spirals occurring in most of the major psychiatric disorders and the correction of time problems associated with these spirals form the key ingredient for effective treatment of the psychiatric patient.

Thus this book provides a new and highly creative approach to understanding and treating the loss of control in acute psychosis, blocks to the future in depression, and the dread of the future in neuroses. It is a book well worth reading for it is destined to influence clinical practice for many years to come.

H. KEITH H. BRODIE, M.D.

James B. Duke Professor and Chairman of Psychiatry
Duke University
President, American Psychiatric Association

Acknowledgments

There are innumerable people that I wish to thank for their encouragement, advice, and support in preparing this book. I cannot mention them all, but I hope they know of my gratitude.

Colleagues who shared in the research projects summarized in this book include Jared R. Tinklenberg, Arthur M. Freeman, III, Helena C. Kraemer, Alfred E. Weisz, Leo E. Hollister, David R. DeMaso, and many others. I also thank the National Institute of Mental Health for granting me research support for these projects. Some of my mentors, to whom I am especially indebted, are mentioned in the Prologue.

This book could not have been written without the unswerving support of H. Keith H. Brodie, Professor and Chairman of the Department of Psychiatry at Duke University. I also am grateful to Patricia B. Webster and David B. Larson for their steadfast encouragement. These colleagues, by helping me lead the Duke teaching program and family-oriented inpatient program at Durham County General Hospital, provided a fertile context for the continual testing of the time-related psychotherapies described in this book.

My wife, Connie, and my sons, Rick and Kurt, have helped in many practical as well as inspirational ways. Also, I owe a great deal to my residents, students, and especially my patients for teaching me so much.

For help in preparing the manuscript, I thank Richard W. Bagge, William T. Carpenter, J. B. Chassan, Harvey Kennedy Clow, Arthur M. Freeman, III, John Giragos, Frederick Hine, Michael Kahn, Helena C. Kraemer, David B. Larson, Jane Messer, Herb Reich, Joseph M. Strayhorn, Ervin M. Thompson, Patricia B. Webster, and Irvin D. Yalom.

I am especially grateful for the meticulous work of Vicki B. Pasipanki and Virginia L. Herold for their help with the final stages of the manuscript, particularly the Bibliography and the Indices.

For permission to reprint segments from published works, I thank the editors of the journals listed below:

The Archives of General Psychiatry, with respect to "Types of Hopelessness in Psychopathological Process," by F. T. Melges, and J. Bowlby, Volume 20, pp. 690–699, copyright 1969, American Medical Association; "Temporal Disintegration and Depersonalization During Marihuana Intoxication," F. T. Melges et al., Volume 23, pp. 204–210, copyright 1970, American Medical Association; "The Personal Future and Self-Esteem," by F. T. Melges et al., Volume 25, pp. 494–497, copyright 1971, American Medical Association; "Temporal Disorganization and Delusional-Like Ideation: Processes Induced by Hashish and Alcohol," by F. T. Melges et al., Volume 30, pp. 855–861, copyright 1974, American Medical Association. *The American Journal of Psychiatry* with respect to "Persecutory Delusions: A Cybernetic Model," by F. T. Melges and A. M. Freeman, III, Volume 132, pp. 1038–1044, copyright 1975, The American Psychiatric Association; "Tracking Difficulties and Paranoid Ideation During Hashish and Alcohol Intoxication," by F. T. Melges, Volume 133, pp. 1024–1028, copyright 1976, The American Psychiatric Association; "Temporal Disorganization and Inner-Outer Confusion in Acute Mental Illness," by F. T. Melges and A. M. Freeman, III, Volume 134, pp. 874–877, copyright 1977, The American Psychiatric Association; "Temporal Disorganization, Depersonalization, and Persecutory Ideation in Acute Mental Illness," by A. M. Freeman, III and F. T. Melges, Volume 135, pp. 123–124, copyright 1978, The American Psychiatric Association. *Science*, with respect to "Marihuana and Temporal Disintegration," by F. T. Melges et al., Volume 168, pp. 1118–1120, copyright 1970, American Association for the Advancement of Science. *The Journal of Nervous and Mental Disease*, with respect to "The Personal Future and Suicidal Ideation," by F. T. Melges and A. E. Weisz, volume 153, pp. 244–250, copyright 1971, The Williams and Wilkins Co. *The American Journal of Psychotherapy*, with respect to "Future Oriented Psychotherapy," by F. T. Melges, volume 26, pp. 22–33, copyright 1972; "Grief-Resolution Therapy: Reliving, Revising, and Revisiting," by F. T. Melges and D. R. DeMaso, volume 34, pp. 51–61, copyright 1980. *The British Journal of Psychiatry*, with respect to "Depersonalization Phenomena in a Sample Population of College Students," by J. C. Dixon, Volume 109, pp. 371–375, copyright 1963, The Royal College of Physicians. *Psychological Monographs*, with respect to "Generalized Expectancies for Internal Versus External Control of Reinforcement," by J. B. Rotter, Volume 80 (no. 609), pp. 1–28, copyright 1966, American Psychological Association.

F. T. M.

Contents

Tables and Figures

Prologue

Time has stopped; there is no time. . . . The past and future have collapsed into the present, and I can't tell them apart.

STATEMENT BY AN ACUTE SCHIZOPHRENIC PATIENT

The above statement was made by one of my first patients 18 years ago, shortly after I began my psychiatric residency. He was a highly intelligent physicist in his thirties who had become acutely paranoid. He had none of the time disorientation typical of organic brain disease. Each day that I consulted with him he would desperately try to communicate his uncanny experiences of time. Back then, the standard textbooks of psychiatry offered no explanation for such unusual time experiences other than Freud's (1915, 1933) rather cryptic statement that unconscious processes were "timeless." I was puzzled yet fascinated, since I had come to psychiatry with an interest in biological rhythms and the neuroendocrine control of timing. Further experiences with this and other patients prompted me to question whether disturbances in time sense and timing give rise to lack of control in psychiatric illness. This launched my career of studying various kinds of time distortions in different forms of mental illness.

EMPHASIS ON THE FUTURE

Over the years I came to realize that the importance of time distortions in psychiatric illness was that they cloud the personal future. That is, time distortions, such as alterations of sequence and rate, distort a person's view of his future and thereby disrupt goal-directed behavior.

I also came to realize that a person's view of his personal future, including his expectations, anticipations, and intentions, affects his experience of psychological time. In contrast to my medical and psychiatric training, which emphasized the search for past causes to explain present behavior, I became impressed with another important perspective for understanding human behavior: *the future influences the present.*

I believe that the effect of the personal future on the present has to be added to the traditional psychiatric approaches of the effect of the past on the present. In particular, it appears that how a person constructs his outlook on his personal future determines, in large measure, the time patterns of his life and the ways in which he derives meaning from life.

The emphasis of this book, then, is on the role of time and the personal future in the understanding and treatment of psychiatric disorders. This emphasis is reflected in the title of the book, *Time and the Inner Future.* The inner future refers to a person's inward view of his future unfolding through time.

THE CENTRAL IDEAS AND THEORETICAL FRAMEWORK

The central ideas of this book are summarized in the following general postulates:

1   Humans are by nature goal-directed organisms.
2   A person attempts to gain control over his personal future through an interplay of future images, plans of action, and emotions.
3   Distortions of psychological time disrupt a person's sense of control over the future and lead to psychopathological vicious cycles (spirals).
4   Correction of the time distortions and the harmonization of future images, plans of action, and emotions restore the sense of control over the personal future.

These general postulates will become more clear as they are developed throughout this book. By emphasizing goal-directed behavior and control over the future, it can be seen that the basic theoretical framework of these integrating postulates is that of cybernetic theory.

The postulates are relevant to clinical psychiatry in a number of important ways. In particular, they are relevant to the understanding and treatment of different degrees of loss of control over the future and ensuing spirals in various types of psychiatric illness. In this regard, it appears that the following broad psychiatric categories can be roughly differentiated according to different future outlooks:

1   In psychoses, there is marked loss of control over the future. As the psychotic peers into the future, future images, plans of action, and emotions are confused and disorganized.

2   In depression, the future seems blocked. The depressed person believes that his plans of action are no longer effective for reaching future images and goals.

3   In neurosis, the future seems uncertain and foreboding. The neurotic person feels that something catastrophic might happen in the future.

Once the future becomes clouded, it often induces a vicious cycle since the person's goal-directed behavior is impaired. As a result, there may be progressive mismatches between future images, plans of action, and emotion. This may lead to further spirals of lack of control over the future.

These spirals may become malignant if there are basic time distortions of the sequence and rate of mental processes. Such time distortions, as will be seen, are common in acute psychosis. The time distortions impair the timing and coordination of future images, plans of action, and emotions. Mismatches are then likely to occur.

Another way to state this is that time distortions alter consciousness and impair reality testing. Moreover, whatever the triggering or underlying cause of the time distortion, once a time distortion is present, it will continue to alter consciousness and impair reality testing until it is corrected.

Blocks to the future, such as hopelessness and grief, are common in depression. There are dysjunctions between future images and plans of action. In neurotic anxiety, there is dread of the future. The neurotic person's future images are colored by catastrophic expectations stemming from the past.

The general postulates also provide a framework for focusing psychiatric treatment on time and the future. The restoration of control over the personal future can be accomplished through the correction of time distortions and the harmonization of future images, plans of action, and emotions. The restoration of control over the future is the key to interrupting psychopathological spirals.

PROCESS VERSUS CONTENT

By using a cybernetic framework, I realize that the book presents a series of time-related paradigms that may be new and unfamiliar to clinicians. By emphasizing temporal paradigms, I may not have given sufficient attention to alternative theoretical formulations. For instance, rather than exploring the relationship of time to behavior, I might have examined the relevance of space to behavior and psychopathology. Spatial factors, such as distance–closeness, inclusion–exclusion, and lower–higher, are certainly relevant to social hierarchies. Yet I believe that the form of behavior is primarily temporal in character, especially the timing and synchronization of sequences. This book is an attempt to explore some temporal factors that appear especially relevant to psychiatry.

In my highlighting temporal processes, the emphasis of this book is on process, rather than content, in psychiatric illness and psychotherapy. The unique content of each individual's experience with time and the future would require a series of in-depth case histories. To be sure, in my mind there are numerous case histories behind the scaffolding presented in this book. I have let them come through in the form of brief clinical quotes, examples, and vignettes, but this does not do justice to the richness of content in experiences of acute psychosis, paranoia, neurotic emotionality, hopelessness, grief, and identity diffusion. It is my belief, however, that psychiatrists and psychotherapists often pay too much attention to content rather than process, to *what* the patient is experiencing rather than *how* he is construing the events of his life. In my view the understanding and treatment of processes lead to changes in how the person is framing the content of his experiences.

The question of how a person is construing the events of his life brings to fore considerations of time and the personal future. How is the person connecting events through time? What does he think the events mean for his future? How do his anticipations affect the ways he is construing past and present events as well as other future events?

Time is both a medium and a perspective. It is a medium through which we live as the future becomes present. As the future becomes present, we become aware of duration and succession. Also, by transcending the present and looking at it from the past or future, we gain perspective on the present. These time processes are fundamental to out construction of reality. If they are disturbed, our view of reality may become distorted.

In considering time processes, it is important to point out that whatever the cause of a time distortion, once it occurs it affects the person's psychological organization. That is, the time distortion disturbs the temporal processes through which the person is construing reality. This pertains not only to distortions of sequence and rate but also to blocks or fearful anticipations of the future. Moreover, the cause of the time distortion may be momentary or intermittent (for example, a seizure discharge), and yet the resulting construction of reality may persist with a life of its own at the psychological level because of the person's attributions about the momentary experience (for example, delusions of special powers).

In this regard, it is possible to look at a time distortion as either a manifestation or mechanism of mental illness (Melges and Fougerousse, 1966). That is, it may be a reflection of other causes, or it may be a disrupting factor once it occurs. In this book, rather than just considering distortions of time and the future as manifestations or epiphenomena, I have mainly taken the view that these distortions disrupt a person's psychological organization once they occur. I have done this largely because time seems to be such a fundamental medium and perspective for human psychological organization, and also to explore the usefulness of this viewpoint as a paradigm.

By emphasizing process, rather than content, and by using cybernetic theory, it is my hope that I have not neglected the humanistic richness of experiences of time and the future. In this regard, the dimensions of time and the future reverberate through the central existential issues of death, freedom of choice, isolation, and meaning (Yalom, 1980). In particular, time as a medium and perspective is a fundamental framework through which we give meaning to death, choice, and isolation.

THE ORGANIZATION AND SCOPE OF THIS BOOK

I have divided the material of this book into five major parts. Part I deals with the basic components of psychological time (sequence, rate, and temporal perspective) and leads to a model of control of the future through future images, plans of action, and emotion. Part II outlines the temporal approach to the psychiatric patient by giving an overview of time and the future in psychopathology and provides some general strategies for the clinician for the assessment of time problems and treatment planning, including the use of time in treatment. Part III deals with loss of control of the future in psychoses. Loss of control from difficulties with sequential thinking provides a paradigm for understanding acute psychoses. Attempts to regain control through over-projections into the future provide a model of paranoid thinking. Part IV deals with blocks to the future in depression, such as hopelessness and grief. Part V deals with the neurotic dread of the future and ways of treating emotional spirals through future-oriented psychotherapy. In Parts III, IV, and V, the influence of distortions of time and the future on psychopathological spirals is first discussed and then treatment strategies are outlined.

Finally, at the end of the book, a concluding statement is given. Also, since some terms relating to time and cybernetic processes may be unfamiliar, a glossary is added for the definition of key concepts as used in this book. Some of the research strategies are summarized in the appendixes. More detailed aspects of the research can be found in the cited references.

It can be seen that the scope of this book is broad as it relates to general temporal factors relevant to the fields of psychiatry and psychotherapy. In giving an overview of findings relevant to a temporal theme, my intent is not to resolve controversies in research but rather to acquaint the clinician with a temporal approach to some common clinical problems. Most of the postulates of this book have been confirmed by clinical and experimental investigations as indicated by the cited references. More references could be adduced, but were omitted for brevity. Yet since the approach is relatively new, the postulates remain as hypotheses in need of further refinement and testing. Also, I have made an attempt to combine investigative sources of information with clinical experience; I believe that the latter offers a wealth of information that often goes beyond what can be scientifically measured with the available instruments for inquiry into the human condition.

Since psychological time and the personal future are by nature subjective phenomena, they are not directly observable and have to be measured in terms of what people report about their emotions, images, and plans and how these experiences change over time. This is a fundamental problem of the scientific inquiry into such key psychiatric phenomena as emotions, attitudes, self-images, illusions, and hallucinations (Melges, 1972). The methods that my colleagues and I have developed for testing hypotheses about these subjective phenomena are outlined in the appendixes.

When the terms mankind, man, he, and his are used in this book, reference is being made to both men and women. This has been done for brevity and to streamline the flow of reading.

THE BACKGROUND FOR THIS BOOK

This book has had a gestation period of about 18 years, during which I studied various disorders of psychological time and the personal future in both clinical and experimental settings. Many of its chapters represent a confluence of experiences that impinged upon me during a particular epoch.

Having been trained in psychiatry at the University of Rochester where John Romano and George Engel emphasized the biopsychosocial approach, I was well grounded in psychoanalysis but also open to alternative theoretical formulations about behavior. During my early years in psychiatry, in searching for relevant ideas about time and behavior, two books impressed me a great deal. These were George Kelly's (1955) *The Psychology of Personal Constructs,* which builds a coherent theory of personality in terms of how anticipations govern behavior, and Miller, Galanter, and Pribram's (1960) *Plans and the Structure of Behavior,* which shows how sequences of thought and action become organized through feedback loops. The influence of these two books will be seen throughout this book, particularly in Part I.

During my early years at Stanford, I was exposed to a host of new ideas and approaches to behavior that made me realize some of the limitations of traditional psychiatric thinking. This was both unsettling and stimulating. While being one of the main teachers of psychodynamic formulations and psychiatric diagnosis, I was simultaneously immersed in a variety of different research approaches to behavior. These included neurophysiological and neuroendocrine studies of timing behavior in monkeys, the neuropsychology of emotions, the effect of psychotomimetic drugs in producing time distortions in normal humans, hormonal factors in premenstrual tension and postpartum psychoses, hypnotic time distortions, and the mistiming of communications in family systems. I thank David Hamburg, who was then Chairman of the Department of Psychiatry at Stanford, for making such a diverse, stimulating academic environment possible. My attempts to synthesize these clinical and experimental approaches to behavior helped me to appreciate the different levels of inquiry that are necessary for understanding human time sense.

In this regard, I became convinced that an extended sense of time is unique to humans. Although I learned a great deal about behavioral techniques while doing research on monkeys in the neuropsychology laboratories of Karl Pribram, I also was impressed with the limited temporal capacity of these infrahuman animals. In one experiment it took me four months of daily work to train rhesus monkeys to wait consistently for 90 seconds before pressing a lever to get a reward. This was a far cry from the vast spans of time that concerned my patients. Largely for this reason I became disenchanted with the relevance of using lower animals to study timing behavior, and I therefore returned to human studies.

During this time Karl Pribram and I were hammering away at a neuropsychological theory of emotion (Pribram and Melges, 1969). We came to realize that many of our arguments stemmed from different viewpoints about the time span encompassed by emotions. His viewpoint, taken largely from his work with infrahuman primates, focused mainly on concurrent emotional states (for example, pleasure and displeasure), whereas my viewpoint, taken largely from my clinical work with humans, centered on prospective outlooks reflected in emotions (for example, optimism and pessimism). We finally combined our viewpoints in the published model. This model generated some of the concepts about the interplay of future images, plans, and emotions as discussed in Part I, especially in Chapter 3.

A few years later, while Karl Pribram was studying Freud's project from the standpoint of modern neuropsychology, John Bowlby spent a year at Stanford. Besides helping me translate some psychoanalytic concepts into information theory while dealing with the phenomenon of hopelessness, John Bowlby reawakened my interest in grief, an interest already kindled by my former teacher George Engel. When Erich Lindemann arrived at Stanford, he furthered my interest in grief. I began exploring various ways to treat unresolved grief, but the final form of grief-resolution therapy did not come to full fruition until I got to Duke and North Carolina, where there seemed to be a high incidence of unresolved grief among my patients. These influences culminated in Chapter 10 on grief-resolution therapy.

Erich Lindemann was a dear friend, my next-door neighbor, and one of my main mentors at Stanford. He was very impressed with the relevance of cybernetic theory to psychiatry, and he strongly encouraged the development of future-oriented psychotherapy (Chapter 12). But he taught me more than knowledge; I learned more than I can express as I watched him struggle valiantly with cancer and his own death.

Erich and I wrote a long manuscript on the relevance of time sense to psychiatry as a background for some clinical symposia we did together. This manuscript, which we never attempted to publish, has served as a springboard for much of my research on time and psychosis. A confluence of experiences gave further impetus to these studies. During the same period that I was doing experimental studies (with Jerry Tinklenberg and Leo Hollister) on time distortions during tetrahydrocannabinol (THC) intoxication in normal human subjects, I was also serving as the main clinical teacher of psychiatry at the Stanford-affiliated Santa Clara Valley Medical Center, which had the only locked wards on the Peninsula. I was again impressed with the marked time distortions in these acutely psychotic patients. Also, faced with over 500 acutely paranoid patients per year, Art Freeman and I became aware of the limitations of some of the traditional views about paranoid processes; this spurred the development of our cybernetic model of paranoid thinking (Chapter 8). Meanwhile, much to my surprise, some very trusting, affable, and normal subjects undergoing THC intoxication (in the range of hashish) became acutely paranoid and looked very much like acute paranoid schizophrenics. This prompted further systematic studies of the role of time distortions in acute psychoses, a paradigm summarized in Chapters 4 and 7.

Like most psychiatrists, I have always been keenly interested in psychotherapy. Even when immersed in research and academic pursuits, I have always had a number of patients in psychotherapy. Perhaps because of my research background, as well as my nature, I may be more of a pragmatist than some psychiatrists; I have been alert to procedures that seem to work within a relatively short period of time. I have been fortunate to find kindred souls in this regard, such as Erich Lindemann, Al Weisz, Irv Yalom, and Bob Goulding. As will become clear, the psychotherapies that I have generated make use of both psychoanalytic and behavioral methods for a combined cognitive approach that attempts to integrate emotion, image, and plan toward the future as a means of interrupting vicious cycles.

Finally, the writing of this book was accelerated by a personal crisis that spurred me to try to draw my ideas together. Rather than pursuing further research, which would have been my natural inclination, I wanted to see what could be integrated at this stage about the relevance of time and the future to psychiatry. Moreover, the personal crisis broadened the scope of the book to include an existential interplay of time, meaning, and the future.

I had to deal with the threat of death at a relatively young age. This threat to the future made time become ever so precious (see Epilogue). It also made me realize the wisdom of a statement of Thomas Wolfe (1952, p. 3): "Every moment is the fruit of forty thousand years . . . and every moment is a window on all time."

FREDERICK TOWNE MELGES

Durham, North Carolina
August 1982

Time and the Inner Future

A TEMPORAL APPROACH TO PSYCHIATRIC DISORDERS

PART ONE

Time
and the Control
of the Future

In Part I of this book, I will outline some important relationships between psychological time and the ways in which people attempt to gain control over their personal futures. It is hoped that these background concepts will serve to introduce how distortions of psychological time may disrupt anticipatory control and lead to psychopathological vicious cycles in mental illness, as developed in later parts of this book.

In Chapter 1, the basic components of psychological time are proposed to consist of sequence, rate, and temporal perspective. Sequence refers to successive events. The rate of events refers to their apparent duration. Temporal perspective refers to larger spans of awareness into the past and future. These basic components of psychological time are introduced in terms of varieties of abnormal and normal time experiences, different conceptions of time, and the brain–mind relationship.

Chapter 2 outlines the relationship between psychological time and the personal future in terms of development, emotions, thinking and anticipation, and possible brain mechanisms.

In Chapter 3, I propose that people commonly attempt to gain control over their personal futures through an interplay of future images, plans of action, and emotions. When this interplay is disrupted by distortions of psychological time, lack of anticipatory control and vicious cycles (spirals) may ensue. This cybernetic proposal sets the stage for the discussion of psychopathological spirals as developed in later parts of this book.

CHAPTER ONE

The Role of Time in Experience and Behavior

The processes of the system Ucs. are timeless; i.e., they are not ordered temporally, are not altered by the passage of time; they have no reference to time at all.

SIGMUND FREUD (1915, p. 187)

In 1915 Freud emphasized that, in contrast to the awareness of time relationships in conscious processes, unconscious processes are characterized by timelessness. In 1933 (p. 74) Freud stated that "too little theoretical use" had been made of the timelessness of unconscious processes since it seemed "to offer an approach to the most profound discoveries."

The understanding of time as it relates to the organization of the mind is highly important in psychiatry and psychotherapy. In this regard, a central aim of insight-oriented psychotherapy is to restore continuity of awareness where there are discontinuities between the past and the present. That is, the therapist helps the patient place his present behavior within historical perspectives by discovering insights about how past events influence present thinking, emotions, and behavior.

Yet the role of time in the organization of the mind goes far beyond connecting the present with the past. How a person anticipates future events appears to govern much of human behavior (Kelly, 1955). Also, the continual restructuring of consciousness entails integrating past, present, and future as the person attempts to time his responses to changes in the environment. Altered states of consciousness, which are common in psychiatric illnesses, often involve distortions in the sense of time (Ludwig, 1966). Disorders of psychological time, such as disturbances in rate, sequence, and temporal perspective, may be involved in the disorganized thinking and misconstrued expectations of a variety of psychiatric syndromes. Thus disorders of psychological time may be involved in the disorganization of the mind, and corrections of the time disorders may be important for treatment.

This postulate will be explored throughout this book. In this chapter I will briefly outline some of the varieties of time experiences, different concepts of time, and the possible relevance of time to understanding relationships between the brain and the mind.

VARIETIES OF TIME EXPERIENCE

Uncanny distortions of the sense of time are often incomprehensible to persons who have not experienced them. Only those who have had an acute psychotic episode or have taken a potent psychedelic drug have an inkling of what these ineffable experiences of time are like. Even for these people the experience often seems so much like a dream that, in retrospect, it is difficult for them to report the nature of the timeless experience. During an acute psychosis, inner time often seems stretched out, sometimes like an eternity, and the past, present, and future seem mixed up in a kaleidoscopic whirl. Intermittently time seems to race ahead at an incredible rate but then suddenly comes to a standstill so that the person feels frozen in time. Frequently the person feels that there are unusual time connections, such as uncanny coincidences, deja vu, and precognition. As I will detail later, these distortions of time sense probably play an important role in the defective testing of reality seen in acute psychosis and during psychotomimetic experiences (Chapters 4 and 7).

For the normal person, perhaps the dream experience resembles to some extent the timelessness of acute psychosis. In dreams, past, present, and future are often condensed and transposed (Gross, 1949). Also, there is a feeling of being carried along through time by circumstances that crop up in an unpredictable way. Unlike the waking state, the dreamer usually does not have a feeling of actively striving for long-term goals but rather is carried along by the flow of time.

The feeling of *deja vu* (from French, meaning ''already seen'') is another common experience that resembles in some aspects the acute psychotic state. In deja vu the person feels that what he is experiencing now has occurred before in the exact same way but he does not know when. Sometimes he gets the eerie feeling that he can predict the future. Some forms of acute psychosis, as we will see, are like a prolonged deja vu.

These uncanny experiences of time during an acute psychosis can take place without the time disorientation typical of organic brain disease (Chapter 4). Besides the marked time distortions of an acute psychosis, there are other types of distortions of time and the future in different forms of mental illness. For example, in mania time seems to race, whereas in depression it seems inexorably slow. In depression there is also the feeling that the future is hopeless. In acute anxiety there is the sense of time urgency in association with the dread of a future event. These alterations of time and the future in psychopathology will be discussed in greater detail in Part II.

Besides the time distortions that take place during mental illness, there are some unusual situations that are associated with changes in time sense in the normal person. One is the "near death experience" (Stevenson and Greyson, 1979). Here individuals have come so close to death that they have experienced dying, only to be saved in the nick of time or to be resuscitated. While they are "dying," such persons report a panoramic life review in which images of their whole life reel before their eyes. The sense of time is markedly altered. Often a whole lifetime is reexperienced in just a few minutes of clock time.

Another unusual situation is that of hypnosis. When normal persons are hypnotized, time can be made to slow down, speed up, or the person can be taken back in time to childhood and reexperience that time of life as though he were back there in time (Chapter 6).

There are other changes in time sense and timing that most normal persons have experienced. These include the jet lag that occurs when crossing several time zones in air flight. This appears to be a disturbance in biological rhythms.

So-called peak experiences are another form of timelessness experienced by normal individuals. During a peak experience, there is an exquisite synchrony between the individual, other people, and the environment (Maslow, 1961, 1968).

One of the most common disturbances in the awareness of time in normal people usually takes place in terms of "having too many things come too fast." In our hurly-burly Western society many people suffer from not having enough time to accomplish what they want to do (Silber, 1971). These people are often prone to what has been called the "hurry-up disease" of our culture, termed *Type A behavior,* in which people are always rushing to meet deadlines (Friedman and Rosenman, 1974). This tendency to always rush and to fill one's time with highly competitive activities has been shown to be correlated with coronary artery disease.

Finally, practically everyone has experienced clock time as either dragging or flying by. During periods of waiting, boredom, or unpleasant emotion, clock time seems to drag. By contrast, during periods of interest, commitment, and creativity, time seems to fly.

Thus the experience of inner time can be quite different from the march of clock time. To gain a greater understanding of the differences, I will now turn to the concept of time—that is, how people think about time.

DIFFERENT CONCEPTIONS OF TIME

In the modern Western world, where people are often tyrannized by the clock, it is easy to forget that the concept of clock time and its measurement is a human invention. Before 1642 A.D., which was the time that Galileo invented the first mechanical clock based on the principle of the pendulum (isochronism), people had no handy way to measure time (Hering, 1962). It is hard for the modern mind to even think of what it would be like to conduct one's daily affairs without recourse to a watch or clock.

Clock time, as it is known today, is rooted in the Newtonian concept of time which holds that time can be measured in terms of uniform motion, with equal units of duration flowing linearly from the past toward the future. This is essentially a spatialized notion of time, based on comparing relative motions in terms of distance traveled. For example, when one looks at a clock, it is the movement of its hands through space over the stationary dial that indicates a change in time. According to Newton's classical mechanics, time equals distance divided by velocity ($t = d/v$). This is only one view of time, one which has been accepted as a convention. The concept is highly dependent on the notion of velocity. The Einstein-Minkowski space-time theory fixed the upper limit of velocity at the speed of light. This gave rise to some paradoxes which were hard to understand for those wedded to the Newtonian concept of time. For example, assuming that the speed of light is the absolute upper limit of velocity, then as one's velocity approaches the speed of light, there is less relative motion and hence time would slow down. This suggests that a man in a spaceship traveling at speeds close to the velocity of light might get younger, while his twin back on earth would continue to grow older as usual.

Paradoxes such as the above jar one's common sense, including one's customary sense of time. Although the four-dimensional space-time of Einstein and Minkowski has revolutionized certain aspects of physics, its practical applications pertain largely to bodies or particles traveling at extremely fast velocities. Einstein himself said that relativistic concepts about space-time had little to do with the "local" time of people in this world. Yet the theory does show that the customary concepts about time can be radically changed. There is no absolute universal time that can be used as a cosmic frame of reference to determine if two events that are a great distance from one another occur simultaneously or if one precedes the other. Although such relativistic concepts about time have little to do with the practicalities of everyday life, including the use of time as an invariant in scientific experiments, it is possible that an equally radical revision of the concepts of biological and psychological time might give new insights into how the brain works.

The concept of time is not limited to duration (that is, time passing by). The English word *time* is derived from several roots that suggest its multiple meanings (Meerloo, 1970). Its original root *ti* means to stretch, and in this way suggests the span of duration stretching over events. But *ti* is also the source of tides, referring to rhythms, as well as the source of temps, referring to changes, as in tempest and temperature. Still another linguistic link is to tidy and tidiness, referring to order and orderliness. Stretching over, rhythms of change, and order are thus condensed in the word *time*.

In its broadest sense time can be considered as a construct that refers to the perception or imputation of changes against some background that is taken to be relatively permanent (Fraser, 1975). For a change to be perceived or imputed, there has to be both succession and duration (Kummel, 1966). That is, when two successive events are separated by an interval, the interval between them is called *duration*. Here duration is defined by succession. The reverse also holds: For two events to be successive, there has to be a time-gap (duration) between them.

When duration and succession are extended backwards from the *now*, or present, the past, or *after-now*, is constructed. Likewise when duration and succession are extended forward, the future, or *before-now*, is constructed (Rescher and Urquhart, 1971). Past, present, and future are the basic elements of what is called *temporal perspective*. The recognition of change usually means that an event emerges from the future, becomes present, and then becomes past. Thus the three basic components of time—duration, succession, and temporal perspective—are closely linked. One of them cannot be conceived of without the other.

The notions of rhythm and order consist of time patterns superimposed on the basic framework of duration, succession, and temporal perspective. That is, rhythm is a repetition of a succession that occurs at regular intervals (durations), like the beat or tempo of a piece of music. A rhythm has order since the nature of the successive intervals is repetitive. Order also can come from a fixed before–after sequence, with one type of successive event regularly followed by another type, as in *AB, AB,* and so on.

The above notions of duration, succession, and temporal perspective are couched within a linear time framework. The Western mind assumes time to be linear, traveling from the past through the present toward the future, like time's arrow. For the Western mind there is also the belief in a progressive upward thrust as one goes from the past toward the future. That is, there is a belief in progress. The Western concept of time as linear can be contrasted with the Eastern or Oriental view of time as cyclical (Needham, 1966). The Oriental philosophers, rather than using an arrow, use a circle to symbolize time. Overall, the direction of the cycles is downward rather than upward. This downward direction is sometimes counteracted by the ultimate belief that, if things get bad enough, there is likely to be the start of another cycle.

There are even some cultures that do not have a language for past, present, and future. In such cultures time is nonlinear. One such culture is the people of the Trobriand Islands (Lee, 1950). The Trobrianders do not assume a timeline of reality. They do not draw inferences from the past or make predictions about what events mean in terms of leading to some future state. For them time appears to be a holistic pattern. It is the pattern that accounts for the events, not one event leading to the next. Lee (1950) points out that this is like knitting a sweater; it is the pattern that generates the parts.

Another culture in which time is nonlinear is that of the Hopi Indians (Whorf, 1956). The Hopi Indians have no words for past, present, and future. For them events that the Western mind would place in the past or future are still present. There is a continual becoming, with past anticipations becoming realized in what Western societies would call present and with present anticipations and preparations ever emerging as future realizations. Rather than dividing reality according to a timeline and saying that "a wave comes into the shore, splashes, and then recedes," the Hopi Indians would refer to the whole process with some word like "slush."

According to Whorf (1956), the way men frame reality depends a good deal on the words and language they have invented within a particular culture. If the world is divided into past, present, and future, then a linear reality is the common frame of reference. By contrast, if there are no words for past, present, or future, then reality becomes construed in terms of nonlinear relationships.

It would be very difficult for the Western mind to describe reality without constructs like past, present, and future, or duration and succession. These constructs are part of our common sense. Even if they are illusions, they have proven useful for the conduct of our practical life. They also provide the backbone for scientific method. The conception of time as linear is necessary for the scientific testing of hypotheses through prediction and accumulation of recurrences. To test a prediction, not only must the past, present, and future be kept distinct, but also there must be precision about succession and duration (that is, about when and in what order the predicted events will occur and for how long the prediction holds). It is this method of testing predictions by attempting to disprove them that has stripped Western culture of many of its former beliefs in magic, animism, and vague prophecy (Popper, 1965).

Cultures that have no concept of linear time appear to be vulnerable to the influence of myths and magic, perhaps because they have no ready method for distinguishing fact from fantasy.

Thus there is little doubt that a linear concept of time is useful. Whether it is the only useful way to conceptualize time is open to question. I will later deal with the possible merits of simultaneous processes, of seeing holistic patterns, like the Trobrianders and the Hopi Indians.

Although the ways in which people conceptualize time and measure it are human constructs and inventions, few would hold that time is merely a figment of the imagination. It refers to a process common to our experiences. Also, all living organisms appear to have a sense of time. That is, infrahuman species show biological timing mechanisms that can obviously function without recourse to human inventions such as the clock. The ability to store information over time is a fundamental characteristic of living organisms (Miller, 1976). Without this ability it would be difficult for an organism to synchronize its responses with periodic changes in the environment so that there is an exchange of foodstuffs, and so on, at the right time (Goodwin, 1976). Biological rhythms are perhaps the most rudimentary timing mechanisms of living organisms. They appear even in tiny creatures whose nervous systems are infinitely smaller than that of the human. For example, the tiny beach crab (*Talitrus*), with only one millimeter of nerve tissue, is able to "calculate" the time of day and the course of an hour (Portmann, 1962). Bees that have been trained to come for food at a certain time in Paris, when transported to New York, keep coming for food according to Paris time, even though the light–dark cycle is completely different in New York (Renner, 1955). Also, at higher phylogenetic levels, besides the persistence of biological rhythms, animals can be conditioned to time itself, indicating that there is some biological way of registering time. That is, an interval of time can serve as a discriminative stimulus which, with reinforcement, can become a conditioned stimulus that evokes a conditioned response; after training, at a later time, the passage of the interval itself can trigger a conditioned response. For this to happen in animals who have no symbolic way to represent time, duration must somehow be perceived and registered at a biological level.

Biological time relationships can differ from those of the physical sciences. Probably the most fundamental difference is the importance of *now* in biological systems (Fraser, 1978). For an organism to synchronize with periodic changes in the environment or with other organisms, what is happening *now* in the other systems has to be taken into account in relation to the *now* of the organism. There are numerous examples of the importance of the *now* for biological adaptation: Bees synchronize their search for nectar with the time that flowers open their petals to the sun; birds migrate southward just before the Northern climates turn colder; the dominant male chimpanzee waits until the female is at the precise time of ovulation in her estrus cycle before he has intercourse with her, thereby ensuring the preservation of the species.

Thus in the biological world the synchronization of various systems takes place around the critical interface of *now*. There is a time and place for everything, as the saying goes. By contrast, the *now* is relatively unimportant in the geophysical sciences. In these sciences contingencies (if *x*, then *y*) hold regardless of when. That is, cause leads to effect regardless if *now* is yesterday or today. By contrast, the difference between a *now* yesterday and today may be vast in terms of different constellations of periodic changes impinging upon biological systems.

There are also fundamental differences between the linear concept of geophysical time, as codified in the clock, and psychological time, the inner time of the mind (Fraser, 1981). These differences will be dealt with throughout this book. At this point, some of the key differences can be summarized as follows:

Geophysical (Clock) Time	Psychological Time
Now relatively unimportant.	*Now* important for coordinating with other systems.
Uniform motion.	Inward tempo can be accelerated or decelerated.
Sequences have a fixed order, once they have occurred.	Sequences can be reversed in the mind.
Unidirectional toward the future.	Multidirectional, backwards and forwards, into past or future.

In contrast to the geophysical notion of units of time flowing equally one after the other from the past toward the future, psychological time can differ from clock time in terms of rate (duration), sequential ordering, and temporal perspective. In psychological time the experience of duration can be prolonged or shortened by accelerating or decelerating inner tempo, sequences can be reversed and reordered, and the mind can go backwards and forwards into the past or future. In this regard, while the invention of the clock has greatly aided our precision in synchronizing activities with other systems, in some respects the clock can be looked upon as a prosthesis or code system through which humans express transformations of time made within the mind.

TIME AND THE BRAIN–MIND RELATIONSHIP

The human mind can be thought of as an organization for making time connections. The mind interrelates past, present, and future largely for the purpose of making inductive inferences about the future (Von Forster, 1965). That is, on the basis of collating past events relevant to the present situation, it computes the nature and likelihood of certain future events. Korzybski (1926) emphasized this special "time-binding" quality of the human mind. Without the ability to replay and transform experiences of the past, present, and future in terms of symbolic representations, language would be impossible except for making gestures to things seen in the present.

Fraser (1975) refers to the human brain as "the organ of time sense." In this regard, Von Monokov and Mourgue (1930), as well as Kappers (1930), emphasized that the central nervous system works according to "time-binding principles," particularly through its registration of the simultaneity of events during learning and development. Pavlov (1927) also highlighted the importance of the temporal contiguity of events (stimuli and reinforcements) for conditioning to take place in the brain. More recently Wallis (1966) and MacKay (1962) have stressed that the brain may process information primarily on the basis of temporal codes and frequency analysis. Along this line John (1976) and Pribram (1971, 1976) suggest that complex processes, such as memory, may work by the superimposition of temporal rhythms transmitted throughout the brain.

Esteemed neurologists and neurophysiologists have noted the importance of neural timing as it relates to behavior but have been baffled by it (Lashley, 1929, 1951, 1958). Indeed, Lord Brain (1963) believed that central issues of the brains–mind problem could be approached by attempting to answer the following question: How can an instant of "brain time" refer to vast spans of psychological time extending into the past and future?

The role of various areas of the brain in contributing to different aspects of psychological time will be outlined briefly in Chapters 2 and 4. For now suffice it to say that when the whole brain becomes diseased, all components of psychological time—rate, sequence, and temporal perspective—become chaotic and behavior becomes markedly disorganized. An intact brain appears necessary for the temporal organization of the mind.

At this stage the central point is that time constitutes a fundamental process of what is called *mind*. That is, time is important for many key functions of the mind, ranging from conditioning to planning.

In classical conditioning there is an optimal time interval for the formation of a conditioned response (Pavlov, 1927). That is, stimuli and reinforcements have to occur together within an interval somewhere between 0.5 and 0.75 seconds in order for a conditioned response to be formed (Fraisse, 1963; Prescott, 1966; Jenkins, 1970). In operant conditioning it is best to have rewards and punishments follow immediately after responses in order to modify behavior (Dollard and Miller, 1950; Skinnoz, 1953).

The capacity to maintain behavior by delayed reward increases as one goes up on the phylogenetic scale. A rat can sustain a delay of about 4 minutes, a cat 17 hours, and a chimpanzee 48 hours (Cohen, 1966). Of course, the capacity of humans for delayed reward is much longer.

One of the most distinctive human characteristics is the capacity to bring together vast spans of time. To quote Boulding (1956, p. 201), "Man is distinguished from the animals . . . by a much more elaborate image of time and relationships; man is probably the only organization that knows that it dies, that contemplates in its behavior a whole life span, and more than a life span."

It is possible that man's capacity for an extended sense of time and temporal relationships is his greatest evolutionary gift. The capacity for language appears to depend on the ability to make temporal discriminations (Efron, 1963a, 1963b; Neff, 1964; Eisler, 1968; Jones, 1976). Also, the perception and inference of a cause–effect relationship, which is fundamental to human thought, depends a great deal on noting before–after sequences (Michotte, 1958; Chisholm and Taylor, 1960). Moreover, the human ability to consider future consequences has given mankind survival skills unprecedented in the animal kingdom.

Thus it appears that many key functions of the human brain relate to its capacity to make extended time connections. These time connections constitute most of what is generally referred to as mind. The mental processes of the human mind entail different ways of making time connections, including classical conditioning, instrumental learning, delayed reward, the attribution of cause–effect relationships, language and symbolism, and the anticipation of future consequences. What is called mind, then, appears to depend on the human brain's capacity to connect segments of time that transcend the immediate perception of present events.

In contrast to infrahuman animals who are largely bound to present stimuli, the human comprehension of reality extends beyond the present into the past and future. While this capacity to collate vast spans of time has given humans coping skills unprecedented in the animal kingdom, it also may make humans especially vulnerable to distortions of reality when there is malfunctioning of the temporal processes.

SUMMARY AND CONCLUSIONS

This chapter has given a general overview of the important role of time in the mind. The major points are summarized below:

1   It is proposed that disorders of psychological time are involved in the disorganization of the mind and that correction of time disorders may be important for treatment.

2   There are a variety of time experiences, ranging from the timelessness of an acute psychosis to the experience of time dragging or flying by in the normal person.

3   In Western societies time is conceptualized to be linear. In this framework the basic components of time consist of rate (duration), sequence (succession), and temporal perspective covering spans of time into the past and future. In contrast to these linear concepts of time, there are cultures which have cyclical and nonlinear concepts of time.

4   Timing and time sense appear to be fundamental functions of living organisms. In lower forms of life timing is primarily manifested in terms of biological rhythms, and at higher phylogenetic levels animals can be conditioned to time itself.

5   Similar to clock time, the fundamental components of psychological time also consist of rate (duration), sequence, and temporal perspective. Although these components are the same as geophysical (clock) time, it is possible for psychological rate, sequence, and temporal perspective to differ markedly from clock time.

6   The capacity of the human brain to integrate time and make time connections plays an important role in what is generally referred to as mind. Many key mental functions are time dependent. These include conditioning, learning, the attribution of causality, expectations and anticipations, and the capacity for language and symbolism. These functions allow humans to transcend the present so that past events can be related to future consequences.

7   It is possible that the human capacity for an extended sense of time is man's unique evolutionary gift, yet it also may make him vulnerable to distortions of reality when the time processes go awry.

CHAPTER TWO

Psychological Time
and the Personal Future

I think it is fair to say that no theory of psychology will ever be complete which does not centrally incorporate the concept that man has his future within him, dynamically active in this present moment.

ABRAHAM MASLOW (1968, p. 15)

The future is dynamically active within a person. Most of the so-called higher brain functions of *homo sapiens,* such as language and symbolism, are related to this capacity to transcend the present and foresee future possibilities. This capacity has enabled humans to be proactive toward the future rather than being like lower animals who are largely reactive and time bound to events happening in the present (Litchfield and Sattler, 1968).

A person's span of awareness into the future is called *future time perspective*. This chapter will highlight the importance of future time perspective in the experience of psychological time. In doing this, I will give a brief overview of the interrelationship between time sense and future time perspective in terms of psychological studies, development, emotions, different temporal modes of thinking, and possible brain processes. These considerations will touch on the following general theme: *The experience of time is closely related to a person's span of awareness into the future.*

In giving an overview of concepts and data relevant to this theme, the discussion will focus on relationships and constructs which provide the background for the role of time and the future in psychopathology and psychiatric treatment, as developed in later parts of this book. For those readers interested in the controversies and complexities of the research, please refer to the cited references and the salient reviews of the literature, such as those by Wallace and Rabin (1960), Fraisse (1963), Fraser (1966), Orme (1969), and Doob (1971).

The clinical relevance of the central theme of this chapter will become clear in Part II. For now suffice it to say that when a person experiences an alteration in time sense, it is likely that his internal processes necessary for making adjustments to goals have gone awry.

TIME SENSE AND FUTURE TIME PERSPECTIVE

The term *time sense* usually refers to how a person is experiencing the passage of time. That is, clock time seems to be going either slow or fast compared to one's estimate of the amount of time passing by. There are various research methods for measuring this comparison of a person's internal estimation of duration with standards of clock time (see Appendix A). A good deal of research indicates that if a person's so-called internal clock is going fast, then outside clock time by comparison seems to be going slow (Hoagland, 1950; Frankenhauser, 1959; Doob, 1971). This speeding of the hypothetical internal clock can occur with rises in temperature, stimulant and psychedelic drugs, and emotional distress in acute mental illness (Melges and Fougerousse, 1966). Thus, in general, the greater frequency of internal changes per unit of clock time makes clock time *seem* to be longer.

However, further research has indicated that the estimation of duration is not just a matter of comparing internal rate with the rate of passage of clock time. Ornstein (1969) has shown that the subjective experience of duration is related not only to the frequency of successive changes but also to the complexity and organization of the stimuli within a person's span of attention. The latter is related to the capacity of immediate memory, which is usually limited to holding in mind about seven elements at a given time (Miller, 1956; Fraisse, 1963). In general, when stimuli are complex or unorganized within immediate memory, there appears to be a greater frequency of successive changes, and duration therefore appears to be prolonged. Also, if immediate memory is impaired, the storage capacity for incoming stimuli is reduced, giving rise to an apparent crowding of incoming stimuli, making internal rate seem fast compared to clock time. The combination of these factors may have clinical relevance since they may account for some of the marked alterations in time sense seen in acute schizophrenia and during psychotomimetic drug intoxication (see Chapter 7).

Thus the sense of time stems from more than a simple comparison of rates of change. Moreover, the three fundamental components of psychological time—rate, sequence, and temporal perspective (see Chapter 1)—appear to be interrelated in a person's experience of time passing by. In general, the rate of successive changes appears to speed up when the person feels pressed to accomplish a goal within a relatively short span of future time (Schonbach, 1959). In such a situation the amount of future time seems relatively short, but the experience of clock time, while it is passing by, seems prolonged. A common example of this is the apparent lengthening of the passage of time toward the end of a close game such as in basketball. By contrast, when there is no urgent goal to be accomplished and future time span appears open and unrestricted, clock time seems to pass by normally (Wohlford, 1964, 1966).

The above proposal has emphasized future time perspective as a context within which the rate of successive changes is appreciated. It should be noted that there are other dimensions of temporal perspective than the span of awareness into the future. For example, there is temporal perspective into the past, which refers to the amount of past time encompassed into one's awareness. Past temporal perspective does not appear to be as important for the sense of duration as future time perspective. Perhaps the reason for this is that as a future event gets nearer to the present, it takes on a greater demand character (Lewin, 1942; Cottle and Klineberg, 1974).

The role of the future in the experience of duration has been neglected in many psychophysical studies of the microstructure of psychological time and of time estimation, but it has been emphasized by some scholars of time. For example, Minkowski (1933) felt that it was difficult to comprehend "lived time" except in relation to the personal future. In addition, in an extensive review of psychological time, Fraisse (1963, p. 210) stated, "The experience of duration . . . arises from a comparison of what is with what will be, i.e., from awareness of the interval separating two events."

In summary, it appears that rate (duration), sequence, and future time perspective are interrelated. A greater frequency of successive sequences within a relatively short future time span is associated with a fast internal rate, making clock time by comparison seem to be going slowly. By contrast, long intervals between sequences within an open future time span appear to be associated with a slower internal rate, making clock time seem to be passing by normally or faster than usual. Moreover, if there is no pressing goal to be accomplished, the person may not be aware of the passage of time since there is no need to pay attention to it. It appears that a person's experience of time is closely related to his span of awareness into the future.

THE DEVELOPMENT OF TIME SENSE AND FUTURE TIME PERSPECTIVE

The development of time sense and future time perspective occurs throughout childhood. Moreover, they appear to develop in relation to one another. That is, as future time perspective becomes more extended and complex, the child's experience and concept of time matures (Wallace and Rabin, 1960).

In the infant the first experience of duration is thought to occur during waiting periods of unmet needs, such as hunger (Fraisse, 1963; Piaget, 1966). According to Spitz (1972), the infant reaching out for the breast or the mother is the prototype of early temporal experience. The interval between "the cup and the lip" during periods of suspenseful waiting is deemed to be the early experience of time (Hartocollis, 1972).

If the mother is predictable in meeting the infant's needs, then the infant develops what Erikson (1959) calls "basic trust." Erikson (1959, p. 141) defines basic trust as the "inner conviction that—after all—sufficient satisfaction is sufficiently predictable to make waiting . . . worthwhile." By contrast, if the mothering figure is unpredictable, unreliable, or absent, there is lack of development of basic trust and the child's development of time sense is impaired. Infants deprived of adequate mothering do not develop a mature sense of time (Bender, 1947; Chambers, 1961; Campos, 1963).

Since the infant has little sense of time and anticipation, he is unable to postpone gratification: the infant "wants what he wants when he wants it." As development proceeds into early childhood, there is an increase in the capacity to delay gratification so that the child learns to wait and expect and, later, to plan (Rapaport, 1960; Singer, 1974). This increasing capacity to delay gratification appears to be related to the growth of anticipatory processes, particularly as mediated by language and more complex visual imagery of future possibilities (Piaget and Inhelder, 1966; Paivio, 1971; Kagan, 1979). It is not until about the eighth year of life that a normal child's language reflects a full understanding of past, present, and future (Ames, 1946). Also, around the eighth year of life there is a decisive increment in anticipatory processes (Piaget and Inhelder, 1966), and the child's concept of time becomes more abstract and operational (Piaget, 1966). In this regard, it is interesting that abstract thinking involves being able to deal with that which is not here and not now in new ways, particularly the capacity to consider future possibilities (Goldstein, 1939; Goldstein and Scheerer, 1941). When the child is less concretely bound to present stimuli and able to extend his thinking to future possibilities, he appears to be more capable of abstract reasoning.

A completely abstract notion of time is not achieved until about age 13 or 14 years (Wallace and Rabin, 1960). Also, future time perspective develops rapidly during adolescence. The adolescent is faced with choices about what to do with his future time and how to make it meaningful.

In this regard, Erikson (1959, p. 123) has pointed out the future becomes increasingly "tangible" for the adolescent who must make choices about physical intimacy, occupation, competition, and psychosocial self-definition. The choices and commitments that he makes are important for the formation of identity. Erikson (1959, p. 89) states that the sense of identity comes from "the accrued confidence that one's ability to maintain inner sameness and continuity . . . is matched by the sameness and continuity of one's meaningful others." These predictable time patterns appear necessary for the development of identity.

Adolescents who have difficulty in making choices and future commitments often experience a diffusion of identity. A key feature of identity diffusion is "time diffusion," where there is a mistrust of time itself with the "disbelief in the possibility that time may bring change, and yet also a violent fear that it might" (Erikson, 1959, p. 126). Time becomes diffused because it brings tension, conflict, and frustration. The tension usually is between the familiarity of the past versus the uncertainty of future directions.

Adolescents who form firm identities are more realistically future oriented than maladjusted adolescents (Cottle and Klineberg, 1974). Moreover, adolescents who are successful in meeting new challenges commonly employ detailed future rehearsals (Teahan, 1958; Goldrich, 1961; Ezekiel, 1968).

Whereas the experience and concept of duration and of past, present, and future becomes fully developed during adolescence, it appears that future time perspective is further altered by later life stages, although there is less systematic research on this (Buhler and Massarik, 1968; Neugarten, 1979). For the young adult a common conflict is between making long-term future commitments and keeping one's options open (Levinson et al., 1978). During middle age, a person commonly reappraises his life in terms of the time he expects to have left to live (Neugarten, 1979). In this regard Sheehy (1974) has called middle age the "deadline decade." Older persons commonly engage in a life review in order to appreciate the meaning of their own and others' lives within an overall temporal perspective. These different time perspectives during later life stages need further research since a person's "behavior is profoundly affected by his view of the time process in which he stands" (Boulding, 1956, p. 201).

EMOTIONS, TIME, AND THE FUTURE

Emotions and the sense of time are closely linked. Emotions serve as signals of time urgency as well as about what is expected to happen in the future (Monat, 1976). This linkage between emotions, time, and the future begins during early development and continues into adulthood.

In the infant the early impression of duration goes hand in hand with emotional experiences. As outlined in the previous section, if a need is aroused in the infant, such as hunger, and this need is not met in time, then the infant shows signs of distress and often cries violently until the need is satisfied (Rapaport, 1960). When the need is met in time, the infant becomes quiescent and may show signs of pleasure. Thus the early experiences of pleasure and displeasure are associated with the interval between the present and the future during states of aroused needs.

This function of emotions as overall signals of expectations of self and others has been emphasized by Freud (1926), Arnold (1960), R. Lazarus (1966), and Beck (1971). In particular, Beck (1971) indicates that various emotions can be differentiated in terms of expected risks or gains. For example, a person's expectation of a gain in his life domain is often reflected as euphoria, a loss as sadness, an interference as anger, and a threat of danger as fear or anxiety.

In this regard, emotions are usually aroused when an ongoing plan of action is interrupted and there is a change in expected reinforcement (Melges and Poppen, 1976). Once aroused, emotions commonly reflect different appraisals of what is likely to happen in the future (Melges and Bowlby, 1969). That is, besides the experience of pleasure or displeasure, which reflect the current state of affairs, most emotions also reflect optimism or pessimism about the personal future (Pribram and Melges, 1969; Melges and Harris, 1970). For example, hope is obviously optimistic, depression is pessimistic, and with anxiety the person is either threatened or uncertain about the personal future. Krauss (1967) describes how anxiety is commonly the dread of a future event.

Once a given emotion is aroused, it usually outlasts the inciting stimulus. That is, unlike transitory thoughts and perceptions, emotions are relatively long-lasting phases of the mind. They are like "fields of awareness" that can bias subsequent thinking, perception, and action. As such, emotions serve to prompt motives (dispositions toward action). As signals about expected outcomes, emotions commonly help the person to maintain or gain control over situations by guiding the reorganization of plans and goals (Melges and Harris, 1970). This thesis will be elaborated in Chapter 3. Also, the power of emotions to reflect distorted expectations and prompt vicious cycles will be detailed in Chapter 11.

Thus as signals of expected outcomes, emotions reflect overall subjective probabilities about reaching valued goals within a desired or necessary time period (Melges and Harris, 1970). That is, a given emotion, such as euphoria or depression, reflects the person's appraisal of the likelihood or unlikelihood of his reaching goals that are central to his existence within a certain time frame. In this way emotions serve as overall signals about the personal future.

Besides serving as signals about the personal future, different emotions also reflect different urgencies about time and are associated with different impressions of time passing by (subjective duration). In general, pleasant emotions are associated with a normal sense of time, whereas unpleasant emotions are associated with a feeling of time urgency and a fast internal rate, making clock time by comparison *seem* to be passing by slowly (Melges and Fougerousse, 1966).

There are a host of studies that indicate a faster internal rate, making clock time seem to go slowly, during unpleasant emotions such as anxiety (Kahn, 1966; Burns and Gifford, 1961; Pearl and Berg, 1963). In addition, during unpleasant emotions, future time perspective is foreshortened (Wohlford, 1964, 1966; Epley and Ricks, 1963; Melges and Weisz, 1971). By contrast, during pleasant emotions future time perspective is longer and is experienced as open and unrestricted. Perhaps the reason for this is that during pleasant states there is little need to accomplish a goal (such as restoring an interpersonal relationship) within a short period of time. That is, there is less time urgency during pleasant emotions.

Thus, in line with the general thesis of this chapter, emotions appear to monitor a person's awareness of the passage of time as it relates to the personal future.

To conclude this section, the relationships between emotion and time sense are portrayed in a quip made by Albert Einstein: "When you sit with a nice girl for two hours, you think it's only a minute. But when you sit on a hot stove for a minute, you think it's two hours. That's relativity."

THINKING AND ANTICIPATION

Now that the role of expectation and anticipation in emotions has been outlined, it should be obvious that there is an interplay between emotion and cognitive processes, including thinking, perception, and memory. This interplay has been stressed by a number of scholars (Beck, 1971; Tomkins, 1963, 1967; Izard, 1977). It appears that the appraisal of outcomes reflected in emotional signals involves an interplay of cognitive processes as they relate to anticipation (Kelly, 1955).

It is beyond the scope of this book to review the vast area of cognition. Nevertheless, some tentative generalizations will be made in order to point to different temporal modes of thinking that appear to be involved in the process of anticipation.

The term *anticipation* usually refers to the process of preparing to respond to a future event in advance of its occurrence. Arieti (1947) makes the distinction between expectation and anticipation: expectation refers to a replay of a past sequence in a similar situation, whereas anticipation goes beyond expectation to future events for which there is no current clue of their recurrence. So defined, expectation is not difficult to explain on the basis of memory, that is, as a replay of past sequences. However, anticipation cannot be so readily explained. It appears to involve the transformation and synthesis of memories (Paivio, 1971; Piaget, 1947).

It is probable that at least three types of memory are involved in anticipation: immediate, short term, and long term (Baddeley, 1976). Immediate memory refers to the tracking of sequences that happened just seconds ago; short-term memory, to events from a few minutes to hours ago; and long-term memory, to events days or years ago. As is well known, memory fades with time (Ebbinghaus, 1913; McGaugh, 1956). In particular, events in immediate memory and in short-term memory become hazy with the passage of time, and for long-term memory people generally have to reconstruct events of the distant past (Bartlett, 1932; Norman, 1970; Neisser, 1966). Bartlett (1932) proposed that the reconstruction of the past is guided by a process of reconstruction, "an effort after meaning." "An effort after meaning" may also take place during anticipation. That is, according to some emotional need to gain control over a future event, a person may begin to collate events of the distant past relevant to the flow of recent events. This process is commonly witnessed during a psychiatric interview (see Chapter 5).

The three types of memory appear to generate the elements about which the person begins to think. In Western society *to think* usually means to organize one's thoughts sequentially toward a goal (Efron, 1967). But such sequential thinking is only one type of thinking (Ornstein, 1972). There is also "primary process thinking," which is not goal directed (Freud, 1911, 1920). In addition, a third type of thinking has been proposed that appears to process visual displays simultaneously (Bogen, 1974).

These proposed types of thinking are presented in Table 1 as primary,

Table 1 Proposed Time Relationships for Different Types of Thinking

Type of Thinking	Relations of Past, Present, and Future	Probes into Future	Examples
Primary process	Timeless	Random hunches	Dreams
Secondary process	Sequential	Prediction	Reasoning: "1st *X*, 2nd *Y*, 3rd *Z*" "If *X*, then *Y*."
Tertiary process	Simultaneous	Holistic patterns	Metaphor: "*A* looks like *C* but both look unlike *B*."

secondary, and tertiary thinking. Each type of thinking appears to operate according to a different temporal mode.

In primary process, relationships between past, present, and future are not kept distinct, and experiences often seem timeless. Dreams and the dynamic unconscious operate according to primary process (Freud, 1901). In dreams events often crop up in an unpredictable way, the dreamer is focused almost exclusively on what is happening in the present, and yet there is often a telescoping of events that during waking would be kept distinct as past, present, and future (Gross, 1949). In this regard Freud (1915) emphasized the timelessness of primary process. It is possible that other characteristics of primary process, such as fluid symbolism, condensations, and contradictions, could stem from timelessness (Melges et al., 1974).

Secondary process thinking is step-by-step reasoning. There is sequential order to secondary process, such as *first do X, second Y, and third Z* (Horowitz, 1970). Contingent sequences also are tested, such as *if X, then Y*. The testing of scientific predictions is rooted in secondary process thinking. In secondary process the sequences are organized toward a goal, as when one makes a point, disproves a hypothesis, or plans a trip. It can be seen that secondary process is the type of thinking with which most people are familiar, particularly since it is emphasized in Western society.

By contrast, many people are unfamiliar with tertiary process thinking, although they may employ aspects of it in everyday living. Indeed, psychiatrists, psychologists, and neurophysiologists are just beginning to define what is meant by tertiary process thinking. The temporal mode of this form of thinking appears to be simultaneous (Table 1). That is, elements of the past, present, and future are seen all at once as holistic patterns which are often captured in metaphors (Jaynes, 1976; Ornstein, 1972). The holistic patterns often represent a synthesis of visual images from which intuitions about the future arise. There is increasing evidence that the right (nondominant) cerebral hemisphere may be primarily involved in simultaneously processing visual displays (Galin, 1974; Carmon, 1978). This will be discussed further in the next section on the brain.

Tertiary process thinking has been proposed to be involved in creativity. In this regard creative thinking commonly employs visual imagery and the simultaneous juxtaposition of antithetical ideas (Rothenberg, 1971, 1976, 1979). This process of simultaneously bringing together seemingly opposite ideas into visual juxtaposition appears to be involved in creative intuitions not only in art and literature but also in science. Metaphors appear to be useful vehicles for this simultaneous juxtaposition (Stein, 1975, 1978; Gordon, 1971).

Of course, there is much controversy about the creative process. Some scholars emphasize the role of primary process in generating a wealth of associations relevant to a problem (Kris, 1952; Neisser, 1966; Arieti, 1976), while others stress the conscious interaction of simultaneous and sequential thinking (Bogen and Bogen, 1969; Rothenberg, 1979). Whatever the case, it appears that creative insights do not usually evolve from linear step-by-step thinking but appear rather suddenly as whole patterns. In this regard, Jung (1955) developed the notion of *synchronicity* to refer to the connection of events that take on special meaning even though there is no cause–effect relationship (Von Franz, 1966). Jung's interest in symbolism and intuition may have antedated what is now popularized as right (nondominant) hemispheric functions, which are thought to involve the simultaneous processing of information.

Whereas expectations that reflect a replay of past sequences could stem from sequential thinking (secondary process), anticipations of future events way beyond the present probably require simultaneous thinking (tertiary process). That is, in order to anticipate the person has to view sequences simultaneously. Possible future sequences are seen together in a pattern. In this way he may get a picture of the future, at least a hunch about it. This speculation will be explored further in Chapter 3.

Of the three types of thinking proposed in Table 1, it is probable that the sense of duration moving from the present toward the future is most closely associated with the sequential, goal-directed thinking of secondary process. Since primary process, as in dreams, is not goal directed and entails little sequential feedback, it is commonly experienced as timeless. Pure simultaneous thinking, as in tertiary process, also may be relatively timeless compared to secondary process. In this regard persons preoccupied with visual imagery (for instance, watching scenery or being flooded with visions during psychedelic drugs) often are unaware of the passage of time. Also, the sense of time is often lost during moments of creativity.

These themes are roughly in line with the general thesis of this chapter: The more a person is consciously directed toward the future, the greater will be his awareness of the passage of time.

In this regard, it should be mentioned that most altered states of consciousness are associated with changes in the sense of time (Ludwig, 1966; Tart, 1969). A common feature of an altered state of consciousness is a diminished awareness of the future (Melges et al., 1971). This can occur during meditative states, in which there is often a rhythmic centering on the present (Goleman, 1977), or during psychotic states, in which the relationship between the present and future becomes blurred (see Chapter 7). It is probable that a diminished awareness of the future induces the feeling of timelessness associated with altered states of consciousness, since secondary process thinking is disrupted. That is, the voluntary goal-directed activity of the mind, commonly felt as conscious mental activity, is diminished (MacKay, 1966).

In altered states of consciousness all components of psychological time— rate, sequence, and temporal perspective—are commonly altered (Melges et al., 1971). These changes in psychological time can occur during hypnosis (Aaronson, 1968), psychedelic drugs (Melges et al., 1970b, 1971, 1974), and sensory deprivation (Goldberger and Holt, 1958; Vernon and McGill, 1963). It appears that distortions of psychological time may be fundamental aspects of altered states of consciousness. This theme will be explored further in Part II of this book.

THE BRAIN: TIME AND ANTICIPATION

The human brain can be considered to be a highly specialized, time-binding organization (see Chapter 1). Although different areas of the brain have unique functions (for instance, visual perception in the occipital cortex), there appears to be no one brain center that is primarily involved with timing and temporal processes. That is, different areas of the brain appear to contribute to the temporal processing in different ways. In this section an overview of some of these different temporal processes will be outlined. The focus will be on broad generalizations that will not do justice to the complexity of the processes.

During phylogenetic development, it appears that the evolution of the central nervous system entails an increasing capacity to handle more extensive spans of time (Cohen, 1966). The human brain, which is the most capable time-binding organization, contains anlage of its ancestral brains, each having a more limited temporal capacity. These ancestral brains can be called the reptilian, or "snake," brain and the mammalian, or "dog," brain. The reptilian brain includes the midbrain, hypothalamus, and cerebellum. The mammalian brain includes the limbic system and parts of the frontal cortex.

The older reptilian brain appears to be involved in biological rhythms, arousal, conditioned reflexes, and the coordinated timing of movements. The midbrain and hypothalamus are involved in arousal and biological rhythms (Magoun, 1964). The suprachiasmic nucleus appears to be particularly important for the regulation of biological rhythms, probably as it relates to melatonin metabolism (Wehr, Muscettola, and Goodwin, 1980). The cerebellum, extrapyramidal system, and thalamus are involved in the coordination and timing of movements (Dimond, 1964).

The mammalian brain is capable of handling longer time periods than the reptilian brain underneath it. Moreover, the more complex mammalian brains can handle longer time spans. For example, in studies of delayed reaction a chimpanzee can wait longer than a cat, which in turn can wait longer than a rat, for a delayed reward (Cohen, 1966). The limbic system, with its connections with the frontal lobe, is involved in emotion and drive states subserving self-preservation and reproduction of the species (MacLean, 1950). Papez's (1937) original hypothesis about the role of the limbic system in emotion was prompted by the idea that this ringlike structure was ideally suited for handling the relatively long-lasting, reverbatory nature of emotions. Reward and pain centers are intimately connected with the limbic system (Olds, 1965). In its role in emotion the limbic system appears to play an important part in the modulation of goal-directed behavior (Pribram and Melges, 1969).

Besides its role in emotion and the monitoring of goal-directed behavior, the limbic system also appears to be involved in the tracking of sequences through time (Flynn, MacLean, and Kim, 1961; Pribram, 1971; Pribram and Tubbs, 1967). Lesions in the hippocampus (a limbic region) give rise to severe deficits in immediate and short-term memory (Milner, 1969). As outlined in Chapters 4 and 7, disturbances in the hippocampus and nearby structures may account for some of the peculiar time disturbances in Korsakoff's psychosis as well as in acute schizophrenia. The inability to track sequences relevant to goals is prominent in acute schizophrenia and psychotomimetic drug intoxication (Chapter 7).

In comparison with the reptilian and lower mammalian brains, the human brain has a more highly developed frontal cortex as well as cerebral cortices. The frontal lobes appear to be important for the maintenance of goal-directed behavior and for planning. If the connections between the limbic system and frontal lobes are cut, or if the frontal lobes are removed, the capacity to plan ahead, project into the future, and inhibit distractions is impaired (Jacobsen, 1935; Milner, 1964; Pribram, 1971). Patients who have had their frontal lobes removed are often indifferent toward the future (Greenblatt and Solomon, 1958; Valenstein, 1973). Since such patients are less concerned about the future, their worry about the future is reduced, but this is at the high price of impairing their ability to plan ahead and to engage in future-oriented problem solving.

The cerebral cortex is most highly developed in the human brain. In the past it was assumed that both the left and right cerebral hemispheres shared equally in producing man's higher functions such as reasoning, language, and creativity. Recent evidence, however, suggests that the left and right cerebral hemispheres contribute in different ways to these higher functions (for review, see Ornstein, 1972; Kinsbourne, 1978; Restak, 1978; and Wexler, 1980). Spurred by the work of Sperry and his colleagues (Sperry, Gazzaniga, and Bogen, 1969) on split-brain human patients who had had the two hemispheres disconnected by cutting the bridge between them (the corpus callosum) for the treatment of intractable epilepsy, it was found that the two hemispheres functioned differently on certain tasks. In a sense there appeared to be "two brains in one head." In right-handed persons the left cerebral hemisphere is dominant for speech, whereas the right cerebral hemisphere is nondominant for speech. This has been known since the discoveries of Broca and Wernicke in the mid-nineteenth century, but recently there have been other discoveries of hemispheric specialization.

One of the most interesting findings is that the left and right hemispheres appear to process time relationships differently (Mills and Rollman, 1980). Time relationships in the left hemisphere are primarily sequential, whereas in the right hemisphere they are largely simultaneous (Carmon, 1978; Ben-Dov and Carmon, 1976). In this regard language (particularly writing and the sequencing of consonants) is processed primarily in the left cerebral hemisphere (Geschwind, 1980). The nature of language is sequential and linear. Human speech requires the coding and decoding of auditory sequences and frequencies (Neff, 1962; Jones, 1976; Siegman and Feldstein, 1979). Patients with aphasia (difficulty in understanding and expressing language) have lesions in the left cerebral hemisphere. In this regard Efron (1963a, 1963b) has emphasized that the basic defect underlying aphasic dysfunction is an impairment of the temporal discrimination of sequences. That is, language appears to depend on this capacity for temporal discrimination.

In contrast to the sequential functions of the left cerebral hemisphere, the right cerebral hemisphere (that is, the nondominant hemisphere in right-handed persons) appears to process information in terms of visual–spatial patterns so that it can be seen all at once. That is, the right cerebral hemisphere appears to bring elements together as holistic patterns rather than stringing them out linearly (Bogen, 1974). In this way when the right hemisphere "sees" a part, it can quickly extrapolate to the whole pattern. For example, when a fragment of a person's face is seen, the right hemisphere can more quickly and accurately recognize the whole face than the left hemisphere. Or from just a few notes of a familiar tune, the whole melody can be grasped quickly by the right hemisphere. The left hemisphere primarily uses words in its sequential processing, whereas the right hemisphere primarily uses visual images for viewing events all at once. Also, there appears to be a close relationship between emotion and the right hemisphere functions (Sackeim, Gur, and Saucy, 1978).

The relevance of these hemispheric-specialized functions to clinical psychiatry is just beginning to be explored (Galin, 1974). The predominant differences have spurred fresh hypotheses about unconscious processes, creativity, deja vu, and the thought process disorder in schizophrenia. For example, as outlined in the previous section, the sequential, goal-directed nature of secondary process thinking would appear primarily related to left hemisphere functions, whereas the simultaneous functions of the right cerebral hemisphere may be related to tertiary process thinking, perhaps as it relates to primary process thinking. In schizophrenia there is some evidence to suggest a relative impairment of left cerebral hemispheric functions, perhaps in conjunction with overactivation of the right hemisphere (see Chapters 4 and 7). In the normal person the interaction between the two hemispheres via the corpus callosum has been proposed to account for original problem solving and creativity (Bogen and Bogen, 1969).

The phenomenon of deja vu has been explained by Efron (1963b) on the basis of different powers of temporal discrimination between the left and right hemisphere. The basic hypothesis is that the left hemisphere receives the same input twice. Since the left hemisphere has greater powers of temporal discrimination, it can more readily pinpoint when an event occurred in time compared to the right hemisphere. In deja vu it is proposed that the left hemisphere receives input directly from the environment and then receives roughly the same input at a later time coming from the right hemisphere after crossing the corpus callosum. Normally the input coming from the right hemisphere is not noticeably delayed in crossing the corpus callosum, but in deja vu the crossover is delayed by a minor seizure in the right hemisphere or its limbic connections. Thus the experience of deja vu is that the person knows that he is in the here-and-now seeing what is happening around him (direct input into the left hemisphere) and feels that what he is seeing has already been experienced the exact same way but cannot pinpoint when (delayed right hemisphere input). In line with Efron's proposal, Mullan and Penfield (1959) found that deja vu and illusions of the familiarity predominantly came from lesions or seizures in the right cerebral hemisphere. The lesions or seizures could accentuate the delay of input crossing over to the left cerebral hemisphere.

It should be emphasized, however, that normally there is a rapid exchange between the left and right hemispheres via the corpus callosum. This prompts the question: What would be the advantages of processing the same ongoing input both sequentially and simultaneously? One possibility, already touched on in the previous section on thinking and anticipation, is that the process of anticipation might be enhanced. That is, by seeing an array of sequences all at once the person may be in a better position to look ahead. Rather than his going through the sequences step by step, an overall picture of the sequences could be seen simultaneously as a pattern. This is somewhat similar to looking at a map to see what lies ahead rather than traveling through all the pathways step by step. Thus the simultaneous imaging of sequences may be basic to the process of anticipation.

The usefulness in visualizing future possibilities will be explored in Chapters 3 and 12. It is proposed that imaging the personal future initiates the organization of sequences of thought and action toward the future.

Of course, there remain many mysteries that revolve around the question of how the brain anticipates. The research strategies presently available for measuring expectancy and anticipation in the brain are relatively crude EEG measures but nevertheless do indicate that the brain does process information with regard to what lies ahead (Restak, 1978). For example, there is the so-called expectancy wave (that is, contingent negative variation) that develops over the frontal cortex as a person readies himself to respond to a predictable stimulus (Walter et al., 1964). Also, there is the P 300 that arises when a regularly expected stimulus does not occur (Squires et al., 1976). What might be taking place deep within the brain during anticipation has been explored in animal brain preparations (Olds et al., 1969). Nevertheless, there is need for much research that focuses on the fundamental question of how the brain anticipates.

SUMMARY AND CONCLUSIONS

The general theme of this chapter is that the experience of time is closely related to a person's span of awareness into the future. This theme is supported by the following considerations:

1 The experience of duration appears related to the interval between the present and an event of concern in the future.
2 During development, the early experience of duration is thought to occur during waiting periods of unmet needs when there is tension between the present and future. During later development in childhood, a more abstract notion of time develops with the increasing capacity to delay gratification and to project into the future.
3 Emotional signals are closely linked to the sense of duration, particularly the interval between the present and an event of concern in the future. Emotions appear to monitor a person's awareness of the passage of time as it relates to the personal future.
4 During goal-directed thinking, a person is usually attuned to the passage of time, whereas there are other types of thinking that are relatively timeless.
5 Although how the brain anticipates remains a mystery, disturbances in brain function are commonly manifested in terms of alternations in the sense of time as it relates to anticipation.

CHAPTER THREE

Anticipatory Control: Futuring, Temporal Organization, and Emotion

It is memory that gives us the power of foresight: We push into the future with images in which we fixed the past. Full consciousness therefore looks both ways, and the most important look is into the future. All biological processes are directed toward the future, but man is distinguished by being consciously directed—his consciousness includes the future.

JACOB BRONOWSKI (1966, p. 80)

Consciousness is largely directed toward the future. This is particularly true in Western society where people attempt to gain control over their futures by anticipating and preparing for future events. The anticipations, in turn, influence much of human behavior (Kelly, 1955). In this chapter I will review the role of the personal future in behavior and also propose some ways that people attempt to achieve anticipatory control over their futures.

Existential writers have emphasized the relationship between the present and future as fundamental for commitment and meaning in life (Minkowski, 1933; Kierkegaard, 1934; Tillich, 1952; Frankl, 1978). In this regard May (1958, p. 69) has stated: "We are never merely the victims of automatic pressures from the past. The deterministic events of the past take their significance from the present and the future." Other psychiatrists and psychologists of diverse theoretical orientations have also emphasized the role of anticipations and life plans in behavior (Adler, 1929; Kelly, 1955; Berne, 1972; Bandura, 1974, 1977).

Nevertheless, for the most part the role of the future in behavior has been neglected. This is somewhat surprising in view of the fact that most people in Western society are future oriented (Cottle and Klineberg, 1974; Trommsdorff and Lamm, 1973). In America, the billions of dollars spent each year on life insurance is a testimony to the future orientation of Western society. Moreover, Tiger (1979) proposes that a future orientation goes beyond cultural determinants and is rooted in a biological predisposition of humans to optimistic pursuits. Yet despite the prominent future orientation of most people, it has not been emphasized in most theories of personality and psychopathology. Allport (1955, p. 51) has described the problem well: "People, it seems, are busy leading their lives into the future, whereas psychology, for the most part, is busy tracing them into the past."

There are a number of reasons for this neglect of the future in studying behavior. One is the belief in Western society that finding past causes is crucial for the explanation of present phenomena. This belief is reflected in the psychoanalytic emphasis on uprooting past causes in order to understand and modify present behavior. Another reason is the avoidance of teleological explanations in the physical sciences, which has influenced people to make the erroneous assumption that such concepts as goal seeking and goal correction must also be avoided in biology and psychology.

Although the early work of Cannon (1932) introduced the concept of homeostasis, the pervasiveness of cybernetic control mechanisms in biology and psychology has only been fully recognized for about the last two decades (Von Bertalannfy, 1968; Bowlby, 1969, 1973). In biology, Pittendrigh (1961) points out that it is difficult to understand a system unless one attempts to understand what it is organized *for*. Neuropsychological theories of the brain have been developed that focus on anticipatory control (Miller, Galanter, and Pribram, 1960; Sommerhoff, 1974). Yet except for the works of Kelly (1955) in psychology and Bowlby (1969, 1973, 1980) in psychiatry, the concept of cybernetic control has not yet been given due prominence in psychology and psychiatry, even though the importance of a general systems approach in psychiatry has been recognized (Grinker, 1967; Gray, Duhl, and Rizzo, 1969; Peterfreund, 1971; Buckley, 1968).

In this chapter I will introduce some basic concepts about cybernetic control as it might relate to psychiatry. These ideas will be expanded in Part II of this book which emphasizes the role of vicious cycles (spirals) in psychopathology. Also, in later parts of this book, treatment strategies for interrupting vicious cycles will be outlined. Future-oriented psychotherapy is designed specifically for this purpose (Chapter 12). In this regard, it should be emphasized that except in terms of reworking the past and present, it is only the future that can be controlled. Thus before developing the concept of cybernetic control, I will first outline the role of the personal future in behavior.

The general theme of this chapter can be stated as follows: *An extended future time perspective, which integrates past and present outcomes toward future goals, is important for the cybernetic control of human behavior.*

THE ROLE OF THE PERSONAL FUTURE IN HUMAN BEHAVIOR

There is considerable research which indicates that how a person construes his future influences his feelings, thinking, and behavior. These studies come from different research traditions, such as behavioral modification, the study of cognition and beliefs, field studies of normal individuals, and clinical psychopathology. In general, the findings suggest that coping and a coherent future orientation go together, whereas failure to cope is often associated with a limited or fragmented future time perspective.

In the behavioral tradition one of the cardinal principles of operant conditioning is that behavior is controlled by its consequences. Since humans have an extended future time perspective, a person's behavior is particularly under the control of anticipated consequences. To quote Bandura (1974, p. 860): "Our choices of action are largely under anticipatory control." It was formerly thought that immediate consequences outweigh remote consequences; there is growing evidence now, however, that this applies mainly to animals and not to humans who can tie the present to the distant future (Mowrer and Ullmann, 1945, 1960; Bandura, 1974, 1977; Mischel, 1961, 1973). Moreover, Bandura (1974) points out that in humans conditioning is fostered by a setting of expectancy. That is, when events are expected to come together in time, and then they do, conditioning and learning are facilitated. In this regard there has been a strong trend in the last decade for behaviorists to make use of cognitive concepts such as anticipation and expectancy.

In the framework of social learning theory, research has shown that future orientation is significantly correlated with internal control of reinforcement. According to Rotter (1966), internal control of reinforcement refers to the belief that a person's destiny is determined largely by one's own skilled action, whereas external control denotes a belief that luck or fate is largely responsible for what happens to the person. The future-oriented person believes in the efficacy of his skilled action in bringing about outcomes (Teahan, 1958; Levine and Spivack, 1959). Both future orientation and internal control have been found to be conducive to coping (Goldrich, 1967; Platt and Eisenman, 1968). On the other hand, the belief that environmental events beyond one's control determine the outcome of the situation is often associated with a lack of future orientation and a failure to cope. If a person believes that there is little he can do to change the expected outcomes of a situation, then he is less likely to strive to change the circumstances in which he finds himself.

A person's expectations about his own efficacy influence greatly how he copes with other people and environmental circumstances. As Bandura (1977) points out, a person can expect that a certain response will produce certain outcomes, but in order to carry out such responses, the person usually has to expect that he is capable of doing them. These latter expectations of self-efficacy influence whether the person even tries to cope with a situation. If he expects that he does not have the resources to cope with a threat as he construes it, he will experience anxiety (R. Lazarus, 1966). On the other hand, if he expects that he can be effective in producing the expected outcome, he will not only try to cope but also will persist in trying to master the situation. In this regard Lewin (1942) highlighted the importance of integrating expectations for short-term and long-term rewards in order to instill morale in individuals as well as in groups. That is, when people can see the connections between what they are doing now in relation to the more remote future, they are likely to have high morale and to persist in their efforts.

Self-control is also related to future orientation. A key aspect of self-control is the capacity to tolerate short-term hardships in the interest of pursuing rewards in the long-term future (Kanfer and Marston, 1963; Kanfer and Karoly, 1972; Klineberg, 1968). This capacity to delay gratification is fundamental to what is called *ego strength* (Blanck and Blanck, 1974; Singer, 1955, 1956). Ego strength can be thought of as the ability to cope, cooperate, compromise, comprehend, coordinate, and create, all of which require future orientation. Measures of ego strength have been found to be significantly correlated with an extended future time perspective (Rabin, 1976).

In the area of cognition and personality, perhaps one of the most articulated theories about the important role of anticipations is Kelly's (1955) theory of personal constructs. Kelly (p. 46) builds his theory on the following fundamental postulate: ''A person's processes are psychologically channelized by the ways in which he anticipates events.'' Essentially, Kelly's theory states that anticipations govern a person's psychological organization. A personal construct is a way in which a person customarily anticipates events. Personal constructs are bipolar ways of framing anticipations. For example, an event (such as an interaction with another person) can be expected to turn out either good or bad, to be strong or weak, or to be active or passive. If an interaction with another person is anticipated to be good–strong–active, the individual is likely to behave differently toward the other person than if the latter is construed as bad–weak–passive. Still another set of preparations comes into play if the other person is construed to be bad–strong–active. In this way the linkages between constructs give a different anticipatory set. Kelly proposes that people continually revise the linkages between their personal constructs by making predictions of which anticipations will go together and then testing whether the predictions hold up or not. In this way people operate much like scientists, although the testing of personal constructs and anticipations is not as precise as validating or invalidating a scientific prediction.

The practical applications of Kelly's (1955) theory of personal constructs have been reviewed by Bannister and Mair (1968) and Adams-Webber (1977). Perhaps the greatest usefulness of this theory is in understanding how each individual sees his world and himself in a unique way, each looking at the world with a different set of anticipations that, according to Kelly, are like a set of colored lenses on one's glasses. That is, the perception of reality is colored by one's anticipatory constructs. In Chapters 11 and 12 I will deal further with the role of personal constructs in interpersonal perception and psychotherapy.

Personal constructs can be thought of as highly individualized beliefs. The function of most beliefs is to serve as guides into an uncertain future (Frank, 1978). Whether a belief system can be modified or not depends somewhat on how far into the future the beliefs extend. Rokeach (1960) shows that those people with an unmodifiable "closed mind" usually have a belief system that pertains to some utopian goal in the far-off future, whereas those with an "open mind" usually use outcomes in the present and near future in order to revise their beliefs.

A flexible set of strategies for dealing with future contingencies has been found to be one of the hallmarks of successful coping (Coelho, Hamburg, and Adams, 1974; Hamburg and Adams, 1967). In dealing with life stresses, such as matriculation to college, the loss of a child, or suffering from severe burns, people who cope well set priorities, actively seek information, maintain hope, plan for alternative ways of approaching a problem, and rehearse plans of action in advance. All of these coping strategies involve a future orientation.

Perhaps one of the most careful field studies of coping behavior is Ezekiel's (1968) study of Peace Corps volunteers before and after their placement overseas. It was found that those volunteers who, prior to their overseas assignments, wrote "future autobiographies" characterized by a detailed mapping out of how they would meet challenges made the most successful adjustment and contribution when they actually went overseas. Success was evaluated by supervisors, peers, and self. The future autobiographies were substantially more predictive of eventual success than a battery of commonly used psychological tests.

While an extended future time perspective is related to coping, internal control, self-control, and ego strength, a lack of future time perspectives or a negative future outlook is frequently associated with a failure to cope. In that regard, the most common general problem that brings people to psychotherapy is demoralization or loss of hope (Frank, 1974). During the course of psychotherapy individuals are initially focused on the past and present, but as they get better they get more future oriented (Smeltzer, 1969). Frank (1974) asserts that the restoration of morale is one of the cardinal functions of psychotherapy.

Many forms of mental illness are characterized by a bleak, foreshortened or fragmented future time perspective. These findings will be reviewed in later parts of this book and will only be touched on here. Hopelessness is a central feature of depression (Melges and Bowlby, 1969). It also is at the core of most serious suicide attempts. A negative outlook on the personal future is highly correlated with a lack of self-esteem. Also, changes in self-esteem have been found to covary through time with changes in future outlook, suggesting that the two processes are dynamically interrelated (Melges et al., 1971). In addition, delinquents and sociopaths commonly have foreshortened future time perspectives. Since they do not consider and weigh future consequences as much as other people, they are especially prone to spur-of-the-moment impulsive acts. Schizophrenics have been found to have an incoherent and disorganized future time perspective (Wallace, 1956). The experience of depersonalization (that is, strangeness about the self) is strongly related to a feeling of lack of continuity between past, present, and future (Melges et al., 1970; Freeman and Melges, 1977).

In summary, it appears that the structure a person gives to his personal future plays an important role in controlling his behavior, thinking, and feeling. In general, those with an articulated future time perspective cope well; those without it are vulnerable to a failure to cope.

CYBERNETIC CONTROL: FEEDBACK AND FEEDFORWARD

In cybernetic theory only the future can be controlled (Kelley, 1968). That is, since the past has already happened and the present quickly becomes past, control over action means control directed at the future.

The term *cybernetic* comes from the Greek word for steersman (Wiener,

1948). A steersman maintains control over his ship by making corrections whenever the ship wanders off course. This process of maintaining control through correcting deviations from a goal is the essence of cybernetic theory (Powers, 1973). That is, through the detection of errors (feedback), deviations from the goal are counteracted.

Feedback refers to outcomes taking place in the present. The extension of feedback into the future has been called *feedforward* (MacKay, 1966; Pribram, 1971). Feedforward refers to expected or anticipated deviations from a goal. On the basis of feedforward a system can prepare to respond in a certain direction. That is, its readiness to respond is biased in a certain direction. For example, if the steersman were tracking an enemy ship, the steersman would feedforward to the predicted course of the enemy ship in order to prepare to make corrections in the direction of his own ship.

Feedforward is commonly added to feedback in situations where a goal is a moving target rather than a fixed reference condition. That is, feedforward is built into most servomechanisms, such as guided missiles; this allows the servomechanism to adjust to future changes in the goal rather than just responding to feedback about deviations from a fixed set point, as with the homeostatic control of temperature via a thermostat (Simon, 1975).

Human beings are particularly prone to feedforward. People commonly forecast outcomes and project into the future. In situations of uncertainty people are even more prone to use feedforward in an attempt to gain control over the future (Pribram and Melges, 1969; Melges and Harris, 1970).

For control to be maintained feedforward usually has to be kept in check by present-time feedback. That is, projections into the future have to be modified by actual outcomes taking place in the present. In the analogy of the steersman, if the steersman placed too much credence in his predictions of where the enemy ship might be in the future (excessive feedforward), then he is apt to make insufficient adjustments for present changes in the enemy ship (feedback). Thus for control to be achieved over the long run, feedback has to be integrated with feedforward.

It should be obvious that this integration of feedback with feedforward has to be timely in order for control to be maintained. For example, if the steersman waits too long before responding to feedback, the ship may have wandered way off course, and it will take much more time and effort to get it back on course. On the other hand, if the steersman responds too quickly to momentary feedback without taking into consideration long-range feedforward, the ship may oscillate frantically in attempting to track minute changes in the enemy ship. The importance of timing in maintaining or losing control is relevant to the wide oscillations in behavior and lack of control seen in psychotic illness (Chapters 4 and 7).

LACK OF CONTROL AND VICIOUS CYCLES (SPIRALS)

Whereas control is achieved through counteracting deviations from a goal, lack of control is usually manifested as the amplification of deviations from a goal (Maruyama, 1963). That is, one change augments another change. This snowball effect is commonly referred to as a vicious cycle. A more appropriate image of this process is that of a spiral, since the deviations from the goal progressively get worse and worse.

Vicious cycles (spirals) usually result from (1) unclear goals, (2) lack of feedback, (3) excessive feedforward, or (4) the mistiming of feedback and feedforward.

In the analogy of the steersman, an unclear goal is exemplified by the steersman being unable to see the enemy ship. Without the goal in sight, the ship is likely to wander off course. Lack of feedback is exemplified by a failure of the ship's instruments to detect how far off target it is; this would hinder making the necessary corrections. Excessive feedforward is exemplified by the steerman's overreacting to the enemy ship's bluff of signaling for air force support, causing the steersman to veer from his original target. The mistiming of feedback and feedforward might occur if the steersman were intoxicated with marihuana (which distorts the perception of time—see Chapter 7). With a time distortion, he might mistakenly perceive a sudden change in the enemy ship's direction (feedback) as occurring at the same time as the bluff signal for enemy aircraft (feedforward); because of the time distortion, the signals might appear to be happening at the same time, thereby augmenting one another and initiating a spiral that leads him astray.

As developed in Part II, vicious cycles are extremely common in psychiatric illness. For example, unclear goals and lack of feedback often underlie identity diffusion and emotional dyscontrol. Excessive feedforward is common to the overworry of anxiety neurosis as well as paranoid overprojections into the future. The mistiming of feedback and feedforward is prominent in acute schizophrenia.

In cybernetic theory, it should be emphasized that a vicious cycle can be initiated by a small change which then augments other changes. With regard to psychiatric illness, this means that the inciting event need not be tremendously traumatic. Rather, it may gain momentum through its interaction with other changes (Wender, 1968). For example, a woman became abjectly depressed after losing her cat. The loss of the cat prompted fears of losing her husband, which tied into catastrophic expectations of losing a person who cared for her, as she had lost her mother when she was a girl. Finding how one change augments another is important for designing treatment, as developed in later parts of this book.

The human proclivity for extensive expectations and anticipations makes people particularly vulnerable to vicious cycles stemming from excessive feedforward. When a person's anticipations prompt other anticipations that, in turn, feed into the initiating anticipations, the anticipations are then likely to become amplified into a vicious cycle. This is especially likely when the feedforward processes are not modified by feedback from the current environment, including other people. In this way a person's view of himself and of the world may become dominated by misconstrued anticipations that are divorced from ongoing reality.

Although most spirals of anticipations feeding into one another represent a lack of control and are therefore termed vicious cycles, it is possible for anticipatory spirals to have a pleasant and growth-producing effect. For example, confidence in one's own social abilities often prompts positive expectations of other people which in turn further augment one's confidence. As developed in Part V, engendering these positive anticipatory spirals is a key step in the psychotherapy of emotional disorders.

In this book I will refer to the growth of plans and goals that a person deems desirable as an *upward spiral*. By contrast, a snowball effect which alienates a person from his goals and is deemed by him to be undesirable will be called a *downward spiral*.

CONTROL OF THE FUTURE: FUTURING, TEMPORAL ORGANIZATION, AND EMOTION

In the previous sections, we have seen that an extended and coherent future time perspective is important for coping and adaptive behavior and that vicious cycles are likely to occur when processes involved in making goal corrections are disturbed. We are now prepared to ask: What are the essential ways that people attempt to gain control over their futures?

This question is central to understanding the temporal integration of behavior (Hearnshaw, 1956). Temporal integration is of great importance for adaptive human behavior, since it means that relevant aspects of the past, present, and future are coordinated and synthesized in order to make timely adjustments for reaching goals (Melges et al., 1970a, 1970b). In this regard, Mowrer (1950, p. 454) states that the essence of integrated behavior is the capacity to bring the future into the psychological present.

In attempting to bring the future into the psychological present, people often initiate this process by visualizing future possibilities. Some people may be only dimly aware of their future images, while others may be keenly conscious of them. The role of visual imagery in thinking, imagination, and behavior has received a resurgence of interest in recent years (Singer, 1974; Horowitz, 1970, 1976). Visual imagery appears to be an important alternative mode of processing information that is different from sequential thinking (see Chapter 2). The process of visualizing future images is exemplified by such terms as envisioning the future, picturing what might happen, sketching a scenario, and so on.

We will refer to this process of visualizing future possibilities as *futuring*. Futuring was chosen as a general term to refer to the generation of future images. It involves expectation, anticipation, and imagination, but specifically refers to the visualization of future images. The way that people see into the distance is by sight. Accurate seeing into the future is called foresight. Although futuring refers to the process of attempting to see into the future, it does not necessarily mean accurate peering into the future, as with foresight. Also, futuring refers to visualizing a relatively extended period of future time, which is in contrast to the more limited time spans suggested by the terms expectation and anticipation. In addition, it is hoped that the term futuring is relatively free of the traditional connotations of the terms expectation and anticipation.

In humans a visual image of the future is often a goal, either a desired or undesired state. It may not be a goal in the precise cybernetic sense of a set point or target, but a future visual image can serve as a reference condition, or template, for guiding subsequent thinking or action. Common examples of this are the golfer envisioning the optimal path and trajectory of the ball before executing his swing, the football quarterback envisioning the emerging patterns of his receivers weaving through the defense before passing the ball, or the businessman attempting to foresee the reactions of others to his strategies and negotiations.

Futuring enables the selection of preferred images (that is, goals) out of the simultaneous display of possible options. The seeing of future possibilities all at once facilitates the selection of goals out of the future images. Also, when a series of future images are seen all at once, they no longer need to be seen as a fixed series. For example, in looking at a map, a person can view alternative pathways simultaneously. Futuring brings a series of future states into the present and thereby makes them simultaneous. Once the options are simultaneous, they can be reordered and rearranged. One no longer has to proceed step by step in order to eliminate options, combine some of them, or synthesize two or three by superimposing them. Thus futuring enables the person to telescope segments of the future into the present, so that what was formerly strung out into the future can be seen all at once and possibly rearranged.

By bringing future possibilities into the present, futuring helps develop a flexible set of plans to deal with the possibilities. By working backward in time from the future to the present, futuring is similar to working backward in problem solving where one proceeds from the unknown to the known in order to find the unknown. This process of working backward has been found to be highly useful in solving problems with an unknown element (Polya, 1945).

Whereas futuring goes from the future toward the present, the process of planning moves from the present toward the future. Futuring is primarily simultaneous; planning involves the step-by-step organization of sequences. Futuring and planning go hand in hand as people attempt to gain control over their futures. What a person imagines in the future influences his plans, and what he plans influences his future images. In this sense futuring forms rough outlines for the generation of plans of action.

Plans of action are hierarchically organized sequences of intended action. According to Miller, Galenter, and Pribram (1960, p. 16), "A Plan is any hierarchical process in the organism that can control the order in which a sequence of operations is to be performed." These authors show how much of behavior becomes structured by plans of action that become progressively organized through a series of feedback loops. They also point to the reciprocal relationship between images and plans. That is, changes in the images are effected by plans for gathering, storing, and transforming information; changes in the plans are made by information drawn from the images.

In human behavior plans of action that extend far into the future are often hierarchically organized as subplans within the time framework of more extended plans. For example, planning to go to college organizes the subplan of taking entrance examinations, and the latter subplan organizes sub-sub-plans down to initial steps such as buying paper and pencil.

In searching for control over the future, the *temporal organization* of plans of action is a common way that people give structure to their futures. Temporal organization may be thought of as the organized sequencing of plans of action—that is, the planning of plans. In contrast to futuring, which involves the simultaneous picturing of options and possibilities, temporal organization consists of the sequential planning of plans. Futuring moves from the future toward the present; temporal organization moves from the present toward the future. In this sense futuring is like looking at a map, whereas temporal organization is like a schedule of intended pathways into the future.

Besides futuring and the temporal organization of plans of action, emotions also play a role in attempting to gain control over the future. As outlined in Chapter 2 and as detailed by Pribram and Melges (1969) in a neuropsychological theory of emotion, emotions are involved in the search for control. When plans of action give rise to outcomes that meet the future images, control is achieved. When control is achieved, the person experiences satisfaction. By contrast, when plans of action fail to produce outcomes that meet future images (particularly the goals embedded within the images), control is not yet achieved, and this is reflected in feelings of dissatisfaction. As previously discussed, the unpleasant emotions are further differentiated according to appraisals of the likelihood of reaching goals (chapter 2).

Thus a person's view of his future is constructed from the interaction of images, plans, and emotions. These are proposed as the essential variables with which people attempt to gain control over their futures. That is, emotions are aroused when there is a discrepancy between the present and some future event of concern; the emotions prompt future images of possibilities; the future images in turn spur the development of plans of action; and discrepancies between images and plans prompt further emotions. To put this succinctly in terms of control, it is proposed that emotions control the images, the images control the plans, and incongruities between images and plans control the emotions.

Since a plan can be considered as an organized sequence of intended action, it is likely that the left cerebral hemisphere is primarily involved in this process of the temporal organization of sequences (see Chapter 2). Also, images are likely to be processed primarily by the right (nondominant) cerebral hemisphere which appears to make use of visual–spatial patterns. It is well known that the limbic system is involved in emotion. In this sense the proposal has at least a rough correspondence with known brain functions. That is, in terms of broad generalizations about the ways in which various areas of the brain appear to process time relationships, we could speculate the futuring primarily involves the visual–spatial, simultaneous processing of the right cerebral hemisphere, the temporal organization of plans of action primarily involves the sequential ordering of the left cerebral hemisphere, and emotions involve the limbic system.

These possible neuropsychological relationships are not essential for the proposal, since the latter is aimed primarily at the psychological level of inquiry. At this level the term *futuring* will generally be used to refer to the dynamic process of generating images of the future, and the term *temporal organization* will refer to the ongoing process of developing and reorganizing plans of action. The word *planning* can be substituted as a rough equivalent of temporal organization, but the latter term is preferred since it refers to the continual revising, updating, and rearrangement of sequences of plans of action.

Thus it is proposed that the main ways by which people attempt to gain control over their futures is by futuring, temporal organization, and emotion. In the normal person there is a synchronized interaction between these processes. This dynamic interplay can be summarized as follows: *Within an emotional context, as images of the future are brought into the present, plans of action are generated to meet the evolving images.*

In the remainder of this book I will deal with some of the practical implications of this proposal for understanding various forms of mental illness as well as for certain types of psychotherapy. The normal synchronization of emotion, futuring, and temporal organization will serve as the point of departure for considering abnormal forms of emotion, futuring, and temporal organization. For example, when an emotion spurs visual images of the future for which there is no ready plan of action, a vicious cycle of emotion prompting images which, in turn, prompt further emotions may ensue, leading to an emotional disorder.

Since the proposal deals with rather easily labeled internal events (for instance, emotion, images, and plans), it facilitates talking to patients in straightforward terms about what they are experiencing. In this sense the proposal is a cognitive-behavioral model. But one should not be misled by its apparent simplicity, since the combinations and permutations of emotion, image, and plan are legion. In addition, other psychodynamic constructs such as ego, superego, and ego-ideal can be reframed in terms of plans and images (Melges and Bowlby, 1969). One important advantage of employing such constructs as emotion, image, and plan is that these terms provide readily communicable words that patient and therapist can share when attempting to understand vicious cycles (spirals) in psychopathology. As discussed in Part II, vicious cycles are most likely to occur when there are disruptions in the normal interplay among emotion, futuring, and temporal organization, thereby distorting a person's view of his future.

SUMMARY AND CONCLUSIONS

The general theme of this chapter is that an extended future time perspective, which integrates past and present outcomes toward future goals, is important for the cybernetic control of human behavior. The major points relevant to this theme are as follows:

1 An extended and coherent future time perspective is associated with coping, whereas a limited and fragmented future time perspective is often associated with a failure to cope.

2 The cybernetic concept of control essentially means control over the future. Control is achieved through feedback (that is, the detection and correction of deviations from a goal) and feedforward (that is, using expected deviations from a goal in order to make corrections in advance).

Lack of control often stems from unclear goals, lack of feedback, excessive feedforward, or the mistiming of feedback and feedforward. Lack of control is manifested as the amplification of deviations from a goal. These vicious cycles (downward spirals) are common in mental illness. A downward spiral is a vicious cycle that progressively alienates a person from his goals; an upward spiral is a growth process involving the ramification of desired goals and plans.

3 In humans anticipatory control over the future comes from the interaction of emotion, futuring, and temporal organization. Emotions, by drawing attention to the tension between the present and future, set the context for the interplay between futuring and temporal organization. Futuring refers to the process of bringing future images into the psychological present in order to select goals from the simultaneous display of future possibilities. Temporal organization refers to the linear sequencing of plans of action toward the goals selected from the future images. Normally, as people search for control, there is an interplay between emotion, futuring, and temporal organization. That is, emotions prompt visual images of the future, the latter in turn guide the formation of plans of action, and discrepancies between images and plans prompt emotions. Within an emotional context, as images of the future are brought into the present, plans of action are generated to meet the evolving images.

4 Disruptions of this dynamic interplay between emotion, futuring, and temporal organization often lead to lack of control over the future, giving rise to vicious cycles (downward spirals) of psychopathology.

PART TWO

The Temporal Approach to the Psychiatric Patient

In Part II, I will outline general strategies for the use of temporal concepts in the understanding and treatment of psychiatric disorders. The general thesis is that time distortions disrupt anticipatory control and lead to psychopathological spirals. That is, problems with time, such as distortions of sequence, rate, and temporal perspective, disrupt the normal interplay between future images, plans of action, and emotions, thereby leading to lack of anticipatory control and vicious cycles (spirals).

The intent of Part II is to serve as a bridge between the basic concepts of Part I and more specific, clinical aspects of the general thesis in later parts of this book, such as loss of control in psychosis (Part III), blocks to the future in depression (Part IV), and the dread of the future in neurosis (Part V). In Part II, the presentation of the general temporal paradigm will progress from theoretical considerations to clinical-assessment strategies and then to the use of time in treatment.

Chapter 4 presents a hierarchical model of time problems as related to some common psychiatric disorders. Problems with sequence are proposed to be more severe than problems with rate, which, in turn, are more severe than problems with temporal perspective. Each of these time problems is commonly associated with different misconstructions of the personal future. The interaction between a time problem and a misconstruction of the personal future often gives rise to a psychopathological spiral.

In Chapter 5, I outline clinical strategies for the assessment of time problems and for the differentiation between problems of sequence, rate, and temporal perspective. Case illustrations are given to show how time problems are detected and how psychopathological spirals might be formulated using this temporal approach.

In Chapter 6, the use of time in treatment is explored. This includes correction of problems with sequence, rate, and temporal perspective, as well as inducing changes in these temporal factors for the purpose of altering a patient's construction of his personal future.

It will be seen that the overall aim of this temporal approach to the psychiatric patient is to restore or enhance anticipatory control and to interrupt psychopathological spirals.

CHAPTER FOUR

Time and the Future in Psychopathological Spirals

A person's processes are psychologically channelized by the ways in which he anticipates events.

GEORGE KELLY (1955, p. 46)

This fundamental postulate of George Kelly's (1955) theory of personal constructs can serve as a point of departure for our temporal approach to the psychiatric patients. There is ample research that supports this postulate (Bannister and Mair, 1968; Adams-Webber, 1979). Essentially, the postulate states that a person's psychological organization depends on how he constructs and revises his views of the personal future. This chapter will explore how a person may become psychologically disorganized if the ways in which he anticipates events become disrupted by problems with sequence, rate, and temporal perspective. *My central thesis is that these problems with psychological time impair anticipatory control and may lead to psychopathological spirals of progressive psychological disorganization.*

Part I explored how time is both a medium and a perspective. As the future becomes present, people live through the medium of succession and become aware of rate and duration. Yet they are also able to gain perspective on this medium by transcending the present and considering past and future events related to the present. In this chapter, we will see how disturbances in time as a medium may hinder the process of gaining temporal perspective and how distortions of temporal perspective may make it difficult to live through the medium of the present.

Distortions of psychological time, such as problems with sequence, rate, and temporal perspective, have been found to be significantly more frequent during the active and acute phases of mental illness (Melges and Fougerousse, 1966; Melges and Freeman, 1977). In these studies, none of the patients had the time disorientation typical of organic brain disease, since such patients were carefully excluded. Thus problems with sequence, rate, and temporal perspective can occur without there being gross impairment of brain function. Moreover, in these studies, as the same patients improved such that their psychiatric illnesses became less severe and less active, their problems with sequence, rate, and temporal perspective also improved. This raises the question, to be explored in this chapter, whether problems with psychological time may not only be a manifestation of psychiatric illness but also a contributing mechanism of psychological disorganization.

In exploring this question, I will be using the cybernetic concepts outlined in Chapter 3 to consider the induction and aggravation of vicious cycles (spirals) when a person's anticipatory control becomes disturbed by problems with sequence, rate, and temporal perspective. In these terms, another way of stating the central thesis is as follows: *Psychopathological spirals are likely to occur when problems with psychological time distort the normal interplay between futuring, temporal organization, and emotion.*

FORM VERSUS CONTENT AND PROCESS VERSUS CAUSE

Although the flow of duration and changes in past, present, and future are central human experiences, it is easy to overlook distortions in the temporal form of a person's existence. This is partly because we tend to focus more on content rather than form, more on things rather than processes (Bronowski, 1966). Also, as outlined in Part I, time is an elusive concept; its dimensions are not as concrete as those of space or the world of things. When a person is talking to us, we tend to focus mainly on the events rather than how the events are being integrated through time. We rarely ask: Is this person in a different time frame than I am? Is he confusing sequences? Is his mind going too fast or too slow? Is he primarily focused on the past, present, or future? Is he confusing these time categories? It is questions such as these that may be highly relevant to understanding the temporal form of mental disorders.

Although it is not widely recognized, aberrations of temporal form in various types of psychopathology were highlighted by a number of pioneers in clinical psychiatry. Lewis (1931, p. 614) concluded that "a disorder of time consciousness . . . is a primary alteration of consciousness and may be found as often as it is looked for in mental illness." Minkowski (1933) emphasized the loss of the "I–here–now" position in schizophrenia so that the person loses the reference point of present reality for interpreting past and future experiences. Minkowski (1933) also underscored the importance of the future seeming blocked and monotonous during depressive illness. Schilder (1936) highlighted time fragmentation in the disintegration of the ego, particularly as manifested in the symptom of depersonalization. Jaspers (1959) and other existential psychiatrists pointed to the dread of the future as central to anxiety disorders. Freud (1915, 1933) noted the timelessness of unconscious processes and believed that this might provide the key to "profound discoveries."

Although current knowledge in psychiatry has advanced considerably in the twentieth century, we are still awaiting discoveries that might be crucial to the treatment of mental suffering. Nevertheless, significant advancements have been made in understanding the interplay of biological, psychological, and social factors that influence a person's emotions, thinking, and behavior. From a conceptual standpoint, psychiatry has come to realize that, for most psychiatric illnesses, it is an error to attempt to isolate a single cause and that it is probable that an interaction of biopsychosocial factors contributes to the emergence and perpetuation of mental disorders (Engel, 1977, 1980). In this regard, it would be an error to think that a certain kind of time disturbance is the sole cause of a certain type of mental disorder. Thus in what follows, I will consider distortions of time and the personal future as contributing or aggravating factors in certain types of mental illness.

In addition, this inquiry will be largely limited to the influence of distortions of time and the personal future on the psychological experience of reality. However, I will mention possible biological or social factors that might impact on these psychological experiences. In many instances, psychiatric knowledge about the exact causes of a time disturbance is insufficient at this point in history. In highlighting temporal aberrations in psychopathology, I wish to point the way for exploring biopsychosocial factors that may be relevant to time disturbances at the psychological level. Nevertheless, as mentioned in the Prologue, the heuristic position taken here is that once a time distortion occurs, whatever its cause, it alters psychological organization. Since time is a pervasive medium and perspective of human awareness, it is likely that alterations of psychological time will disturb psychological processes.

In considering psychological processes, it is possible to look at a time distortion as either a manifestation or a mechanism of illness. For example, a biochemical abnormality may give rise to a seizure in the brain that is manifested psychologically as a time distortion, such as a jumbling of mental sequences. It then may become a mechanism for explaining disorganization at the psychological level of inquiry. For instance, the jumbled sequences may be experienced as deja vu at the psychological level (see Chapter 2), and this experience of deja vu may affect the person's subsequent psychological processes regardless of the original cause of the jumbled sequences. In this example, the experience of deja vu may prompt the person to believe that he has uncanny powers of prophecy, and this belief may become a grandiose delusion. As previously mentioned, my point of view is to consider a time distortion as both a manifestation and a possible mechanism of illness.

Nevertheless, I should emphasize again that, within our cybernetic framework, I am considering mutual causality and the interaction of factors, rather than implying that problems with time and the personal future are the sole causes of mental disorders. It is difficult to express the interaction of processes in the English language which, as outlined in Chapter 2, tends to couch events as linear sequences that suggest a one-way causal direction. In instances where I use such words as *since, then, because, induce, produce, influence, stems from, and as a result of,* I hope that the reader will be tolerant and know that I am referring to sequences that are imbedded within a system of interacting factors.

VICIOUS CYCLES AND PSYCHOPATHOLOGY

A vicious cycle is a deranged process that gets worse and worse over time. I refer to these vicious cycles as downward *spirals* (see Chapter 3). These spirals are extremely common in psychopathology (Wender, 1968). Some of these spirals can be understood in terms of cycles of reactions and counterreactions that occur according to real time. For example, the rebellious adolescent rebels against his strict parents who then become more strict prompting the adolescent to rebel even more. The attempts to solve the problem become the problem (Watzlawick, 1978).

Other spirals are not so easily understood as cycles of reactions and counterreactions. For example, why does a chronically depressed person persist in self-defeating behavior rather than seeking rewarding experiences? Or why does the paranoid patient search for threats when the finding of such threats is apt to make him more paranoid? In short, why is it that some forms of abnormal behavior fail to be self-correcting?

One answer to such a question, I propose, is that the person may have a distortion of psychological time and/or is misconstruing his personal future. The time problem may be a distortion of sequence, rate, or temporal perspective. In addition, the individual's construction of his personal future may be such that it seems beyond his control, blocked, or dreaded. The time problem may induce distortions of future outlook, which, in turn, may aggravate the time problem, which may then further distort the personal future. In this way, a vicious cycle, or spiral, ensues.

In the case of the chronically depressed person, for example, the time problem consists of slowing (psychomotor retardation) and the distorted future outlook is that of hopelessness. The slowness makes the person feel hopeless about getting sufficient rewards, and the hopelessness prompts the person to give up, slowing him down even further. Or in the framework of mutual causality, it is possible for the hopelessness to come first and induce slowing of mental rate, which prompts the person to feel ineffective and may lead to further hopelessness. That is, it is possible for a distortion of the personal future to initiate a time problem. For example, in the case of the paranoid person, a future threat may prompt an over-focus on the future, which accentuates the search for other future threats, which, in turn, are interpreted as confirming the necessity of being overly focused on the future (Melges and Freeman, 1975).

Thus I propose that an interaction between a time problem and a misconstruction of the personal future often gives rise to psychopathological spirals. The time problems consist of abnormalities of sequence, rate, or temporal perspective (the span of awareness into the past or future). The misconstructions of the future are usually in the form of distorted future images, plans of action, or anticipatory emotions. In terms of the cybernetic concepts presented in Chapter 3, my central thesis is that *psychopathological spirals occur when problems with sequence, rate, and temporal perspective disrupt the normal interplay between future images, plans of action, and emotions.*

The time problems can be thought of as disrupting present-time *feedback.* For example, a person who has trouble keeping track of sequences is apt to find it difficult to compare present-time outcomes with what he is currently intending to do. With a confusion of sequences, the feedback is apt to be poorly integrated with his current sequences of actions and thoughts. If a person's mind is going too fast or too slow, feedback may be excessive or diminished. The misconstructions of the personal future can be thought of as impairing the process of *feedforward.* That is, as outlined in Chapter 3, the person's anticipatory control becomes impaired by disruptions in the interplay between future images, plans of action, and emotions. For example, the person's plans of action may recurrently mismatch with his future images, giving rise to negative emotions. Moreover, the problems with feedback and feedforward may compound each other. This is particularly likely when there is mistiming of feedback and feedforward. In this situation, present outcomes are not integrated with future projections. For example, an apprehension about a future event may distort the perception of present outcomes. Thus problems with time and the personal future may induce mistiming of feedback and feedforward and induce vicious cycles (spirals). Lack of anticipatory control stems from the temporal incoordination or mismatching of future images, plans of action, and emotions.

A HIERARCHY OF PROBLEMS WITH TIME AND THE PERSONAL FUTURE IN PSYCHOPATHOLOGY

With this background, let us now examine the central thesis in terms of two postulates:

1 *Distortions of psychological time and the personal future are involved in psychopathological spirals.*
2 *Different psychopathological spirals are related to different types of distortions of psychological time and the personal future.*

To explore these postulates, I have listed different problems with time and the personal future in relation to some common psychiatric syndromes in Table 2. This will provide a rough framework for introducing these possible correspondences in this chapter. The next chapter will offer some clinical guidelines for the assessment of problems with time and the personal future. This general temporal approach to the psychiatric patient will serve as an overall framework for dealing with more specific issues in greater depth in Parts III, IV, and V. It should be pointed out that the correspondences of Table 2 are presented as a model of possibilities that represent a blend of clinical and research findings. That is, Table 2 is a way of organizing information as a framework that hopefully will spur further investigations.

The time problems listed at the left of Table 2 may be defined briefly as follows: Time disorientation refers to pervasive problems with sequence, rate, and temporal perspective such that the person is unable to orient himself to clock and calendar time. The temporal disintegration of sequences refers to impaired sequential thinking with an inability to order sequences toward goals. Rate and rhythm problems refer to the acceleration or slowing of mental processes. Problems with temporal perspective refer to imbalances of the span of awareness or focus on the past, present, or future. Desynchronized transactions refer to interactions between people that are mistimed, out of phase, or at cross purposes.

The time problems listed at the left of Table 2 are hierarchically ordered with the most severe problem at the top and the least severe at the bottom. The

Table 2 Different Problems with Time and the Personal Future in Psychiatric
Disorders

Time Problem	Personal Future	Psychiatric Disorder
1. Time disorientation	Confused	Organic brain disease
2. Temporal disintegration of sequences	Fragmented	Schizophrenic disorders
3. Rate and rhythm problems:		
Increased rate	Over-expanded	Mania
Decreased rate	Blocked	Depression
4. Temporal perspective problems:		
Over-focus on future	Threatened	Paranoid disorders
Over-focus on past	Dreaded (uncertain)	Anxiety disorders
Over-focus on present	Disregarded	Antisocial personality
5. Desynchronized transactions	Ambivalent	Adjustment disorders

hierarchical order indicates that the more severe time problems often include the less severe forms of time problems but usually not vice versa. That is, in Table 2, time problem 1 often includes time problems 2 through 5; time problem 2 often includes time problems 3 through 5; and so forth. But time problem 5, although often occurring as the result of more severe time problems listed above it in the hierarchy, can occur by itself. In general, this hierarchical model proposes that problems with sequence are more severe than problems of rate, which are more severe than problems with temporal perspective. Moreover, problems with sequence are proposed to induce problems with rate and temporal perspective, and rate problems are proposed to induce problems with temporal perspective. It is rare for the reverse order to take place. Problems with temporal perspective are not likely to induce major alterations of rate and sequence, nor do problems of rate induce major difficulties with sequence. As will become clear, however, it is possible for problems with sequence to become aggravated by problems with rate and temporal perspective.

In later sections of this chapter, I will discuss more fully the relationship of the time problems listed in Table 2 to major clinical syndromes in psychiatry. At this point, I will continue to explain the hierarchy by outlining the nature of each time problem.

1 *Time disorientation* is the most severe time problem in which the person is unable to relate to customary time markers such as the clock and calendar. In time disorientation, it is common for all components of psychological time—sequence, rate, and temporal perspective—to be deranged. Because of these pervasive problems, a person with time disorientation, as in organic brain disease, is likely to have the remainder of time problems listed in Table 2, such as the temporal disintegration of sequences, rate and rhythm problems, problems with temporal perspective, and desynchronized transactions. Moreover, because of the pervasive problems with sequence, rate, and temporal perspective, the patient's outlook on his personal future is confused (Table 2). He usually has marked loss of control over his personal future, since he has difficulty with ordering his future images, plans of action, and emotions with reference to a timeline extending into the future. He has lost his moorings in time.

2   The *temporal disintegration of sequences* refers to the breakdown of sequential thinking. The person has difficulty with keeping track of sequences. Since this is an intermittent problem, a person with temporal disintegration usually does not have the pervasive problems with time typical of time disorientation. Nevertheless, the intermittent problems with tracking sequences may be accompanied with episodic difficulties with rate, temporal perspective, and desynchronized transactions with other people. The reason for this, it is here proposed, is that adequate ordering of sequences is necessary for the temporal organization of plans of action (see Chapter 3). Moreover, if sequences become confused or omitted, the rate of mental events may accelerate or slow down, since the succession of events and the rate of events are interdependent (see Chapter 2). Moreover, with difficulties in sequential thinking, the larger sequences of temporal perspective (past, present, and future) are apt to become confused or telescoped. Finally, the temporal disintegration of sequences would make it difficult for the person to organize sequences of interactions with other people, and his transactions with them are apt to become desynchronized. A person with the temporal disintegration of sequences, such as a schizophrenic patient, usually does not have time disorientation but does have intermittent difficulties with the other time problems listed in Table 2.

3   *Rate and rhythm problems* refer to the acceleration or slowing of mental events, thought to be induced by phase shifts in circadian rhythms. These problems usually occur without there being time disorientation or the temporal disintegration of sequences. (There are some exceptions, as discussed in a later section and in Chapter 5.) The acceleration of mental events, as in mania, may induce problems with temporal perspective, such as an overly expanded view of one's personal future (Table 2). In addition, the flood of mental events and the person's fast pace of behavior may prompt desynchronized transactions with others who have difficulties in keeping pace with the person. On the other hand, the slowing of mental events, as in depression, may prompt the person to have a constricted or blocked awareness of his

future, and the person's slowed pace may incite desynchronized transactions since he lags behind others. Thus rate and rhythm problems usually occur without time disorientation and the temporal disintegration of sequences, but are often complicated by the other time problems listed in Table 2, such as problems with temporal perspective and desynchronized transactions.

4 *Problems with temporal perspective* refer to imbalances in the integration of spans of awareness directed to past, present, and future. These imbalances usually take the form of an over-focus on the past, present, or future, an abnormal span of awareness into the past or future, or the relative exclusion of one or more of these frames of reference. I propose that these problems are common in neurotic and personality disorders in which the temporal context through which one lives is often misframed. Problems with temporal perspective can occur without time disorientation, the temporal disintegration of sequences, and rate and rhythm problems, but are often complicated by desynchronized transactions with other people (Table 2). One reason for the desynchronized transactions, I propose, is that the temporal context of interpersonal expectations is often distorted by the problems with temporal perspective. For example, a person who is over-focused on the past may distort his current and future relationships with others in terms of the distant past.

5 *Desynchronized transactions* refer to transactions with other people that are mistimed, out of phase, and at cross purposes. These can occur per se without any of the other time problems listed in Table 2, yet all the other time problems are usually accompanied by desynchronized transactions with other people. That is, it is possible for desynchronized transactions to occur without there being any marked problem with sequence, rate, or temporal perspective, as with an adjustment disorder such as marital discord or a family feud. Nevertheless, as mentioned, problems with temporal perspective often prompt desynchronized transactions when the parties involved are operating from different sets of expectations governed by different time frames.

With this introduction to the hierarchy of time problems presented in Table 2, the discussion is now prepared to deal with the nature of the time-related psychopathological spirals that occur in some common psychiatric syndromes. Table 2 provides a format for visualizing two kinds of spirals that I will emphasize: (1) *Spirals that occur between the time problems*. This refers to the potential of the more severe time problems to include or give rise to the less severe time problems listed *from top to bottom* in Table 2. Since the more severe problems of sequence and rate often are biologically determined, as will become clear in later sections and chapters, the influence of these more severe time problems on disrupting temporal perspective and transactions with others has a biopsychosocial direction. That is, biological factors affect psychological function, which, in turn, affect one's social transactions with others. (2) *Spirals that occur between a time problem and a misconstruction of the personal future.* That is, the time problem may prompt a misconstruction of the future, which, in turn, augments the time problem and further distorts the personal future. These spirals can be visualized by reading *across* Table 2 from left to right. They occur largely at the psychological level of organization. As will become clear, distortions of the personal future often initiate imbalances of temporal perspective and desynchronized transactions.

In considering the latter spirals that occur between a time problem and a distortion of the personal future, I am making a distinction between time as a *medium* through which one lives in the present and the personal future which is an important *perspective* or temporal context for framing one's existence in time. The time problems affect how one lives through the medium of the present, and the alterations of the personal future affect the anticipated framework or channel toward which one is going. This is analogous to the steersman of a ship who currently is traveling through troubled waters but is also looking ahead. What he sees ahead can either offset or compound his current problems. For example, if it looks calm ahead, the troubled waters around him do not look so bad; however, if it looks stormy ahead or if he cannot get a clear picture of what is ahead, his current problems are apt to seem worse.

Thus it is here proposed that the time problem both induces and can be aggravated by the distorted future outlook, which, in turn, can further aggravate the time problem. For example, in the time disorientation of organic disease, pervasive problems with sequence, rate, and temporal perspective induce confusion about the personal future, and the latter augments the time disorientation since the person does not know where he is headed. Or in the case of temporal disintegration of sequences as seen in schizophrenia, the temporal disintegration induces the personal future to be experienced as fragmented, and this fragmented personal future augments the patient's sequential difficulties since the temporal context in which the sequences can be ordered is now disorganized. These potential spirals between problems with time and the personal future in some common psychiatric syndromes can be visualized by reading across Table 2, and will be discussed separately in later sections of this chapter as well as in subsequent chapters.

Obviously, not all forms of psychopathology are covered in Table 2. For example, alcohol addiction cannot be conveniently classified in terms of any one of the major time disturbances in Table 2. Nevertheless, alcohol does produce time alterations. Alcohol has been found to make clock time seem to pass by quickly and to provide a "time-out" from duties and deadlines imposed by social and work schedules (Newell, 1971; MacAndrew and Edgerton, 1969). Moreover, addiction to alcohol involves a time-dependent vicious cycle: after withdrawing from alcohol, the person experiences withdrawal symptoms and then drinks more alcohol to quell these symptoms. Many other forms of addiction follow a similar pattern whereby the solution to the problem of withdrawal becomes the problem. Also, the problem often spreads to produce psychological and social conflicts which prompt further drinking. In what follows, it should be kept in mind that the potential of a vicious cycle, once started, to involve biological, psychological, and social areas is a common phenomenon.

TIME DISORIENTATION AND ORGANIC BRAIN DISEASE

Time disorientation is a classic sign of organic brain disease. It is manifested by the patient being unable to tell the date, month, or even the year (Orme, 1966). Missing the date by more than three days is generally accepted as indicative of time disorientation. In organic brain disease, disorientation to time appears earlier in the course of illness than disorientation to place or person. It can be subtle at first, such as not being able to tell how long one has been in the hospital or how long one has spent with the interviewer. Strategies for assessing time disorientation are presented in Chapter 5. At this point, I will deal with the spiral accompanying time disorientation and its appearance in some common organic mental disorders.

As previously noted, time disorientation is just a sign of pervasive problems with sequence, rate, and temporal perspective. These general and pervasive time problems induce confusion about the personal future (Table 2). The confusion about the personal future may augment the problems with sequence, rate, and temporal perspective. For example, one patient wanted to call her daughter who had written her a note to call her at 3 P.M.; the patient called her daughter in the morning, not realizing that she had to wait until 3 P.M. or thinking that it was this time because of her time disorientation; when her daughter did not answer the phone, the patient became worried and frightened that something had happened to her daughter; when she was told that it was not yet 3 P.M., she felt that other people were playing games with her and she became upset with what they were doing to the clocks. Here the confusion about the future event prompted her to become even more disoriented to time.

In organic brain disease, vicious cycles often occur because of progressive degrees of disorganization of goal-directed behavior. As sequence, rate, and temporal perspective become disorganized, the person becomes more disoriented toward the future; and the disorientation toward the future strips the person from a comprehensible timeline for organizing his goal-directed behavior. In a sense, this disorganization of goal-directed behavior can be understood as difficulties in remembering the future—that is, what the person intends to do, or even that he has a future. Although the clouding of the future obscures the temporal context in which rates of sequences are adjusted to meet goals, there is a saving grace: If the person forgets the future, he has less anticipatory fear. This lack of future awareness may help prevent spirals of anticipatory fear to become grafted upon the general disorganization.

Of course, the past and present also are often obscured in organic brain disease because of impaired memory. Impaired memory is a central feature of organic brain disease, such as a delirium or a dementia. The impaired memory makes it difficult for the person to locate where he is in time. When a person is dislocated in time, he has great difficulty in making appropriate adjustments to changes in his social and physical environment.

Clouding of consciousness is typical of a delirium. A delirium is an acute global impairment of the brain, usually caused by toxic or metabolic factors (Engel and Romano, 1959). Distractability, emotional liability, illusions, and hallucinations (especially visual) are common in a delirium. In a delirium, the person cannot sustain attention to environmental events. When he does perceive ordinary external events, such as a door slamming shut, he may overreact with fear, perhaps since the event is not apprehended within the context of the time flow of previous happenings. Since events cannot be placed in time, they seem unfamiliar and jarring. As outlined in Chapter 2, since consciousness depends on the integration of past, present, and future, I propose that the general clouding of consciousness seen in a delirium probably stems largely from an inability to locate oneself in time. Whatever the case, the marked disorganization of behavior in delirium clearly demonstrates that intact behavior is highly dependent on the adequate temporal processing of information.

A dementia usually develops insidiously and is not characterized by the acute clouding of consciousness typical of a delirium. In a dementia, there is a generalized decrement in higher brain functions, such as memory, abstract reasoning, and judgment. Usually there is a greater impairment of short-term memory as compared to long-term memory. The impairment of short-term memory is associated with disorientation to time (Benton, van Allen, and Fogel, 1964). A demented person's disorientation is greater when he is placed in unfamiliar surroundings. His disorientation to time is usually first detected by his inability to order events chronologically when asked to give a history of his problems.

Besides the diffuse brain diseases of delirium and dementia, time disorientation also can occur with focal brain disorders, particularly those involving the limbic and frontal lobe areas. In these focal brain disorders, there is usually no clouding of consciousness, but the person shows gaps in his temporal awareness. Examples include the amnestic syndrome, herpes simplex encephalitis, psychomotor epilepsy, and frontal lobe disorders.

In the amnestic syndrome (formerly called Korsakoff's psychosis), there is impairment of both short-term and long-term memory but no impairment of immediate memory. The intact immediate memory probably accounts for the lack of clouding of consciousness in these patients and their ability to at least carry on a superficial conversation. However, these patients have great difficulty in recalling events that occurred three to five minutes before (Williams and Zangwill, 1950). Their memory for *when* events occurred appears to be more impaired than for *what* events occurred (Talland, 1960, 1968). These patients can be easily led astray because of the gaps in their awareness as to what went before, as though they were driving without a rearview mirror. The amnestic syndrome is usually caused by prolonged alcoholism with resultant thiamine deficiency that destroys areas of the diencephalon and limbic system, such as the mammillary bodies and hippocampal complex. The peculiar inability to index when recent events occurred in time deserves further study, since it might shed light on areas of the brain that are involved in locating sequences in time.

Irritation or lesions of the hippocampal complexes produce marked deficits in immediate or ''working'' memory and may give rise to psychotic syndromes (Douglas, 1967). In this regard, many psychotomimetic drugs, such as LSD, psilocybin, and tetrahydrocannabinol, produce seizures predominantly in the hippocampi and nearby structures in the temporal lobe (Adey, Bell, and Dennis, 1962; Miller, 1979). All of these psychotomimetic drugs produce marked alternations in the sense of time.

A seizure disorder can produce transient gaps of awareness that momentarily disrupt a person's orientation to time. Changes in time sense have been found to occur during an epileptic attack (Holubar and Machek, 1962). In addition, many of the psychic phenomena of psychomotor epilepsy include uncanny time experiences, such as deja vu, feelings of predestination, mystical coincidences, and the telescoping of past, present, and future (Bear and Fedio, 1977; Monroe, 1978; Karagulla and Robertson, 1955). The seizures of psychomotor epilepsy usually stem from abnormal electrical discharges in the temporal lobe and limbic system. During brain surgery, direct stimulation of the deep structures of the temporal lobe commonly produce uncanny time experiences (Penfield, 1955; 1958; Stevens et al., 1969). As discussed later, the uncanny time experiences associated with dysfunctions of the limbic system and temporal lobe may have relevance to distortions of reality during the active phases of schizophrenia.

Disorders of the frontal lobe impair a person's orientation toward the future. These disorders can come from tumors, infarcts, or surgical excision of the frontal lobes. After frontal lobectomy, a person is often indifferent toward the future and tends to be focused primarily on the present (Petrie, 1952; Orme, 1969; Greenblatt and Solomon, 1958). Although patients with frontal lobotomies may show little change in standard intelligence tests, tests that involve planning ability and the temporal integration of information, such as the Porteus maze, are impaired (Riddle and Roberts, 1978). Although these patients are less anxious since they are unconcerned about the future, this benefit is at the high cost of losing powers of anticipation necessary for coping and problem solving. Largely for this reason, frontal lobectomies have been abandoned as a method of treatment.

In summary, time disorientation is commonly associated with diffuse organic brain syndromes, particularly when there is clouding of consciousness as in a delirium. In addition, focal lesions or irritations in subcortical areas of the brain can produce transient gaps in temporal awareness or unusual time experiences that disrupt the person's orientation to the time flow of events around him.

TEMPORAL DISINTEGRATION OF SEQUENCES AND SCHIZOPHRENIC DISORDERS

The next time problem listed in the hierarchy of Table 2 is called the *temporal disintegration of sequences*. Temporal disintegration means that the person has difficulties with sequential thinking so that it is difficult for him to coordinate sequences toward a goal (Melges et al., 1970a, 1970b). Unlike diffuse organic brain disease but somewhat similar to focal seizures, these difficulties with tracking sequences are usually intermittent. That is, the person has brief episodes of impaired sequential thinking interspersed with normal functioning. I propose that these intermittent sequential problems are prominent in the group of schizophrenias and may account for many other symptoms of an acute psychosis, as detailed in Chapter 7.

During these episodes of impaired sequential thinking, there also may be problems with rate and temporal perspective. This is because the gaps between a succession of events governs the rate of mental events (see Chapter 2). In addition, the larger sequences of temporal perspective (past, present, and future) may become jumbled with impaired sequential thinking.

It is here proposed that these episodes of impaired sequential thinking induce the person to experience his personal future as intermittently fragmented and lacking coherence (Table 2). The fragmented and incoherent future time perspective, in turn, robs the person of a consistent timeline for ordering his mental sequences, thereby augmenting his problems with sequential thinking. In this way, the temporal disintegration of sequences becomes aggravated by the incoherent personal future, and the escalated sequential difficulties further fragment his personal future. A vicious cycle ensues.

The impaired sequential thinking can take place without the time disorientation typical of organic brain disease. I propose that there are two reasons for this. One is that the sequential difficulties are intermittent, thereby allowing the person to register and orient himself to clock and calendar time during his periods of normal functioning. The other reason is that, rather than short-term and long-term memory being affected as in organic brain disease, the difficulties with sequential thinking may be related to problems with immediate or "working" memory. I will explore this below as well as in Chapter 7. Whatever the case, the episodes of impaired sequential thinking make it difficult for the person to direct his thinking toward a goal.

This inability to direct one's thinking toward a goal is fundamental to what is called the *formal thought disorder* of the group of schizophrenias. A formal thought disorder means that thinking processes are disturbed; the deranged processes often give rise to bizarre thought content, such as delusions. Research has shown that the induction of temporal disintegration in normal subjects gives rise to delusional thought content (Melges et al., 1974).

The schizophrenic patient's difficulty with coordinating sequences toward a goal is commonly manifested as *loosening of associations*. Bleuler (1911, pp. 14–15) introduced the term loosening of associations to describe schizophrenic speech in which "associations lose their continuity" and the "most important determinant of the associations is lacking—the concept of purpose." This impairment of goal-directed thinking takes place in the absence of clouding of consciousness (as in a delirium) and without diffuse deficits in short-term and long-term memory (as in a dementia). Loosening of associations is manifested as irrelevant speech, in which the person shifts from topic to topic, that has no apparent connection. Derailments or interruptions in the train of thought are frequent. Difficulties with keeping track of sequences over time appear to account for loosening of associations (Melges et al., 1970a). That is, when a person cannot keep track of what he just said or what he intends to say, his thoughts are apt to wander in disconnected directions.

The intermittent nature of these problems with tracking and coordinating sequences has not been sufficiently highlighted in the research literature, although most clinicians who work closely with schizophrenic patients are well aware that their problems are not constant or continuous (Callaway, 1970). For example, except during the very active and florid psychotic phase of schizophrenia, these patients are capable of conducting daily routines and responding to time cues such as when to eat, sleep, meet with their doctor, and group together for a fire drill. Yet they appear to require rather structured external time cues in the physical environment or from an interviewer for them to maintain coherent goal-directed behavior and thinking. When these external time cues are lacking, it is not uncommon for a schizophrenic patient to lose his train of thought four to five times during a five-minute open-ended conversation.

Schizophrenic patients are usually aware of their difficulties with tracking sequences and, when prompted and given enough time to respond, can describe these difficulties (Chapman, 1966; Detre and Jarecki, 1971). For example, to quote a schizophrenic patient of McGhie and Chapman (1961): "My thoughts get all jumbled up. I start thinking about something but I never get them. Instead I wander off and get caught up with all sorts of different things that may be connected with things I want to say but in a way I can't." Here is another example from one of our patients: "I can't keep up with my thoughts, and I lose track of what I'm thinking about."

There are, of course, a number of competing theories about the formal thought process disorder of the group of schizophrenias. This is to be expected in attempting to solve the riddle of schizophrenia, which constitutes a major health problem. Nevertheless, many of these theories and related research can be conveniently conceptualized as difficulties with tracking sequences over time. In this regard, Arieti (1974) emphasizes impaired "seriatim functions" in schizophrenia in which step-by-step thinking is disrupted. Meehl (1962) uses the term "cognitive slippage" to refer to the process whereby thoughts slip out of context. Shakow's (1963) findings of "impaired mental set" indicates that schizophrenics have difficulty in sustaining attention over time. A number of investigators have highlighted impaired immediate or "working" memory in schizophrenia so that the person becomes vulnerable to distraction and to losing his train of thought (McGhie, Chapman, and Lawson, 1965; Callaway, 1970; Braff, Callaway, and Naylor, 1977). In a major review of various hypotheses about disturbed thinking in schizophrenia, Lang and Buss (1965) concluded that the most parsimonious and substantiated hypothesis is that there is some kind of interference with the schizophrenic's immediate memory. Interferences with immediate memory would impair the person's ability to hold in mind and coordinate sequences toward a goal (Melges et al., 1980a; Callaway and Naghdi, 1982).

A number of studies, using a variety of approaches, have demonstrated that schizophrenic patients have difficulty with integrating information over time.

Weinstein, Goldstone, and Boardman (1958) found that schizophrenics are unable to ''take advantage of past experience in conceptualizing current frames of reference.'' Lhamon and Goldstone (1973) found that schizophrenics show an impaired utilization of information to be collated over time. Salzinger (1972) highlights the schizophrenic's distractability to immediate stimuli. Balken (1943) found that, on Thematic Apperception Tests, schizophrenics ''cling desperately and without awareness to the present,'' presumably because they have difficulty in distinguishing past, present, and future.

More recent research continues to point to a deficit in the temporal processing of information in schizophrenia. Steffy (1978) found that an early cue impairs performance on reaction time in schizophrenics, and this impairment is greater at longer intervals. Mo et al. (1978) have found a weakness and instability of time expectancy in schizophrenia. Collins et al. (1978) found a lack of temporal integration of visual information in schizophrenics. Saccuzzo and Braff (1981) have shown that early information processing in schizophrenia is deficient. Moreover, the inability to maintain a temporal context may explain the schizophrenic patient's difficulties in communication, such as poor editing of information irrelevant to the shifting temporal foci of a conversation (Cohen, 1978; Rochester, 1978). Moreover, there is evidence that the antipsychotic drugs, such as chlorpromazine, improve the temporal processing of information by enhancing the span of comprehension and the ability to maintain a mental set (Spohn et al., 1977; Zahn, Carpenter, and McGlashan, 1978; see Chapter 7).

Besides the time problem of difficulties with tracking sequences, future time perspective in schizophrenics has been found to be disorganized and incoherent (Wallace, 1956; Dilling and Rabin, 1967). Their ways of anticipating events appear to be inconsistent and vacillating (Bannister and Mair, 1968; Bannister and Fransella, 1966; Adams-Webber, 1979). In addition, during the very acute stages of schizophrenia, there is marked temporal disorganization of plans of action such that the individual has difficulty with coordinating plans toward goals; and this improves as they are treated and become less ill (Melges and Freeman, 1977).

It is here proposed that the temporal disintegration of sequential thinking induces the fragmentation of future time perspective, which, in turn, aggravates the problem with sequential thinking, since there is an inconsistent or intermittently disrupted timeline for ordering the sequences (Table 2). This may prompt a spiral of progressive temporal disorganization of plans of action.

It is now well recognized that the research about the broad category of schizophrenia must at least distinguish the active, acute phases of this illness from the inactive and more chronic forms. In this regard, research indicates that the more actively psychotic phases of schizophrenia are associated with greater degrees of temporal disintegration and time distortions (Melges and Fougerousse, 1966; Melges and Freeman, 1977). During the actively psychotic phases, it appears that these individuals have difficulty in distinguishing the *now* from the *then*. This temporal indistinction between past, present, and future appears to be related to overt psychotic symptoms, such as delusions of alien control and hallucinations. In Chapter 7, I will deal more explicitly with research that suggests an interrelationship between temporal indistinction and specific psychotic symptoms. The inability to tell the now from the then may stem from extreme difficulties with keeping track of sequences.

There are other signs and symptoms of schizophrenia that may be related to the temporal incoordination of sequences. These include blocking, withdrawal from others, and emotional incongruity. Blocking in schizophrenia refers to the cessation of thought so that nothing is going on in the mind, not even a search for a forgotten item of information. Blocking usually lasts from 10 to 120 seconds. Chapman (1966) has emphasized the similarity between schizophrenic blocking and psychomotor epileptic attacks. He also proposes that these intermittent interruptions in the train of one's thinking prompt the schizophrenic patient to feel uncertain about carrying on social conversations. As a result, to avoid the embarrassment of being unable to talk with or comprehend others, the patient may withdraw from social contacts. Moreover, if the schizophrenic only has a fragmented appreciation of an ongoing social situation, his emotional responses may seem out of touch with what is going on interpersonally. This lack of emotional harmony, called *incongruity of affect* (Bleuler, 1911), thus also may be related to difficulties with keeping track of information over time.

Besides schizophrenia, difficulties with keeping track of sequences also can occur in organic brain disease, particularly during a delirium. The diagnosis of schizophrenia cannot be made unless one first rules out a delirium or other types of organic brain disease. Especially during the acute phases of these illnesses, both schizophrenic and delirious patients are, in a sense, lost in time. From a temporal standpoint, the main difference between these two syndromes is that time disorientation in terms of not knowing the day, month, or year is much more frequent in organic brain disease as compared to schizophrenia. Also, in organic brain disease the impairment of memory usually hinders immediate, short-term, and even long-term memory, whereas in schizophrenia immediate memory is primarily affected (Saccuzzo and Braff, 1981). Moreover, the immediate memory impairment in schizophrenia is usually intermittent and is associated with episodic tracking difficulties compared to the pervasive and persistent tracking difficulties of organic brain disease (Chapter 7). In each syndrome when there is marked temporal disintegration of sequences, whether these are episodic or persistent, psychotic symptoms such as hallucinations are more frequent (Chapter 7).

It should be pointed out that manic or depressed patients rarely have difficulty in distinguishing sequences. The manic patient's thoughts may race, and he often jumps from subject to subject with a flight of ideas, but when stopped and asked, he almost always can recover his intended train of thought. Also, even though the severely depressed patient's thinking is slowed with difficulty in concentrating and inefficient short-term memory, rarely does he confuse sequences of the past, present, and future.

If further research continues to indicate that the temporal disintegration of sequential thinking is a useful way to conceptualize the cognitive deficit in schizophrenia, it will be important to look for underlying neurochemical factors involved in this deficit. In this regard, there is a growing body of evidence that suggests a dysfunction of the left cerebral hemisphere in schizophrenia (Gur, 1979; Wexler and Heninger, 1979; Weinberger et al., 1979; Wexler, 1980). As outlined in Chapter 2, the left cerebral hemisphere appears to be involved primarily in the processing of sequences, as in language. It could be that some kind of subcortical disorder, such as a minor seizure in the limbic system or a disharmony of cerebellar and extrapyramidal functions might produce intermittent dysfunctions of the left hemisphere in schizophrenia. These exciting possibilities await further research.

By way of conclusion, the experience of timelessness is quite common during acute schizophrenia. This experience can be awesome, uncanny, and frightening. To quote a schizophrenic patient of Jaspers (1963, p. 87): "Time had failed and stood still . . . time did not lie before or after me but in every direction . . . I seemed to myself a timeless creature." I will deal with such uncanny experiences in greater depth in Chapter 7. At this point I will just give a flavor of what they are like. The mind may race while the passage of clock time seems inexorably slow. Childhood memories become as vivid and real as the present. Fantasies of the future also seem real. The person loses his grip on the here-and-now as the past and future telescope into the present. The person feels lost in a kaleidoscopic swirl of times past, present, and future. Lost in time, as though in a dream, he cannot tell the real from the unreal.

In summary, it is here proposed that these timeless experiences may stem from problems with tracking sequences. These sequential difficulties fragment time as a medium and perspective of experience. In schizophrenia, when both the present and the future become fragmented, the person becomes vulnerable to being invaded by his past as though it were happening now. This not only impairs his goal-directedness but also ushers in an ever-widening spiral of problems. Since his sequential thinking is impaired, he is unable to organize his plans of action temporally in order to cope with his problems. In short, since he has difficulty in coordinating his plans of action with his future images and emotions, he becomes vulnerable to vicious cycles of episodic dyscontrol.

RATE AND RHYTHM PROBLEMS IN MANIC-DEPRESSIVE ILLNESS

In the hierarchy of time problems presented in Table 2, the next time problem consists of difficulties with rate and rhythm. I propose that problems with rate and rhythm are primarily characteristic of manic-depressive illness, although they may occur as part of the general time disorganization of organic brain disease or as secondary to the temporal disintegration of sequences. However, in manic-depressive illness, these rate and rhythm problems occur without time disorientation or the temporal disintegration of sequences.

In mania, the rate of mental events is accelerated; in depression, it is slowed. This induces two contrasting types of spirals. In mania, the accelerated rate induces over-expansion of the personal future with a host of future images and plans. Often the future becomes so expanded that the person rushes headlong into a myriad of projects and rarely takes the time to complete a plan of action in the preseent. His pace is so fast that he has trouble synchronizing with other people. As a result, he often becomes frustrated and angry, and this may increase his mental rate further. By contrast, in depression, the slowed rate often induces a constriction of the personal future, and the person may become hopeless about his capacity to accomplish his goals, especially when he realizes that he is lagging behind others and slowing them down. His hopelessness may prompt him to give up striving, and this further slows him down. In contrast to the rapid thinking and hyperactivity of the manic patient, the depressed patient thinks slowly, has difficulties with concentration, and even moves slowly. The latter is called psychomotor retardation. Thus an accelerated tempo with an expanded future is characteristic of mania, whereas a slowed tempo with a blocked or hopeless future is common during the depressive phase of manic-depressive illness as well as in other types of severe depression.

In Part IV, I will deal more explicitly with the spiral of hopelessness that can occur in different types of depression (Chapter 9), including unresolved grief (Chapter 10). Slowing and blocks to the future are central aspects of all types of severe depression. At this point, I will focus on rate and rhythm problems in manic-depressive illness.

In this regard, manic patients often report that their "thoughts are racing," whereas depressed patients report that their thoughts are "slowed and sluggish.'' Time-estimation tests are consistent with this contrast between mania and depression. That is, in mania, internal tempo is fast (Mezey and Knight, 1965; Orme, 1966), whereas in depression, internal tempo is slow (Mezey and Cohen, 1961; Melges and Fougerousse, 1966; Wyrick and Wyrick, 1977). The pervasive slowness of thinking during severe depression probably contributes to impaired concentration and sluggish performance on short-term memory tasks (Braff and Beck, 1974). It also may contribute to inefficient goal-directed thinking so that the person becomes temporally disorganized (Kirstein and Bukberg, 1979). In depression, it is here proposed that temporal disorganization is characterized mainly by a dysjunction between plans and goals; that is, the depressed patient believes that his plans of action are insufficient to meet his goals.

The temporal disorganization that occurs in depression is different from that of organic brain disease and in the group of schizophrenias. In depression, rather than confusion or disintegration of sequential thinking, there is a gap between one's future images (goals) and plans of action. Plans of action are deemed insufficient to meet goals. This thesis will be explored more fully in Chapter 9. Rarely does the depressed patient mix up sequences. His thinking may be slow and inefficient, but he usually does not confuse sequences. One exception, of course, is the so-called pseudo-dementia that accompanies very severe depressive illness, especially in the elderly, in which the person's thinking is so slow that he appears demented.

Practical guidelines for clinically differentiating the time problems of organic brain disease and schizophrenia from that of depression and mania will be given in Chapter 5. At this point, it should be noted that manic patients rarely confuse sequences. They may have a flight of ideas with tangential thinking, but when prompted they almost always can recover their train of thought. The one exception is so-called delirious mania in which, it is here proposed, the rate of successive sequences becomes so fast that the sequences become blurred.

Thus in terms of the cybernetic concepts presented in Chapter 3, mania can be viewed as an accelerated rate of future images and plans of action accompanied by optimistic emotions about the likelihood of the plans meeting the future images. But this optimistic feedforward may become so excessive that it overrides feedback from present outcomes. By contrast, severe depression can be viewed as the slowing of the rate of future images and plans of action with pessimistic emotions about the likelihood of plans of action being sufficient to meet valued goals. This pessimistic feedforward may override such feedback as rewards occurring in the present.

Why do these alterations in the rate of functioning occur in manic-depressive illness? There is mounting evidence that problems with biological rhythms may be involved in manic-depressive illness (Wehr and Goodwin, 1981). The hypothesis is that if one's body clocks are not synchronized and kept in check by each other, some clocks may become out of phase and run faster or slower than others. In short, disorders of biological rhythms may induce rate problems.

As with other animals, humans demonstrate a number of biological rhythms that keep them in phase with periodic changes in the environment, such as changes from night to day or from season to season (Sollberger, 1963; Richter, 1965; Halberg, 1968; Luce, 1970, 1973). The relevance of biological dysrhythmias to behavioral disorders is an exciting frontier in psychiatry (Stroebel, 1976; Orme, 1969).

One exciting possibility is that manic-depressive illness represents a biological dysrhythmia (Jenner, 1968; Kripke et al., 1978; Stroebel, 1980). The lifetime pattern of manic-depressive illness indicates that there are cycles of mania, depression, or both, with intervening intervals of psychological health. During the normal intervals, it is well known that these individuals can be highly productive and lead constructive lives. The predisposition to cycles of mania or depression is inherited. The initial episodes of illness appear to be stress induced, but thereafter the cycles appear to take on a life of their own, appearing without definite precipitating stresses. Although there is wide variability between individuals, a person with recurrent bouts of mania or depression (bipolar illness) has an average of about 14 episodes of illness during his lifetime; a person with recurrent depressions (unipolar illness) has about five episodes per lifetime. Although the overall pattern of illness is cyclic, the cycles are usually irregular; this makes it difficult to predict just when a person with manic-depressive illness will have another episode.

It is not known as yet just what triggers the onset of mania or depression. However, there is recent evidence that a phase shift in circadian rhythms may be involved (Wehr, Muscettola, and Goodwin, 1980). A circadian rhythm consists of a phasic change over approximately a 24-hour period. The sleep–waking rhythm is a circadian rhythm that normally synchronizes rest with periods of darkness and activity with periods of light. In manic-depressive illness, the evidence thus far suggests that there is a phase advance of certain biological rhythms. That is, there is an earlier peak of activity, temperature, norepinephrine secretion, and rapid-eye-movement dream frequency than would occur normally. It is possible that when these rhythms are no longer synchronized with other biological rhythms, they begin to take on a life of their own, unchecked by the other biological rhythms.

In this regard, one striking characteristic of mania is the lack of need for rest and the inability to sleep, with many patients getting only one to two hours of sleep per night during a manic phase. It is as though their activity cycle is running free, unchecked by the sleep cycle. In severe depression, there also is lack of sleep, and most depressed patients complain of insomnia, especially early morning awakening accompanied by a sluggish feeling that they still need to sleep. This sluggishness is most prominent in the morning and tends to wear off as the day goes on. This diurnal variation of mood is characteristic of depression. The pattern also suggests a disorder of biological rhythms. In this regard, a cumulative shift of phasic rhythms could explain why some depressed patients are insomniac, while others have excessive sleep or hypersomnia (Stroebel, 1980).

There is evidence that drugs used to treat mania or depression may have an effect on circadian rhythms. Lithium carbonate, which is used to treat mania, has been found to slow biological clocks (Englemann, 1973; Johnsson et al., 1979). On the other hand, drugs used to treat depression, such as the tricyclic antidepressant medicines, appear to accelerate certain biological clocks (Wehr and Goodwin, 1979; see Chapter 6).

It should be noted that, besides manic-depressive illness, there are other behavioral disorders that may be related to biological rhythms. The most common is premenstrual tension (Moos et al., 1969; Melges and Hamburg, 1976). About 20% of women suffer considerable irritability and emotional lability during the premenstrual and menstrual phases of their monthly hormonal cycles. These phases appear to be periods of vulnerability, since approximately 40% of suicide attempts and psychotic breaks take place during these phases in women. Other biological dysrhythmias may be associated with periodic catatonia (Gjessing and Gjessing, 1961) and some psychosomatic disorders, such as peptic ulcer (Luce, 1971).

TEMPORAL PERSPECTIVE PROBLEMS IN NEUROTIC AND PERSONALITY DISORDERS

Temporal perspective refers to the span of awareness into the past or future. It also refers to the focus on the past, present, or future. Problems with temporal perspective pertain to imbalances in a person's span of awareness into the past or future with an overriding focus on the past, present, or future. These imbalances of temporal perspective, as outlined in the hierarchy of time problems in Table 2, are commonly associated with neurotic and personality disorders. They occur in these disorders largely due to learning and styles of coping, and are not secondary to more basic cognitive problems with sequence or rate. However, problems with temporal perspective, as previously discussed, often accompany time disorientation, temporal disintegration, and rate and rhythm problems.

I propose that these problems with temporal perspective bias the nature of a person's anticipations so that he becomes vulnerable to certain types of spirals. This is in line with Kelly's (1955) fundamental postulate that the ways in which a person anticipates events govern his psychological processes. One way to conceptualize this is to consider the interaction between an imbalance of temporal perspective and a way of anticipating the personal future. Such an interaction is outlined briefly in Table 2. It is here suggested that spirals of psychopathology can occur when an imbalance of temporal perspective prompts a particular way of viewing the future which, in turn, aggravates the imbalance of temporal perspective.

Table 2 lists three general types of imbalances of temporal perspective: an over-focus on the future, an over-focus on the past, and an over-focus on the present. This is a gross over-simplification, but it will serve to introduce the kinds of spirals that may stem from such imbalances. More detailed accounts will be given in later chapters. I propose that these predominant foci may give rise to spirals since information from other frames of reference (past, present, or future) is excluded or misconstrued.

Let us begin with over-focus on the future since this problem often complicates loss of control in schizophrenia and mania and gives rise to paranoid thinking as a defense against loss of control. That is, it is often a more severe problem that can become psychotic and is not traditionally conceived as a neurotic problem. My proposal, however, suggests that there may be a "paranoid neurosis," so to speak, since the processes that eventuate in paranoid thinking are commonly misconstrued anticipations fueled by anticipatory fears (see Chapters 8 and 11). In particular, these paranoid processes are discussed at length in Chapter 8, which deals with how they may become augmented by sequential difficulties as in paranoid schizophrenia. But in this section the discussion is not dealing with paranoid schizophrenia, but rather with paranoid personalities.

Although an orientation toward the future and an extended span of awareness into the future is usually conducive to coping (see Chapter 3), it is possible for a person to be overly focused on the future to such a degree that his style of relating to other people is largely in terms of searching for and counteracting future threats to one's security. That is, there is an over-concern with future threats. This may prompt a future–future interaction that begins to spiral, especially when present and past outcomes are neglected. The over-focus on the future sensitizes the person to perceive or interpret his personal future as threatening, and the latter in turn prompts him to focus even more on the future. I propose that these over-projections into the future are common during paranoid disorders. In attempting to deal with a future threat, the person becomes suspicious of others' motives and makes predictions about their plans, but his predictions often increase his sense of threat, making him even more paranoid (see Chapter 8).

An over-focus on the past, especially when coupled with the dread of the future, is common in anxiety disorders, such as phobic and obsessive-compulsive neuroses. As discussed more fully in Chapter 11, it is here proposed that emotional spirals in neurotic disorders commonly involve the dread of the future which has become misconstrued by catastrophic expectations stemming from the past. The catastrophic expectations often are that one will be rejected or controlled by other people, much like a helpless child relating to critical or domineering parents. The neurotic individual may not be fully aware of the past source of his catastrophic expectations that prompt his dread of the future. Instead, he is often preoccupied and over-worried about uncertainties of the future (Krauss, 1967). His dread and uncertainty about the future prompt him to avoid interpersonal situations in the future, such that he will not learn how to deal with them realistically. As he avoids the future, he becomes more vulnerable to being thrown back into the past, thereby coming further into the grip of catastrophic expectations conditioned by earlier experiences usually in childhood. In this way, a spiral of anxiety ensues: the dread and avoidance of the future plunge him deeper into distorted expectations of the past, which, in turn, prompt him to dread his personal future even more.

Although anxiety is the core emotion in most neurotic disorders, there are other negative emotions, such as anger, guilt, and depression, that can become part of the neurotic spiral of anxiety and the dread of the future. For example, the person may dread the future because he is fearful about becoming angry, and this may be rooted in the catastrophic expectation that he will be controlled and dominated by others if he becomes angry. These other emotional spirals are discussed in Chapter 11.

We all react to the present and future in light of past experiences. Yet past experiences may distort present perceptions and future expectations in such a way that a person reacts to a situation at hand as though it were out of his past (Spiegel, 1981). This inappropriate transference of the past onto the present and future is commonly at the core of the emotional overreactions of neurotic emotionality. In particular, the neurotic individual reacts to people in his current environment as if they were figures from his past.

Anniversary reactions are classical examples of how the reactivation of the past can distort the present and future. In an anniversary reaction, the person suffers a recurrence of grief (or its bodily manifestations) at the time of year of a previous loss (Hilgard and Newman, 1959, 1963; Mintz, 1971). The person may be unaware of the source of his distress. For example, a young man with severe chest pain went to the emergency room, fearing that he was dying; he had forgotten that his father had died of a heart attack exactly one year before.

In this regard, unresolved grief can distort the future such that it seems hopeless and devoid of meaning. Chapters 9 and 10 deal with the effect of loss of a close person on a person's view of the future and how this sometimes eventuates in a spiral of hopelessness. It is here proposed that a person vulnerable to becoming depressed has a narrow view of his personal future such that if someone close to him dies or he fails to achieve an important goal, he feels he has lost everything.

An over-focus on the present is common in antisocial personalities, formerly called sociopaths. In Chapter 9, I propose that this predominant present-orientation is a form of chronic hopelessness about the future, and prompts the person to disregard future consequences. The impulsive acts of antisocial personalities are often conditioned by seeking immediate gratification without regard to future consequences.

The role of a predominant present-orientation in other types of personality disorders has been highlighted by Miller (1964). In this regard, Hartocollis (1978) proposes that many of the wide swings in emotion and behavior seen in borderline personalities may stem from a fragmentation of temporal perspective, so that the person becomes overly consumed by whatever he is feeling or thinking at the moment.

Thus problems with temporal perspective may induce distorted ways of viewing the personal future which, in turn, may aggravate the imbalanced temporal perspective, leading to spirals of misconstrued expectations.

It should be noted that these problems with temporal perspective represent distortions of the temporal *form* of thinking and feeling that are often spurred by fearsome *content*. That is, aversive past experiences, such as being rejected or controlled, contaminate the person's future outlook, thereby altering the temporal form of the ways in which he anticipates events. Once the abnormal temporal form is induced, whatever the nature of the triggering content, the altered form may persist as a way of viewing the future that is conducive to subsequent misconstructions. In this regard, as pointed out in Chapter 2, unpleasant emotions tend to foreshorten future time perspective. Although this may assist the person in dealing with the current situation, it may also limit awareness of alternatives down the line. Enlarging or revising temporal perspective has therapeutic implications, as discussed in Chapter 6 and in Part V.

DESYNCHRONIZED TRANSACTIONS AND ADJUSTMENT DISORDERS

The last time problem listed in the hierarchy of Table 2 is called *desynchronized transactions*. This means that the interactions between two or more people are out of phase, mistimed, and/or at cross purposes. Although this is not necessarily a distortion of psychological time, it can stem from any of the time problems previously discussed and is often the problem most conspicuous at the time a patient seeks or is brought for psychiatric help. That is, the patient at least has an adjustment disorder marked by social conflicts and interpersonal difficulties within his family or work situation.

It should be obvious that any of the time disturbances discussed in the previous sections can contribute to the desynchronization of transactions. That is, time disorientation, temporal disintegration, rhythm-rate problems, and problems with temporal perspective can disrupt the flow of interpersonal communications and transactions. Nevertheless, desynchronized transactions need not necessarily arise from pathology within individuals but can occur between people because the *interaction* is "sick," not the individuals.

Mismatched expectations of other people and ambivalence are at the root of most desynchronized transactions. The problems are aggravated when there is failure to communicate and negotiate the differences in the expectations. This may give rise to a variety of devious social ploys ("games") as indirect ways to undercut or free oneself from the expectations of others. In this regard, neurotic individuals are prone to desynchronized transactions and "games" since they often distort their current relationships with other people in terms of catastrophic expectations stemming from the distant past.

Chapter 11 highlights the role of ambivalence in desynchronized transactions. Ambivalence refers to simultaneous positive and negative feelings. Although the term usually refers to feelings of love and hate toward other people, it can also refer to both positive and negative feelings about one's interpersonal future. At the simplest level, if a person is ambivalent about his interpersonal future, he is likely to be hesitant and unsure about his future transactions with others. This may prompt him to avoid clarifying expectations that would facilitate his synchronizing with others. At a more complex level, ambivalence may reflect the expectation that getting close to another person carries the threat of being controlled by the other person. This may prompt a recurrent vicious cycle of interpersonal rifts since as the person gets closer, he becomes more threatened by being controlled and then finds some way to distance the other person. This cycle of getting closer and then distancing from others is common in desynchronized transactions (Chapter 11). It may lead to a spiral of progressive alienation from other people.

SUMMARY AND CONCLUSIONS

The purpose of this chapter was to give an introductory overview of the role of time and the personal future in psychopathological spirals. The central thesis was that psychopathological vicious cycles are likely to occur when problems with psychological time disrupt the normal interplay between future images, plans of action, and emotions, thereby leading to loss of anticipatory control. Two postulates were set forth relating to this thesis:

1   Distortions of psychological time and the personal future are involved in psychopathological spirals.
2   Different psychopathological spirals are related to different types of distortions of psychological time and the personal future.

In exploring these postulates, I proposed a hierarchical model of problems with time and the personal future as presented in Table 2. Using this model, I dealt with two common types of spirals:

1   The potential of more severe time problems to encompass less severe time problems. For example, problems with sequence often induce problems with rate and temporal perspective as well as desynchronized transactions.
2   The interaction between the time problem and the individual's construction of his personal future. For example, in depression, the slowing of mental rate both induces and is aggravated by hopelessness about the future.

The nature of these psychopathological spirals in some of the major clinical syndromes of psychiatry was outlined in terms of interactions between the following time problems and misconstructions of the personal future:

1   Time disorientation and confusion of the personal future in organic brain disease
2   The temporal disintegration of sequences and the intermittent fragmentation of the personal future in schizophrenic disorders
3   Rate and rhythm problems and an overly expanded or blocked future in manic-depressive illness
4   Temporal perspective problems as related to a threatening, dreaded, or disregarded personal future in neurotic and personality disorders
5   Desynchronized transactions with other people as related to ambivalence about one's interpersonal future in adjustment disorders

Since time is an important medium, as well as a perspective of human awareness, distortions of time and the personal future are likely to alter psychological processes, particularly the ways in which people anticipate events. I propose that this sets the stage for vicious cycles (spirals) to ensue. With a time problem, once a spiral is initiated, whatever its triggering cause, it may take on a life of its own and continue to escalate, since there is lack of timely feedback or feedforward that normally would reestablish regulatory control. That is, the person's anticipatory control becomes disrupted by the problems with time and the personal future. The spirals ensue since there is a lack of coordination or frequent mismatches between one's future images, plans of action, and emotions.

CHAPTER FIVE

The Clinical Assessment of Time Problems

A disorder of time consciousness . . . is a primary alteration of consciousness and may be found as often as it is looked for in mental illness.

AUBREY LEWIS (1931, p. 614)

This chapter will present some practical strategies for the clinical assessment of time problems and related psychopathological spirals. The theoretical rationale for this temporal approach to the patient was outlined in Chapter 4 (see Table 2). The purpose of this chapter is to outline how this hierarchy of time problems can be applied to the clinical examination of psychiatric patients. The chapter will serve as an introduction to clinical aspects of these time-related spirals. I will expand on some of these themes in later parts of this book. Research strategies for the assessment of time problems are given in Appendix A. The clinical approaches discussed in this chapter are in part based on these research strategies.

The reason special attention is paid to the assessment of time problems stems from the proposal that disorders of sequence, rate, and temporal perspective are likely to impair anticipatory control by disrupting the interplay between future images, plans of action, and emotions (see Chapters 3 and 4). That is, the time problems are likely to impair anticipatory control and lead to psychopathological spirals. I believe that the assessment of time problems helps to plan treatment for the correction of the time problems so that the psychopathological spirals can be interrupted. Methods for the correction of time problems and the use of time in treatment are discussed in Chapter 6 and in later parts of this book.

THE GOALS OF ASSESSMENT

The overall approach is to determine the nature of a psychopathological spiral by assessing the interaction between a time problem and a misconstruction of the personal future. This approach usually entails the following stages:

1 *Assess problems with sequence and rate before assessing problems with temporal perspective.* Assess the more severe time problems first. In clinical practice, this means that aspects of the mental-status examination should precede a lengthy psychiatric history.

2 *Assess the personal future.* Determine how the patient is misconstruing or distorting the personal future. The assessment of the personal future often sheds light on problems with temporal perspective, such as imbalances of or abnormal spans of awareness of the past, present, and future.

3 *Formulate the nature of the psychopathological spirals.* According to the hierarchy presented in Table 2, this involves generating working hypotheses about (a) the possible influence of one time problem upon another, such as sequential difficulties giving rise to problems with rate and temporal perspective, and (b) the possible interaction between a time problem and the patient's misconstruction of the personal future. Considerable detective work is necessary to discover the idiosyncratic nature of a particular individual's spiral. The hypothesized dynamics should suggest specific interactions that potentially could be treated.

4 *Plan treatment in a biopsychosocial direction.* In general, biological treatments should precede psychological and social treatments. This is based on the following rationale: If the person's cognitive functions are disturbed by problems with sequence or rate of mental events, these should first be corrected so that the patient can profit more from psychosocial interventions. In addition, I believe that at least some degree of individual psychotherapy should precede social interventions, such as family therapy, since a person who is more psychologically intact is in a better position to begin altering his family relationships.

I will exemplify these goals and stages of assessment in terms of some clinical cases of problems with sequence, rate, and temporal perspective. Guidelines for timing in the psychiatric interview and for the assessment of the personal future and interpersonal transactions will be presented at the end of this chapter.

ASSESSMENT OF PROBLEMS WITH SEQUENCE

Chapter 4 outlined how problems with sequence are the most severe time problems and occur in either organic brain disease as time disorientation or in the group of schizophrenias as the temporal disintegration of sequences. The differential diagnosis of time disorientation and the temporal disintegration of sequences is portrayed in the following case histories:

Case A

A 52-year-old, unmarried woman who had been employed as a bank administrator was brought by friends to a psychiatric hospital because she was wandering in the streets and being overly friendly with strangers. When asked why she was brought to the hospital by her friends, she replied, "Because it's my birthday." When asked if she had ever been in the hospital before, she replied, "Yes, I think so. . . . When I was born."

On mental-status examination, she was attractively dressed and neat. She related to the examiner in an overly friendly manner. At one point, she greeted him with a hug, feeling that he was an old friend. She could sustain a superficial conversation about social amenities. The rate of her speech was slow and halting. She politely avoided answering questions about time orientation and doing cognitive tasks, saying that she never paid attention to dates and that she was "no longer a school girl doing numbers." When pressed about when she came into the hospital, she answered, "Oh, sometime recently. . . . This year, yes, this year." She could not give the month or exact date. She failed miserably on such tasks as the serial subtraction of sevens and threes and made many mistakes as she tried to count backwards from 25. Even though she registered and spelled the examiner's name immediately after this information was given her, she could not remember it three minutes later. When asked to name some of her favorite flowers in her greenhouse, she replied, "Very pretty ones. . . . Yellow ones, red, pretty red flowers." When asked if she had ever seen the examiner before, she claimed that he has been one of her customers at the bank where she worked.

On the hospital ward, she was observed to sit in the milieu with other patients and have an almost constant but vacuous smile on her face. When she walked, she was slightly ataxic. She frequently could not find her way back to her room. She persevered about the "nice birthday party" other people were giving her. When asked about her future plans, she stated she wanted to wait "for my next birthday." On several occasions, she became acutely upset and frightened at night in her unfamiliar surroundings. On another occasion, 15 minutes after eating breakfast she became angry that she had not been served breakfast, and then became upset and puzzled that people were fooling her when she was told she had eaten it.

History from friends and relatives revealed that the patient had been a top-notch executive in a bank and had previously been very efficient and accomplished in mathematics. They reported no history of substance abuse or alcoholism. There were no previous psychiatric admissions or anything to suggest schizophrenia. Since the hospital work-up revealed no hypothyroidism, folic acid or B12 deficiency, or space-occupying lesions in her brain, a further search of her apartment was made for toxic substances, such as bromides or alcohol. A stash of vodka bottles was found in a closet.

A presumptive diagnosis of an incipient amnestic syndrome (Wernicke-Korsakoff's psychosis) was made. The patient was treated with intramuscular thiamine injections. Three weeks later, her dementia had partially cleared, and the patient was no longer disoriented to time.

It can be seen that the assessment of Case A entailed the following stages:

1 The time problem was that of time disorientation with pervasive problems with sequence, rate, and temporal perspective. The time disorientation was detected during the initial psychiatric contact, prompting the psychiatrist to conduct the mental status examination before obtaining a lengthy history.
2 The personal future was markedly confused. The patient's future images were vague and obscure, her plans of action were disorganized, and her emotions were superficial and impoverished but could become labile when she was in unfamiliar surroundings and lacked temporal cues from the environment, such as at night.
3 There were two psychopathological spirals:
   (a) The pervasive problems with sequence were associated with slowing of mental rate and marked problems with temporal perspective. The latter was exemplified by her thinking that the people around her were there for her birthday, which, in fact, was months ahead.
   (b) The time disorientation was associated with marked loss of control of the future, which, in turn, aggravated her time disorientation. For example, shortly after eating breakfast she again was waiting to eat breakfast, and then became further disoriented when she was told she had already eaten breakfast. She had lost her moorings in time.
4 The treatment was mainly biological (thiamine injections), but also the

milieu therapy on the ward attempted to make the temporal cues of her psychosocial environment as structured as possible to aid her orientation to time.

Case B

This 32-year-old, married mother of two children was brought to the psychiatric hospital by her husband nine days after delivering a baby boy. The patient was in a confused and bewildered state, claiming that she herself was a baby or that she was about to deliver another infant. Her husband carried her into the psychiatrist's office, since the patient claimed that her "legs were too small" for her to walk.

On mental-status examination, the patient curled up on the couch in a fetal position, rocking back and forth with a dazed look on her face. The flow of her speech alternated between being hesitant and blocked, to a torrent of non sequiturs about her being the Christ child or the Virgin Mary. At one moment, she cried out that she wanted to "go pee-pee and poo-poo," but several minutes later when the secretary entered the room to ask about insurance papers, the patient sat up and searched her purse for the papers, giving the correct information to the secretary. When asked what date it was, the patient looked blank and then uttered, "There is no time." She then stared at a clock on the wall and murmured "tick-tock, tick-tock," giggling to herself.

Since the patient appeared suspicious and distrustful, the psychiatrist asked her husband to sit next to her and acknowledged how difficult it is to trust a stranger. The psychiatrist then suggested that she might have moments of partial trust during which she might be able to give answers to some questions that would be important for helping her. "When you feel you can trust me just a little, please tell me about what time of day it is." The patient looked out the window, noting the position of the sun in the sky, and stated, "It's mid-morning." She was at least roughly oriented to time.

"Are you having trouble following what I am saying?" The patient nodded affirmatively. "Do you often lose your train of thought?" The patient nodded yes. "Can you keep track of what you are thinking about?" The patient nodded negatively. "Do thoughts slip out of your head, like you can't grasp them?" The patient nodded affirmatively. "Can you tell me more about that?" Hesitantly, the patient began to reply, "I can't think straight. . . . My mind goes blank. . . . I've got a baby's brain. . . . I want to cry, I'm a baby, Mommy, *Mommy*. . . . Birds don't cry, bottles bambi baby milk." The psychiatrist then stated, "I'll talk real slow so you can understand me; you tell me if I talk too fast, okay?" The patient nodded yes.

"Is your mind going fast or slow?" The patient replied: "Fast then slow, like a yo-yo, . . . stops." "Can you tell the present, right now, from the past and future?" "Sometimes, but then it all gets mixed up . . . like I'm somewhere else in time." The patient then sat up, looked alert, and addressed her husband, "Will you pick Bobby up when he gets out of school this afternoon?" Suddenly she appeared in contact. The psychiatrist proceeded, "Tell me more about your problems with thinking." She replied, "I wish I could hold onto my thoughts. Can you help me do that?" The psychiatrist reassured her that she could be helped, she looked relieved, but several minutes later she was again dazed, mumbling that her baby was dead, her mother was going to kill her, and that the end of the world was upon us all.

History from her husband revealed that the patient had two previous psychotic episodes, the first seven years ago after the birth of her son and another five years before, after a miscarriage. Between her psychotic illnesses, she had functioned well as a librarian, although she had difficulty in being warm and responsive to her son. There was no evidence of substance abuse, and the patient was not taking any medication.

Past history indicated that her own mother was very dominating and rejecting. The father was institutionalized for a chronic mental illness. When the patient was age nine, she was abandoned by her mother and thereafter raised in an orphanage.

The patient was diagnosed as having a schizophrenic illness complicating the postpartum period. She was initially treated in the hospital with phenothiazine medication. After she was able to keep track of her thoughts, the patient was given individual therapy centering around her ambivalent identification with her rejecting mother, since this appeared to tax her commitment to the mothering role. Her infant was then brought into the hospital, so that she could gradually get accustomed to assuming the mothering role as the nurses carefully helped her to feel comfortable with the baby. In addition, the husband and wife were treated conjointly to clear up miscommunications and plans about their parental role. The patient was discharged from the hospital one month after admission. She did well except for a three-day period where "thoughts began slipping out of her head," at which time the psychiatrist reinstated a higher dose of phenothiazine medication, and this again improved her tracking difficulties.

After the patient had recovered from her illness, she was interviewed about her problems with thinking and the time distortions during her acute psychosis. She reported that the experience was like a dream in which elements of the past and future seemed to telescope into the present, like "everything was happening at once." Using an analogy to a library, she likened her psychotic state to a "library that had lost its indexing system." This was particularly severe when she was compelled to do something for which she felt inadequately prepared, such as tending the baby and quelling his crying: "When he'd cry, I felt like it was me crying. . . . I'd lost my self and become him."

The assessment of Case B went through the following stages:

1   The time problem was that of the temporal disintegration of sequences. She had intermittent difficulty with keeping track of her thoughts. This was manifested in her speech as loosening of associations. She also had secondary problems with rate, such as thought racing and thought blocking. In addition, she had problems with temporal perspective, in that she would intermittently confuse past, present, and future. However, even though she had intermittent sequential problems, she was not disoriented to clock and calendar time.

2   The personal future was fragmented. She could not carry out her mothering role. At times, she felt that she was the baby. Her future images were incoherent, her plans of action were disorganized, and her emotions often were incongruous and inappropriate to the present and future.

3   The psychopathological spirals consisted of:
    (a)   The difficulty with tracking sequences appeared to give rise to secondary problems with rate and the telescoping of past, present, and future.
    (b)   Her sequential difficulties were augmented by her inability to get a consistent picture of her future directions, thereby further impairing the sequential ordering of her thoughts and acts toward goals.

4   Treatment was planned in a biopsychosocial direction. That is, phenothiazines were given to correct the tracking difficulties (see Chapters 6 and 7). After the patient could keep track of sequences, she was given individual therapy about the mothering role which was socially supported by the nursing staff and the conjoint sessions with her husband.

Comment: It can be seen that both Case A and Case B had problems with sequence. The main difference was that the sequential problems were pervasive and persistant in Case A, becoming manifested as time disorientation. By contrast, Case B's sequential difficulties were intermittent, and she could orient herself to clock and calendar time. It should be noted, however, that there are cases of schizophrenia in which the patient has been severely psychotic for weeks on end, obtaining little information relevant to orienting oneself to time. Nevertheless, these patients, unlike those with organic brain disease, are capable of reorienting themselves to time once given the information.

Mild degrees of tracking difficulties do occur with panic and anxiety states, but these occur infrequently (once or twice in 10 minutes) as compared to the high frequency of losing one's train of thought during active schizophrenia (as much as 20 times in a 10-minute period). Also, prolonged sleeplessness can induce tracking difficulties. When in doubt, it is best to wait after the patient has had at least four hours of sleep before documenting the degree of tracking difficulties.

ASSESSMENT OF RATE AND RHYTHM PROBLEMS

As outlined in Chapter 4 (see Table 2), rate and rhythm problems are common in manic-depressive illness. Accelerated rate is typical of the manic phase and slowing of rate characterizes the depressed phase. Slowing of mental rate also can complicate other types of severe depressive disorders. The assessment of these time problems is portrayed in the cases discussed below.

Case C

This 38-year-old mother of two children was brought to the psychiatric hospital by her husband because she had been staying up all night writing poetry and painting pictures for about two weeks. The patient felt that there was nothing wrong with her and that her husband had brought her for help since he was not manly enough to take care of her heightened sexual needs. She reported that she was "blessed" with unusual mental powers, such that her mind was working much faster than other people's. She felt she could read other people's minds by noting nuances of facial expression. She had a host of projects and plans about which she had unbridled optimism. For example, she believed that she was destined to become a great artist and that her creations would be an "oracle of the future."

On mental-status examination, she was a plump, jolly person who bantered humorously with the psychiatrist. She pranced around his office, making interpretations of each painting on the wall and attempting to psychoanalyze the psychiatrist through the paintings he had in his office. Her speech was extremely rapid. She reported that her thoughts were going extremely fast, "delightfully so." She reported an abundance of internal "pictures" racing through her mind. She claimed that she had "perfect recall" and never lost her train of thought. When asked a question, she would seize on it, addressing the issue for a minute or so with an outpouring of associations and then branching into a number of tangents. Nevertheless, when asked, she could recover the original thrust of the topic under discussion and could recall the question asked before she had split off on a flight of ideas. When asked to slow down and talk about her sick grandmother as slowly as possible for three minutes, she spoke on this subject at a normal rate for about 20 seconds and then began to speed up again, talking about how "grand" her mother and all mothers had been, only to catch herself later when she realized that she had been asked to talk slowly about her grandmother. When the psychiatrist told her that she had to talk more slowly for him to understand her, she became irritated and complained that he was "too slow and not smart enough" for her. When the psychiatrist glanced at his watch, she incorporated this into her conversation and began to talk about time. In testing her ability to estimate clock time, she was asked to tell when 30 seconds had elapsed: she produced only 9 seconds, indicating that her internal rate was much faster than clock time (see Appendix A).

History revealed that seven years previously she had become severely depressed and required electroconvulsive therapy. Four years previously, according to her husband, she had an episode of talking very fast and then became quite paranoid. She was hospitalized at a state hospital with the diagnosis of paranoid schizophrenia (probably a misdiagnosis). Since that time, she was noted to have rather marked mood swings that usually occurred in the early spring of the year. These began as a period of sluggishness with early morning awakening, followed after a few weeks by marked sleeplessness, hyperactivity, and talkativeness. These previous episodes subsided without psychiatric therapy.

Past history indicated that the patient had a reasonably happy childhood with a nurturant mother and father. However, when the patient was 23 years old, the father became acutely depressed and committed suicide. There was an aunt who had been diagnosed as having manic-depressive illness.

This patient was diagnosed as having manic-depressive illness and to be in the manic phase. She was initially treated with haloperidol, followed soon afterwards with lithium carbonate. The nursing staff had to make out a half-hour structured schedule of activities for her in order to contain her hyperactivity. The patient was aware of her extreme talkativeness, and asked other patients in the milieu to confront her and help her stop her "motor mouth." She received these confrontations with good humor, saying, "I just can't stop myself from talking." After 11 days of lithium therapy, her accelerated rate of talking and activity began to slow down. Her production of 30 seconds improved to 22 seconds, suggesting a slower mental rate. She and her family were educated about manic-depressive illness and the use of lithium. She had recovered by one month and was tapered off lithium nine months later. She and her family were instructed to watch for signs of thought racing and lack of need for sleep as signs for them to call the doctor. She reliably did this in the subsequent spring, and lithium was reinstituted early in the course of a manic episode and presumably prevented a full-blown manic attack from materializing.

The assessment of Case C went through the following stages:

1   The time problem was that of an accelerated rate of mental events. There also was a biological dysrhythmia manifested by lack of need for sleep and a suggestion of a seasonal pattern to her illness.
2   The personal future was expanded. There were a host of future images, the plans of action were accelerated, and the emotions were euphoric, reflecting optimism about the anticipated matches between her plans and goals.
3   The following spirals were detected:
    (a)   The accelerated rate induced an expansion of future time perspective, that, in turn, appeared to prompt an even greater quest of future pursuits.
    (b)   The patient's accelerated feedforward into the future was insufficiently checked by present-time feedback from others about her unreasonable plans and projects and her need to slow down.
4   The treatment was planned in a biopsychosocial direction. Lithium carbonate was given to slow the patient's mental rate (see Chapters 4 and 6). The psychosocial interventions were largely educational.

Case D

This 33-year-old, married father of one son was admitted to a psychiatric hospital after he had been driving at reckless speeds for most of the night, dangerously flirting with the idea of ending his life in a crash. He finally drove home and plunged to the floor, crying out for help from his wife, who then brought him for psychiatric help.

On admission to the hospital, the patient, a burly, ruddy-faced man, sat slumped in a chair and spoke slowly in monosyllables. He was fully oriented to clock and calendar time. He reported that he was "at the end of his rope" and that he had lost all hope. He felt extremely inadequate: "I'm not the man I used to be." Although he had difficulty concentrating and making decisions, his answers to questions were to the point and he reported no tracking difficulties. He complained that his mind was slowed down. Clock time seemed to drag endlessly for him. He had little interest in living and had to be persuaded to give a gun he had in his car to a policeman.

History revealed that this was his first psychiatric contact. Seven months previously, an arsonist had burned the automobile repair shop that he and his father had struggled to build as a family business. Since his father's death four years previously, the patient felt committed to develop the business to become the finest in the area for repairs of foreign cars. He had succeeded in this goal. He was a perfectionistic mechanic who was reputed to be the best in the area. When the arson occurred, he felt compelled to find and wreak revenge on the arsonist. He believed that this was how a "man like my father" would seek justice. He also felt he must get revenge to prove to his six-year-old son that he was a man and strong father. For months on end, he contrived traps for the arsonist, but failed to find him. He became dejected. Three months prior to admission, he suffered from early morning awakening and felt lethargic. His work output slowed down, and yet he felt he must meet the expectations of his numerous customers. Although he had previously been dominant and extremely "macho" with his wife, his passivity prompted her to begin nagging him. He found this intolerable. He disengaged from sex and could not be sexually aroused. This upset his wife even more.

There was no family history of manic-depressive illness or other mental illnesses, although his father was a heavy drinker.

This patient was diagnosed as having a depressive disorder of the reactive type that had become so severe that he was showing biological signs of depression. Since his mental slowing and early morning awakening with lethargy persisted after one week of hospitalization, he was placed on antidepressant medication. In addition, he was given considerable milieu support, including ample opportunities to ventilate his anger about the arsonist during individual and group therapy. By the third week of hospitalization, his mental slowing and diurnal variation of mood had improved. Nevertheless, he still felt compelled to wreak revenge on the arsonist. Since his quest for revenge appeared related to his identification with his father, a variant of grief-resolution therapy (Chapter 10) was used in order for him to obtain permission from the image of his dead father not to seek revenge and focus instead on being a good father to his son. After a very emotionally moving dialogue with the image of his father in which he did get this permission, he felt tremendously relieved. That evening he went home and made a symbolic gesture of his new directions: he took down the American flag that had been draped across his father's coffin, and was now hanging in his son's room. He told his son that he was "clearing out the road ahead" for both of them. Two weeks later, he was discharged from the hospital. He returned to work and reengaged in life, feeling that he had a "new lease on life."

The assessment of Case D went through the following stages:

1   The time problem was that of mental slowing. There also was a biological dysrhythmia manifested by early morning awakening and diurnal variation of mood (morning lethargy that would improve later in the day).

2   The personal future was blocked. The patient had lost one of his main commitments in life when his shop had been burned down. He felt hopeless about his future. Bound to his identification with his father, he felt compelled to seek revenge on the arsonist; failing that, suicide seemed the only way out. His future images were constricted, his plans of action were slowed, and the disparity between his goals and plans was reflected in depression.

3   The following spirals were detected:
  (a)   The block of his future eventually induced him to give up, and this was complicated by mental slowing, which, in turn, made him feel inefficient and ineffective, prompting further hopelessness.
  (b)   His hopelessness appeared to induce a constriction of future time perspective in which he foresaw few alternatives other than revenge or suicide.

4   Treatment was planned in a biopsychosocial direction. Initially, antidepressant medication was given to improve his mental rate and normalize his biological rhythms (see Chapters 6 and 9). Psychological interventions included ventilation of his anger and grief-resolution therapy for helping him to undo his bind with his father about seeking revenge. In addition, the wife was brought in for conjoint sessions to facilitate his readjustment.

Comment: It can be seen that both Case C and Case D had rate and rhythm problems. The main difference between these cases was that rate was accelerated in the manic case and slowed in the depressive disorder. Another difference was that there was no clearcut precipitating stress in Case C, in which the rate problem appeared to be part of a biological cycle as is typical for manic-depressive illness, whereas there was a precipitating stress for Case D. In the latter, the block of the personal future appeared first, and this eventually led to mental slowing.

Rate problems can occur in other types of mental illness than affective disorders, but they are not as prominent. In acute schizophrenia, as noted in Case B, there often is an oscillation of mental rate that appears secondary to sequential difficulties. During anxiety and anger, mental rate can speed up momentarily (see Chapter 2), but this acceleration is not as sustained as in manic illness, and also there are other concomitants of anxiety and anger that aid in making this distinction. In dementia, as in Case A, mental rate often is slow and halting, but these patients usually have time disorientation which is absent in depression. In addition, passive–aggressive behavior can be manifested as slowing of responses as a way to thwart others through procrastination, but the obstinate and willful quality of passive–aggressive behavior usually is easily distinguished from the severely depressed patient's inability to voluntarily increase his rate.

ASSESSMENT OF PROBLEMS WITH TEMPORAL PERSPECTIVE

As outlined in Chapter 4 (Table 2), problems with temporal perspective involve imbalances of focus on the past, present, or future. There also may be abnormal spans of awareness into the past or future. These problems with temporal perspective are common in neurotic and personality disorders. In neurotic and personality disorders, there may be a predominant focus on the past, present, or future with a relative exclusion of other temporal frames of reference. By contrast, the normal individual primarily uses the present and short-term future in order to integrate information from the past and to revise his beliefs about the more distant future (Shostrum, 1968; Rokeach, 1960).

Since individuals are often unaware of the temporal form of how they are construing reality, it is difficult for them to report accurately as to whether they predominantly focus on the past, present, or future. Thus for the detection of problems with temporal perspective, there is no good substitute for a free-flowing psychiatric interview (Melges, in press). The interviewer should focus not only on content (what the person is saying about whom in relation to himself) but also on the temporal form of the person's statements and replies to questions (whether he focuses predominantly on the past, present, or future and to what degree he excludes one or more of these temporal frames of reference). In addition, how the person is construing his personal future in terms of anticipated transactions with other people often sheds light on the nature of a particular individual's imbalanced temporal perspective. These interviewing tactics will be discussed in later sections of this chapter. For now, I will present three cases to illustrate different imbalances of temporal perspective.

The first case (Case E) portrays an over-focus on the future with the exclusion of past information relevant to the preoccupation with the future. This case is a rather specific paranoid reaction with "neurotic" dynamics involved in it; the case is not typical of the more generalized form of paranoid disorders discussed later in Chapter 8. In Case F, I portray the predominant focus on the present in an antisocial personality; this present-centeredness is discussed more fully in Chapter 9. Case G portrays an over-focus on the past in a neurotic patient who repeatedly misconstrues the personal future and relationships with others in light of preoccupations with the past. This neurotic process is discussed more fully in Chapter 11.

Case E

This 51-year-old, married woman was brought to a psychiatric hospital in an extremely agitated condition, stating that she was "afraid somebody is going to kill me."

On mental-status examination, she was oriented to time and had no tracking difficulties. Her mental rate was neither slow nor fast. She was extremely suspicious. She would not sit down and insisted that she remain at the doorway of her room so that she would not be trapped. She denied hallucinations and illusions. Even though fearful and paranoid, she was able to relate fairly well to the examiner, especially when he sat down within her room and she was allowed to control the situation by standing above him and being close to the door. She was perplexed at why she was so frightened of being killed and reported that her fears were like an uncanny premonition she could not dismiss, even though she wanted to "forget about it" so she could return to work as a saleswoman.

History revealed that the patient had a prior psychiatric admission to a state hospital five years previously, shortly after her 23-year-old son had been killed in an automobile accident on October 22. The time of her present admission to the hospital was October 11. When the psychiatrist noted that this was 11 days prior to the anniversary of her son's death, the patient became visibly upset but refused to talk about the loss of her son. The more that this issue was probed, the patient became more paranoid and frightened.

The past year was complicated by the fact that her father-in-law had moved into her home to live with her husband and herself. The father-in-law had recently suffered from a cerebral vascular accident and required a good deal of care from her. He also had become bellicose and cantankerous, often rejecting her care and striving to maintain his independence. Although she was quite irritated with the father-in-law, she felt forbidden to talk about her anger by her husband who demanded that she maintain a facade of caring and nurturance toward his father. Nevertheless, she frequently found herself exasperated at the father-in-law and entertained wishes to "kick him out of the house.'' When she became aware of these wishes, she would become very upset, and the threat of her somehow being killed would increase at these times.

Through gentle probing, her psychiatrist discovered that, on the evening before her son had left the home and was killed in a crash five years before, the patient had become angry at the son's rebellious behavior and had ''kicked him out of the house.'' The patient cried in agony when she mentioned this. Yet she was too upset to deal further with the psychological significance of this event as the anniversary day of her son's death approached. As this day came nearer, the patient became increasingly paranoid, believing that she was indeed going to be killed.

This patient was diagnosed as having a paranoid disorder. She was not schizophrenic. Medication was not helpful. For her treatment, the psychiatrist and the staff decided to wait until after the anniversary of her son's death to see if she would then be in a better position to deal with her fears. It was predicted that she would become less paranoid after this anniversary had passed. This prediction was confirmed. On October 23, one day after the anniversary, the patient was decidedly less paranoid. Her suspiciousness gave way to depression. Several days later, she was able to talk about the loss of her son. She cried profusely. Further grief-resolution therapy (see Chapter 10) enabled her to see the connection between her wish to ''kick the father-in-law out of the house'' and the similar statement she had made to her son shortly before he was killed. In effect, she had blamed herself for her son's death and felt that she deserved to be killed for this. Two weeks later, when she received forgiveness from the image of her son as she entered a dialogue with him in the funeral home as part of grief-resolution therapy, her guilt feelings dissipated and she felt tremendously relieved.

Further family work helped her to deal directly with her anger about the father-in-law. The husband consented to having the father-in-law live in an adjoining trailer to their home, and the husband started to participate in the caregiving. Within two months, the patient had returned to work and was functioning well as a housewife. On follow-up one year later, the patient reported that she could look at her son's picture without ''falling to pieces'' since she now realized that his death ''was not my fault.''

The assessment of Case E went through the following stages:

1 The time problem was that of an over-focus on the future with the avoidance of a past event relevant to the future impending event. That is, this patient's paranoid fears that she might be killed were related to the

reawakening of her blaming herself for her son's death because she "kicked out" her son, which was the same thing she wanted to do with her father-in-law. Yet she remained over-focused on the future threat of retaliation for her wishes and could not deal with how the past was related to this future threat.

2   The personal future was threatening. The patient had an uncanny premonition that somehow she was going to be killed. Her future images centered around this threat, her plans of action were geared to preventing this threat from occurring, and her emotions were primarily fears and anxieties that other people might trap and harm her.

3   The following spirals were detected:

(a)   Her over-focus on the future prompted her transactions with others to become desynchronized, which, in turn, made her feel even more threatened about her future. For example, she felt alienated from her husband and she was distrustful of others who wanted to help her.

(b)   The impending threat to her personal future prompted her to search for other threats about people attempting to control or harm her, which, in turn, heightened her sense of threat (see Chapter 8).

4   Treatment was planned in a biopsychosocial direction. Biological treatments were of little help, and thus the main treatment was individual psychotherapy and family therapy. These psychosocial interventions focused on disentangling the connection between her guilt about her son's death and her guilt about her anger toward her father-in-law. In effect, she was shown how she was misconstruing a future event in terms of an avoided past event that was contaminating her present situation with her father-in-law. By restoring a more balanced temporal perspective on her problems, this spiral of interconnected events was interrupted.

Case F

This 15-year-old boy was institutionalized for murdering a friend for no apparent reason. He and his friend had been in his parent's bedroom, playing with the stepfather's gun. Holding the gun, the lad suddenly was overcome by a feeling of power and began scaring his friend by pointing the gun at him. As the friend began to cower in fear, the lad felt even more powerful. He suddenly pulled the trigger, shooting his friend in the face, and then fired four more shots.

His parents were not home. He dragged the body downstairs and then under the house. He then went about his business as usual, remaining in the home and not reporting the event to anyone. When his friend turned up missing, he denied knowing his whereabouts. About two weeks later, because of malodor, the body was discovered underneath the house and the boy confessed to shooting his friend.

On mental-status examination, the patient was oriented to time, had no tracking difficulties, and no problems with rate. He related to the psychiatrist in a distant, callous manner, and showed little concern for the murder of his friend or for what might happen to himself. His emotional responses were superficial and shallow. He evinced little concern about the prospect of being separated from his parents and for being institutionalized for a prolonged period.

History revealed that the boy had been abandoned by his father at age three. His mother was alcoholic. He had been sent to a number of foster homes, but never had a sustained relationship with any parental figure. He was repeatedly in trouble with legal authorities for thievery and truancy. Lately, he had partaken of smoking marihuana, but he denied drug taking of any type prior to the murder. In the previous year, his mother had remarried and had obtained permission from authorities to have her son return to live with her. Six months prior to the murder, the lad was beginning to relate to his stepfather, who began to take an inordinate interest in his stepson. Three months prior to the murder, the lad learned that his stepfather was bisexual when he made some passes at the stepson while drinking. The lad denied that this had any connection to the murder and denied any hint of homosexual activities or fantasies with his friend. He also denied being angry at his friend. His explanation for the murder was, "I guess I got carried away. . . . I just felt like doing it."

This lad, who was imprisoned at the time of the psychiatric examination, was diagnosed as an antisocial personality. Treatment within the confines of the prison had to be planned in terms of his learning to relate to and trust his counselors. This was a long and tedious process. In addition, the mother and stepfather had "raised his hopes" about finally having a father, but he had found his stepfather's bisexuality to represent a kind of betrayal, making him feel futile and foolish about ever wanting to hope for a meaningful relationship with a father figure.

The assessment of Case F went through the following stages:

1   The time problem was an imbalanced temporal perspective with an almost exclusive focus on the present. The present was unhinged from the past; future consequences were neglected. The impulsive murder appeared to be a spur-of-the-moment act.

2   The personal future was neglected. In addition, this lad felt that he had been foolish to hope for a meaningful relationship with a father figure; he was foolish to have hoped, especially in light of his past disappointments with parental figures.

3   The following spirals were detected:

   (a)   His exclusive focus on the present led to impulsive acts that alienated him from others and led to an even greater focus on what he could get away with in the present.

   (b)   His penchant for neglecting future consequences was challenged by the arousal of hope for a father figure, but when he felt betrayed in this hope, this again confirmed his modus operandi of not looking to the future.

4   Treatment was planned in a psychosocial direction. This consisted of containment of his impulsive behavior and the fostering of identification, and later, family therapy was conducted to help widen his temporal horizons.

Case G

This 49-year-old, married mother of three grown children came to a psychiatric hospital in an agitated and desperate state. She was anguished by a number of complaints: "My husband is having an affair. . . . My son has left his wife, and my granddaughter will never have a father. . . . My father left me when I was little. . . . Nobody cares for me."

On mental-status examination, the patient was a bleached-blonde woman who looked considerable younger than her stated age. She was oriented to time, had no tracking difficulties (except for occasional thought scattering when she became acutely anxious), and had no rate problems. She related to the examiner in a dependent, whining manner. She was extremely anxious and became increasingly upset when she felt she was not being given sufficient attention. The patient denied having a suicidal plan, although she had entertained the idea of taking an overdose of pills to spite her husband. Even though recent events with her husband and son appeared to be precipitating stresses, the patient had difficulty focusing on these events and would repeatedly delve into traumatic events of her childhood, particularly the separation from her father as described below.

History revealed that the patient had discovered her husband's affair with another woman about five months prior to admission to the hospital. For the 26 years of their marriage, the patient and her husband had "stuck together for the children's sake," but now the children were grown and had left home. The patient's 22-year-old son had been living close to his parent's home, but two months prior to admission had decided to leave his wife (a close friend of the patient), and the patient was dismayed by this. The son's defiance of his mother was perplexing to the patient since he had been "at least one male I thought would do what I wanted." The patient recently berated her son for abandoning his daughter who was two years old: "She will never have a Daddy, like I never did."

Past history indicated that when the patient was age six, her father had left home to live with another woman. She repeatedly bemoaned, "He rejected me; he never loved me." The patient was left to be raised by her mother, with whom she had a poor relationship. During her adolescence, the patient was quite promiscuous: "I guess I was just looking for love." A pregnancy out of wedlock forced her marriage to her present husband, who reported that he had stayed in the marriage "out of guilt," fearing that his wife, as she had threatened, would "fall apart and do herself in" if he left her outright.

This patient was diagnosed as having a neurotic anxiety disorder and a histrionic personality. No medications were given. She was treated with various types of psychotherapy. Individual psychotherapy was aimed at helping her disentangle her relationship with her husband with her past fears of being abandoned by her father. She also was helped to dis-identify with her granddaughter. In addition, conjoint sessions with the husband were aimed at clarifying their ambivalence toward each other. The husband reported that he felt guilty about his affair, but felt "driven away" by his wife since she seemed to nag him incessantly: "I think she beats me for the anger she's had at her father."

The assessment of Case G went through the following stages:

1   The time problem was that of an over-focus on the past which colored many of her relationships of the present and future. That is, since she felt rejected by her father during childhood, she expected to be rejected by men in the present and future and desperately feared that this would happen.

2   The personal future was uncertain and dreaded. With her husband's affair and her son's separation, it appeared that her catastrophic fears of being rejected and abandoned might materialize. Her future images were recurrently misconstrued in light of her past rejection, her plans of action were uncertain, and the emotion was primarily anxiety. There also was considerable ambivalence about her relationships to men.

3 The following spirals were detected:

    (a) The over-focus on the past prompted ambivalent relationships with her husband, which, in turn, induced their transactions to become recurrently desynchronized; this in turn catapulted her back into her past fears of being rejected. Moreover, her attempts to prevent this rejection from her husband by nagging him and making him feel guilty prompted further ambivalence and rejection from him.

    (b) The patient recurrently misconstrued her personal future with her catastropic fears of being rejected. She took her husband's affair as "proof" that she was "unlovable," although she later admitted that she had "pushed him away" in order to test whether he was like her father. Also, the patient identified with her granddaughter, seeing herself being abandoned as though she was the daughter of her son. In a sense, she seemed to desire the role of the victim and went out of her way to get recognition for this role.

4 Treatment was planned in a psychosocial direction. That is, psychotherapy was aimed at interrupting the above spirals. Individual psychotherapy was conducted to help her tease apart her father from her husband, and herself from her granddaughter. She also was helped to disengage from the victim role (Chapter 12). Marital therapy was given to remove the transference of the past onto their current interactions, to help them learn constructive ways of handling ambivalence, and to open more positive exchanges unfettered by misconstructions of the future and binding expectations.

Comment: It can be seen that Cases E, F, and G each had a different type of imbalanced temporal perspective and a different misconstruction of the personal future. Case E was primarily focused on a future threat while neglecting past information relevant to that threat. Case F was primarily focused on the present while neglecting the past and especially future consequences. Case G recurrently misconstrued the future in terms of a catastrophic event that occurred in the past.

In each of these cases, the misconstructions of the future appeared to impair transactions with other people. These disrupted and desynchronized transactions, in turn, appeared to aggravate the misconstructions of the future.

The discovery of these intrapsychic and interpersonal spirals in these cases required sensitive interviewing tactics with individuals and with families. Guidelines for these assessment strategies are discussed below.

TIMING AND THE PSYCHIATRIC INTERVIEW

Good interpersonal timing and a clear picture of what to do when are highly important for an effective psychiatric interview. This pertains to the first interview and the mental-status examination, as well as to all interviews through the course of therapy. The interviewer who knows what he is after and where he is going, and yet is flexibly sensitive to emotional nuances, instills hope and establishes rapport with the patient. Since most patients who come for psychiatric help have lost control over their futures or are out of synchrony with other people, the instillation of hope and the gaining of rapport are important first steps that counteract these problems.

As suggested by the cases discussed above, more extensive interviewing is necessary to discover imbalances of temporal perspective and misconstructions of the future, as in neurotic and personality disorders. In the initial contact with a patient, the mental-status examination (or parts of it) is often conducted early in the course of assessment in order to detect problems of time disorientation, the temporal disintegration of sequences, and rate and rhythm problems. These problems can be delineated further with a complete mental-status examination and other tests (Melges, 1975; see Appendix A). In general, it is wise to detect and correct these more severe time problems before engaging in an extensive psychiatric history about the patient's psychodynamics and misconstructions of the future.

I will not cover details of the psychiatric interview, since these have been discussed elsewhere (Melges, in press; Engel and Morgan, 1973; MacKinnon and Michels, 1971). Rather the focus will be on keys to timing the interview. I have found these guidelines useful for teaching medical students and psychiatric residents about interviewing.

During the first interview, it is highly important for the interviewer to engage the patient warmly while compassionately searching for his existential dilemmas (Havens, 1974; Margulies and Havens, 1981). Assume that the patient is well intentioned, in need of help, and is facing real problems—that is, real to him. By contrast, an interviewer who is cold and aloof and who does not empathize with the patient's existential dilemmas often loses the patient by failing to combat the patient's demoralization. In this regard, combating demoralization and raising hope are central to all forms of psychotherapy (Frank, 1974). To do this, genuineness, empathy, respect for the patient, and nonpossessive warmth are necessary qualities of the interviewer. These characteristics have been found to be qualities of good therapists, regardless of their theoretical orientation (Meltzoff and Kornreich, 1970; Strupp, 1978; Lazarus, 1978).

To engage the patient existentially, a key background question for the interviewer to ask himself as he directs questions to the patient is, ``Why now?'' That is, why is it that the patient has come for psychiatric help at this time? What has changed in his life? How is he seeing his future differently now? What expectations and anticipations are impinging upon him at this moment in time? What does he want to change? How does he want others to change? What is uppermost on his mind? What does he fear the most in the future?

Although the question "Why now?" is seemingly simple, it enables the interviewer to relate to the complexities of the patient's life from the patient's point of view. These complexities include how the person is seeing himself in relation to others through his past, present, and future. The "Why now?" question provides a window into these timelines. Also, if the patient has prominent difficulties in constructing these timelines of the past and future as they relate to the question of "Why now?" there may be basic problems with sequence or rate, and this calls for an early shift into the mental-status examination.

When dealing with all the existential complexities of a person, how does the interviewer tell what is important? That is, out of the wealth of information available, are there any guidelines for telling what is important and most relevant to the question of "Why now?"

I propose two flexible plans for discovering what is likely to be most relevant to the question of "Why now?" (1) Search for common precipitating stresses, such as changes in the patient's goals, object relations (relationships with other people), expectations, and self-image. (2) Use nonverbal clues in order to discover which topics are emotionally salient to the patient. That is, look for changes in the patient's posture, affective tone, countenance (facial expression), and tempo of his speech and movement. When the interviewer notes changes in these nonverbal clues, it is likely that the patient is talking about something that is emotionally significant to him. *The use of nonverbal clues to discover what is emotionally significant to the patient is the key to timing an interview. These nonverbal clues signal when to go further into certain areas.*[1]

As is well known clinically, nonverbal communications often reveal what concerns the patient even though he may not be aware of it (Harper, Wiens, and Matarazzo, 1978). In a sense, nonverbal communications provide a special language for emotions. The nonverbal clues serve to emphasize what is emotionally important to the patient. For example, the patient may sigh and agitate his foot when saying, "My mother and I have no problems; we've

---

[1] For teaching purposes, the precipitating stresses are summarized by the mnemonic GOES, which represents goals, object relations, expectations, and self-images. The nonverbal clues are summarized by the mnemonic PACT, which stands for changes in posture, affective tone, countenance, and tempo. The interviewer goes for the GOES by noting changes in the patient's PACT.

always been close." The interviewer, without necessarily commenting on the nonverbal clues, might then probe: "Tell me more about your closeness to your mother."

One reason that it is important to highlight the patient's emotional emphases, whether they are verbal or nonverbal, is that emotions reflect how the person is interrelating his future images and plans of action (see Chapter 3). That is, I propose that unpleasant emotions signal discrepancies between the person's future images and his plans of action. By emphasizing the emotional flow of the interview, the interviewer can then search for the nature of the future images and plans that concern the patient at the moment.

To further aid the search for images and plans, there is another useful guideline: When the patient becomes silent, look at the direction of his gaze. Generally, when he is looking to the right, he is thinking sequentially about something; when he is looking up to the left, he usually is visualizing an image. These changes in direction of gaze are presumed to represent activation of the left cerebral hemisphere (that is, looking to the right) or the right cerebral hemisphere (that is, looking up to the left). This interviewing strategy is discussed by Bandler and Grinder (1975). For our purposes, the direction of gaze provides rough clues to when a patient is dealing with a plan or an image (see Chapters 2 and 3). For example, when the patient looks to the right, the interviewer can ask, "What are you thinking about or planning?" When he looks up to the left, the interviewer can ask, "What are you picturing?" This can be a useful way to access the flow of plans and images of the patient's inner future. It also helps the interviewer to empathize with the patient's construction of his future.

The temporal form of an interview has been given insufficient attention. Most psychiatrists appear to start with the present, then go into the past, and then come back to the present, with little focus on the future. My general approach is to begin asking about the present and recent past, then go into the future, and then focus on past factors relevant to the present and future. Although research is needed on this, I believe that this is the optimal timetable during beginning interviews if the focus is on interrupting psychopathological spirals.

Of course, in discussing almost anything with a patient, the interviewer has the option of focusing on the past, present, or future. Shifting to a different time frame of reference is often useful in prompting the patient to gain perspective (see Chapter 6). Moreover, it helps the patient to enlarge and order the timeline of his life extending from the past through the present toward the future. When the patient feels that the interviewer understands the timeline of events in his life, this helps establish rapport. Moreover, a patient's inability to shift focus to the past, present, or future, even when prompted to do so, often suggests an imbalanced temporal perspective.

In the course of an interview, there are temporal clues to detect rapport. Besides a comfortable flow of conversation and speech, the synchrony of body movements and postures is a good indicator that rapport has developed (Scheflen, 1964, 1968; Harper, Wiens, and Matarazzo, 1978). For example: If the interviewer scratches his head or crosses his legs and the patient does the same shortly thereafter, this suggests that rapport is developing; or if the patient slumps down and holds his head and then the interviewer leans forward and down toward the patient, this suggests a certain degree of empathy and rapport. This synchrony of body movements, colloquially called "good vibes" or when people "click," can be used to gauge the degree of rapport before the interviewer probes into conflictual topics. In this regard, it is important for rapport to have developed and for the patient to feel supported before the interviewer probes into emotionally charged topics.

If there is a lack of synchronous movements between interviewer and patient, this suggests that rapport has not yet developed. Moreover, a discordant synchrony of interpersonal movements may be a clue to the diagnosis of organic brain disease or schizophrenia. With schizophrenia, in particular, the patient's body language appears to be out of step with the interviewer. By analogy, if the interviewer is waltzing, the patient seems to be jitterbugging, and when the interviewer shifts to jitterbugging in an attempt to adjust his rhythmic movements to that of the patient, the patient seems to start some newfangled dance. This lack of synchronous body language often gives the interviewer a strange and uncomfortable feeling that there is something incongruous and unpredictable about the patient. (This strange feeling of being unable to get on the same "wave length" of the patient may account for what has been called the "praecox" feeling in interactions with schizophrenic patients.) When this eerie feeling occurs, it behooves the interviewer to look more precisely for incongruities between the patient's modes of expression, such as dysjunctions between his movement, speech, and emotion. In short, the patient's movement, speech, and emotion are incoordinated. The interviewer can then begin probing for more definite signs of schizophrenia.

In summary, there are various timing strategies that facilitate the development of rapport and the gathering of relevant information during a psychiatric interview. These include the background question of "Why now?" as one searches for precipitating stresses while looking for nonverbal emphases of what is emotionally important to the patient, a focus on the present and future in order to guide inquiry into relevant aspects of the past, the construction of a timeline extending from the past through the present toward the future, and an awareness of synchronous as well as dyssynchronous interpersonal modes of expression.

INTERVIEWS OF THE FUTURE

The above timing strategies facilitate the discovery of what is presently troubling the patient. These present concerns have to be placed in a context of past predispositions and future expectations for their full understanding. That is, the patient's present stresses may precipitate a crisis because (1) they reactivate unfinished conflicts of the past (such as the fear of rejection in Case G) and (2) they induce troublesome expectations (such as the threat of retaliation in Case E).

In attempting to discover the dynamics of a person's problems, most psychiatric interviews traditionally have focused on the interaction between precipitating stresses and past predispositions. Future expectations and anticipations often have not been sufficiently assessed. Although these expectations may be rooted in the past, there often is not a symmetrical isomorphism between past events and future expectations (see Chapter 2). That is, the nature of a person's expectations is construed out of a host of past memories, some of which the person selects and combines in unique ways as he fashions his future expectations. The discovery of conflicts between a precipitating stress and a person's expectations provides an alternative way of formulating psychodynamic processes other than just focusing on past–present interactions. This approach is particularly useful for discovering psychopathological spirals (Chapter 4).

In interviews about the future, the overall approach is to use a series of open-ended questions that help the patient to crystallize the nature of his *future images, plans of action, and emotions.* As proposed in Chapter 3, these are the basic elements through which an individual fashions his personal future.

In inquiring about a future situation, the interviewer should ask about desired and dreaded future images, what he plans to do or not do, and what he feels about the likelihood of his plans meeting his future images. Mismatches between the person's future images and his plans of action are likely to be reflected in negative emotions, such as anxiety, guilt, sadness, or anger. It often is useful for the interviewer to first get a general idea about what the person *feels* about the future situation, and if there were negative emotions, then to probe for the nature of the mismatch between the future images and the plans of action. This seemingly simple triad of future images, plans of action, and emotions can help the interviewer to get to the root of rather complicated sets of expectations concerning future situations. In addition to this free-flowing approach, it is useful for the interviewer to employ some more specific strategies for helping the patient clarify his expectations.

Thus I will outline some guidelines for interviewing the personal future in order to discover the nature and form of a person's expectations. These guidelines will be discussed in terms of interviewing about (1) contingencies, (2) purposes, (3) polarities, (4) future wishes, (5) decision making, (6) time projections, and (7) binding expectations with others. To illustrate these approaches, some examples from the previously discussed cases will be given.

Contingencies

In inquiring about contingencies, an obvious question is, "What if?" For example, in Case E, this man was asked, "What if you don't find the arsonist and never get the revenge you seek?" The patient replied that he felt that he would feel "less of a man." Case G, when asked, "What if your husband leaves you for this other woman?" replied that she would then feel almost totally "unlovable" and confirmed in her conviction that men are unreliable and rejecting like her father. It should be noted that these implied contingencies, though understandable, are nevertheless overgeneralized cognitive misconstructions of the future that can be treated psychotherapeutically (Chapters 6 and 12).

Purposes

Another obvious yet useful question is, "What for?" A patient's inability to give a clear answer of what they are striving for often suggests unconscious motivations. This includes the seeking of an emotional state that serves as a kind of payoff in confirming hidden images of the self in relationship to others. For example, in Case G, after the patient noted that she became recurrently anxious when she nagged her husband and then he withdrew from her, she was asked, "Even though you know that this makes you anxious, can you tell me what you are doing this for?" Upon pondering this question, the patient eventually reported that it had something to do with "proving" herself to be "unlovable." This was further explored as her quest to confirm her image of herself as a victim who was rejected by men. In Case E, the question of "What for?" was more of a background question that helped reveal that her excessive focus on the impending anniversary of her son's death was an attempt to punish herself for "kicking him out of the house" prior to his automobile crash.

Polarities

The personal future usually is viewed in terms of sets of polarities (see Chapter 2). That is, as proposed by Kelly (1955), each person has idiosyncratic ways of anticipating events in terms of bipolar constructs such as good versus bad, strong versus weak, and active versus passive. These polarities are like sets of colored lenses that frame and bias the nature of a person's anticipations. In interviewing about the personal future, after obtaining information through open-ended questions, the interviewer can help the patient crystallize and juxtapose these polarities by statements and questions containing the word *yet*. The word *yet* helps to bring to fore the unexpressed or dormant pole of the person's anticipations.

For example, in Case D, the patient was asked, "Does it seem as though you want revenge, *yet* you fear you will not be man enough to get it?" Case F was asked, "Does it seem like you want a father, *yet* you are afraid that you again will be disappointed?" The following interpretive statement was made to Case G: "You want your husband's love, *yet* you also seem to push him away." In each of these instances, the juxtaposition of these polarities opened further discussion of the bipolar ways that the patient was construing the personal future.

More sophisticated methods for the assessment of bipolar ways of anticipating events are given by Kelly (1955), Bannister and Mair (1968), and Adams-Webber (1979).

Decision Making

Most psychiatric patients are in conflict about future choices and commitments. Many are confused about how to make decisions. The interviewer can help them sort out the relevant future considerations by having them deal separately with anticipations about (1) pragmatic gains or losses for the self, (2) utilitarian gains or losses for significant others affected by the decision, (3) self-approval or disapproval, and (4) approval or disapproval from significant others. Patients often are unaware of the interplay and conflicts between these expectations (Janis and Mann, 1977).

For example, later in therapy Case D was toying with the idea of not rebuilding his automobile repair shop that had been burned in the fire and of seeking an eight-to-five job in another company as a mechanic. In terms of the above parameters, (1) he felt that he would lose income but have slightly more time for himself, (2) he felt that he would have less money to support his wife and son, (3) he believed that he would have greater self-approval since he no longer was attempting to meet up to the image of his father, and (4) he felt that his wife would disapprove of him for not having his former independence.

This helped him to begin to revise his feelings of self-approval which did not need to depend on whether he alone carried on his father's business. He eventually made a compromise by going to work for another company as he gradually built up his business again and lightened his responsibility in it by obtaining partners.

Future Wishes

A person's wishes for changes in the future often reveal how he expects change to come about. That is, changes in the future may come from luck, magic, the action of others, or one's own actions (Chapters 2 and 9). To begin probing the nature of a person's wishes, the following questions often are useful: "Can you tell me three wishes for yourself that you hope will come true? If they come true, how and when do you expect they will happen?"

One of Case G's wishes was that her husband would leave his other woman and begin to love her again. She was at a loss to explain how this would come about except by some kind of "miracle" or if she made him feel guilty enough for his affair. This obviously has the wrong approach and helped to focus therapy on her changing her own behavior rather than passively waiting for an external change or attempting to change her husband through guilt that drove him farther away. In addition, she wanted immediate change and initially could not see the necessity of the long haul of rebuilding the marriage.

Future Time Projections

These often reveal whether the patient sees his future as a replica of the past or whether he wants to change. The patient can be projected ahead into many different time frames, such as one month ahead, one year ahead, or five years ahead. It is best for the patient to close his eyes and attempt to visualize the future time span as though it were happening now (see Chapters 6 and 12). This gives greater experiential substance to the future as compared to when patients speculate and talk about their futures. It should be emphasized that if a patient cannot visualize himself or his situation being different in the future, it is unlikely that future changes will occur (Chapter 12).

When Case F was projected to one year ahead, he reported no images at all and claimed that the task was silly since he "never thought that far ahead." When pressed further to think about it, he stated, "People will just be messing over me." He thought this would be true for 10 years into the future, even if he had been released from prison.

Initially, when Case D was first admitted to the hospital, projections to one year ahead were troublesome for him since he saw himself as either having committed suicide or still seeking revenge. Later, after treatment, he saw himself fishing with his son, feeling good about himself as a father. In this way, future time projections can serve as a measure of therapeutic progress.

Binding Expectations

Binding expectations refer to a person's belief that he must obey parental dictates in order to survive. The binding expectations may not be directly stated by the parents, but are often mediated through identification and reinforcement from the parents. In this regard, the interaction of identifications and reinforcements from parental figures comprises a core aspect of what is traditionally called "unconscious influences." This interaction programs the person to behave in certain ways in the future. The child within the person once decided to obey and go along with what his parents appeared to want for him so that he could survive (Goulding and Goulding, 1978, 1979). As an adult, these binding expectations often continue to determine the person's destiny in life by "scripting" him to feel, think, and act in certain ways (Berne, 1961, 1972). That is, the person enters his future as though he were reading a script written by his past.

For example, in Case D, the patient was heavily identified with his "macho" father who had repeatedly instructed and reinforced his son to be strong and masculine. The patient was bound to this expectation of himself and, in line with it, felt compelled to wreak revenge on the arsonist in order to preserve his masculine image and to pattern himself after his father. By contrast, Case F showed a lack of identification with a father figure, and had incorporated few expectations of himself and was given to impulsive acts in the present.

The nature of these binding expectations frequently come through in dreams where often there is a telescoping of past, present, and future (see Chapter 2). For example, Case D had a dream that his father was chasing him in order to find out whether he had killed the arsonist.

In concluding this section, it should be pointed out that there are many factors which shape the nature of a person's expectations than those mentioned above. A free-flowing interview, guided by a predominance of open-ended questions so as to allow the patient to report these influences from his point of view is the best way to make sure that important areas have been covered.[2]

---

[2]For teaching purposes, the mnemonic SCRIPTED serves to introduce medical students and residents to important areas that shape a person's picture of his personal future. SCRIPTED represents social networks (family and friends), conflicts (internal and external), reinforcements (rewards and punishments), identifications (parental models and mentors), payoffs (what the person expects to get from his transactions with

TIMING AND FAMILY INTERVIEWS

I believe that families should be interviewed as soon as this can be conveniently arranged. There are essentially four reasons for this: (1) Families often provide a wealth of information that is unavailable from interviewing the person identified as the ''patient.'' (2) The family's support is needed in order to help in the understanding and treatment of the identified patient. This support may consist of being educated about severe forms of mental illness, such as organic brain disease, schizophrenia, or depression, as well as helping the family members to streamline their communications and transactions with one another, as often is necessary for the full treatment of neurotic and personality disorders. (3) The family members themselves are often in need of support by the time one of their members has become an identified patient. In many instances, the family has gone through long and exhaustive struggles before one member comes for psychiatric treatment. (4) The direct observation of how family members transact with one another is the best way to study the nature of interpersonal expectations and desynchronized transactions.

This section will concentrate on how the interviewer can observe and analyze the timing of transactions between family members. This approach is useful for determining the nature of desynchronized transactions between people. Desynchronized transactions occur when interpersonal behavior and communications are mistimed, out of phase, or at cross purposes. As outlined in Chapter 4, these desynchronized transactions can result from any of the time problems listed in Table 2. That is, they can result from severe time problems, such as time disorientation in organic brain disease (Case A), the temporal disintegration of sequences in active schizophrenia (Case B), and rate and rhythm problems as in mania (Case C) and severe depression (Case D). This section, however, will concentrate on subtle interpersonal desynchronizations of sequence, rate, and temporal perspective that often occur in neurotic and personality disorders and adjustment disorders.

For a patient with more severe time problems, family members are usually interviewed separately from the patient in order to obtain information and to educate them. Later, after the patient has improved, the family and patient are brought together in order to streamline communications and to plan for future contingencies. However, the usual approach with neurotic and personality disorders is to interview the identified patient and the family members together as early as possible in the course of evaluation and treatment.

---

other people), transactions (whether the person primarily plays the role of victim, persecutor, and rescuer), emotions (feeling states that are recurrent and familiar to the person), and defenses (ways of distorting information in order to maintain a particular self-image or to reduce negative emotions).

Initially, the family members are asked to come in for an interview to help with the treatment of the identified patient and then, if appropriate and warranted, the focus of treatment may be shifted to the entire family when there are prominent interpersonal binds and desynchronized transactions contributing to maladjustments between people.

In normal and effective family transactions and communications, there is a synchrony of the flow of interpersonal sequences, rates, and shifts in temporal perspective between people. This synchronous interaction occurs at the verbal and nonverbal levels of communication. Moreover, in general, there is congruence between these verbal and nonverbal modes of expression, or if there is incongruity, an attempt is made to decode and resolve the incongruous messages being given. By contrast, in desynchronized transactions between people, there are frequent mismatches in interpersonal sequences, rates, and shifts in temporal perspective. These may occur at the verbal or nonverbal levels of communication. Moreover, there are frequent incongruities between the verbal and nonverbal modes of expression that often are left dangling, with few attempts to decode and resolve the incongruous messages being given.

I will illustrate the temporal pattern of these desynchronized transactions by citing some examples from the exchanges between wife and husband in Case G. The focus on this dyad simplifies my approach which, of course, becomes more complicated when many family members are present and the interviewer must simultaneously track a host of exchanges between people. The focus is also on the timing of transactions, and it should be obvious that there are myriads of other factors involved in interviewing families.

In Case G, there were frequent *mismatched sequences* of communication between the wife and husband. These occurred at the verbal as well as nonverbal level. For example, the wife pined at her husband, saying, "You don't love me; you don't care for me." In reply to this, the husband looked down at the floor, sighed, and mumbled, "Well, I'm here, aren't I? That must say something." The wife retorted, "You're here out of guilt; I don't want you to feel guilty; I want you to love me for *me*." The husband turned away from her, mashing his cigarette in an ashtray, "But I do feel guilty." The wife pleaded, "You shouldn't feel guilty; you should love me." The husband slumped in his chair, looked down at the floor again, and said, "I do love you." This did not register with the wife: "I don't feel it; I don't *feel* your love." In these examples, it can be seen that the husband was giving a double message nonverbally, while the wife was not acknowledging what the husband was verbally saying about his feelings. When the psychiatrist asked the husband to look at his wife when he spoke and asked the wife to repeat back what the husband had said, the point-for-point sequences of the communications improved.

This couple also showed *mismatches of rate*. As the wife would escalate the rate of her speech, the husband would slow down and sometimes not even respond, which in turn angered the wife who would then attack him for withdrawing. The psychiatrist countered this by asking the wife to speak as slowly as possible about her anger, while the husband was to speak as fast as possible about his guilt.

There also were *mismatches in temporal perspective*. As previously outlined in the history of Case G, the wife was predominantly focused on the past and tended to misconstrue many events of the present and future in terms of her past rejection by her father. On the other hand, the husband, who functioned well as a business executive, had a fairly balanced temporal perspective with a slight focus on the future. These differences in temporal perspective prompted each of them to frame the reality of their transactions in terms of different segments of time, with the wife primarily focused on the past and the husband focused on the future. For example, the husband declared, "I'd like to get things straightened out and start having some good times with you again." The wife replied, "But I can't forget how you *never* loved me when we were first married; you married me because I was pregnant; you didn't love me." The husband replied, "Why should that matter now? We've lived together for 26 years, and things were okay until the children got grown. Let's build toward the future." The wife then brought in a host of past grievances, saying that she could "never forgive" him. The husband looked mystified, dismayed that he could not move her toward a more future focus.

It is evident that husband and wife held considerable ambivalence toward each other. As detailed in Chapter 11, ambivalence often prompts desynchronized transactions. A common factor in ambivalence is that, as people get closer to one another, they become threatened by being rejected or controlled by the other person, much like a child relating to parents who can reject or control the child. This was true for this couple. As the wife got closer to her husband, she felt that she might be rejected as she once was by her father when she was a child. On the other hand, as the husband got closer to his wife, he felt that she might control him as his mother had controlled him when he was a boy. Many of their miscommunications in terms of mismatches of sequence, rate, and temporal perspective could be viewed as subtle attempts to distance one another in an effort to diffuse the threats of rejection and control that came with getting closer.

In interviewing families, an awareness of the timing of the transactions is crucial for the family members to begin learning new ways of communicating. The interviewer often has to backtrack and get the family members to see what happened to whom at what times in a recent series of transactions. This requires a supportive but "take charge" attitude on the part of the interviewer who must know what he is doing and demonstrate his effectiveness by quickly interrupting spirals and nonproductive escalations between family members. In this way, perhaps more so than with interviews of individuals, assessment and therapy become quickly interwoven in family interviews.

In general, interviews of families require high levels of skill since each family member's personal dynamics and personal future has to be quickly assessed and simultaneously processed as the family members interact. Yet this usually offers a wealth of information about binding expectations and misconstructions of each other's personal future that has rich potential for engendering therapeutic changes.

SUMMARY AND CONCLUSIONS

In this chapter, I have presented some case histories in order to illustrate the clinical assessment of time problems. The overall approach is to determine the nature of a psychopathological spiral by assessing the interaction between a time problem and a misconstruction of the personal future. This approach usually goes through the following stages:

1 Assess problems of sequence and rate before assessing problems with temporal perspective. (a) If there are problems with sequence, differentiate between time disorientation in organic brain disease and the temporal disintegration of sequences in active schizophrenia. (b) Having ruled out sequential difficulties, if there are prominent problems with rate, the diagnosis is likely to be an affective disorder with accelerated rate in mania and slowed rate in depression. (c) If there are no problems with sequence or rate, then assess the patient for imbalances of temporal perspective and desynchronized transactions with others.

2 Assess the personal future. To do this, evaluate the nature of the patient's future images, his plans of action, and his emotions. In acute psychosis, there is loss of control of the future; in depression, the future seems blocked; in neurosis, the future seems uncertain and often is dreaded.

3 Formulate the nature of the psychopathological spirals. These spirals often involve (a) the influence of one time problem upon another time problem and (b) the interaction between a time problem and a misconstruction of the personal future.

4 Plan treatment in a biopsychosocial direction. That is, to interrupt a spiral, it is pragmatic to initiate biological treatments when indicated and then proceed to psychosocial interventions.

Evaluation and continual monitoring of changes in the patient occur during all the above four essential stages of assessment. To do this, sensitive interviewing skills are necessary that are enhanced by the following timing strategies:

1   The use of nonverbal clues to discover what is emotionally significant to the patient and when to go for certain precipitating stresses that are given emotional emphasis.
2   Interviews of the personal future to determine the form and content of the patient's expectations and anticipations.
3   An analysis of desynchronized transactions between family members in terms of mismatches of sequences, rates, and temporal perspectives.

CHAPTER SIX

The Use of Time
in Treatment

Again and again I have had the impression that we have made too little theoretical use of this fact, established beyond any doubt, of the unalterability by time of the repressed. This seems to offer an approach to the most profound discoveries. Nor, unfortunately, have I myself made any progress here.

SIGMUND FREUD (1933, p. 74)

Freud noted that the repressed does not change with time. That is, unlike the capacity of conscious material to be modified by experiences over time, that which is relegated to the unconscious does not change unless it is brought into awareness. Our psychic past is with us regardless of how much time has intervened between our experiences as children and our adult life. The timelessness of the unconscious gives it the uncanny power of influencing us forever unless we find some way of modifying it.

It is here proposed that these unconscious influences from the past are more likely to emerge when anticipatory control is disrupted by problems with sequence, rate, and temporal perspective. That is, as the person loses control over his personal future, he becomes more vulnerable to being influenced unduly by his past. The interplay between future images, plans of action, and emotions becomes contaminated by expectations fueled by distant memories that have little relevance to the realities of the present and future.

In Chapter 4, I presented a hierarchy of time problems that disrupt anticipatory control. In Chapter 5, I dealt with practical strategies for the clinical assessment of these time problems. In this chapter, I will round out this general temporal approach to the patient by giving an overview of the various ways that time can be used in psychiatric treatment. The purpose of this chapter is to introduce some uses of time and the personal future for the treatment of psychiatric disorders that are discussed more fully in subsequent parts of this book.

The central theme of this chapter is that *alterations of sequence, rate, and temporal perspective can be used for the treatment of psychiatric disorders*. In addition, the time structure of therapy and whether there is a predominant focus on the past, present, or future account for some key differences between various types of psychiatric treatment and psychotherapy.

TYPES OF TIME INTERVENTIONS

Although it is not explicitly recognized, many forms of psychiatric treatment consist of time interventions. These time interventions consist of alterations of sequence, rate, and temporal perspective. I will here review some of these time interventions that can be brought about at the biological, psychological, or social levels.

In keeping with my general temporal approach to psychiatric disorders as outlined in Chapters 4 and 5, the correction of problems with *sequence* is mainly indicated for time disorientation or the temporal disintegration of sequences; the correction of problems with *rate* is mainly indicated for affective disorders such as mania and depression; and the correction of problems with *temporal perspective* is mainly indicated for neurotic and personality disorders. Nevertheless, aside from these corrective measures, I will outline ways to alter sequence, rate, and temporal perspective for the treatment of a wide variety of behavioral disorders. It is here proposed that these alterations of sequence, rate, and temporal perspective often help the patient reconstruct his views of reality by changing the temporal pattern of his modes of comprehending and interpreting reality.

Alteration of Sequence

In altering sequence, the therapist either restores the capacity for temporal organization of sequential thinking or helps the patient to restructure if–then contingencies.

With the pervasive problems with sequence in organic brain disease, it should be obvious that, whenever possible, the correction of toxic, metabolic, and space-occupying lesions should be carried out in order to restore adequate sequential thinking and proper orientation to clock and calendar time.

At the biological level of treatment, the capacity for timing and sequential ordering of information appears to be aided by the phenothiazine and other antipsychotic drugs (Spohn et al., 1977; Zahn, Carpenter, and McGlashan,

1978; see Chapter 7). These drugs are therefore helpful to schizophrenic patients who have difficulties with tracking sequences over time. In the future, it is hoped that there will be better drugs, with fewer side effects, that will enhance the capacity to track sequences over time. In this regard, it may prove fruitful to explore drugs that improve immediate or working memory, such as fragments of the ACTH molecule (DeWied, 1976).

As outlined later in Chapter 7 (see Table 3), there are other psychotic symptoms, such as depersonalization, delusional ideation, and hallucinations, that appear to diminish concomitantly when the temporal disintegration of sequences is corrected (Melges and Freeman, 1977). A useful way of titrating the dose of antipsychotic medication is to follow the degree of difficulty with tracking sequences.

At the psychological level of treatment, many psychotherapeutic interventions are aimed at changing habitual if–then sequences. For example, for patients who suffer from lack of motivation, behavior modification techniques can be used to alter the pattern of contingencies so that the patient is rewarded (or rewards himself) for desired behaviors (Premack, 1959). To enhance self-reinforcement, an improbable response (for example, studying) can be patterned so that it is followed by a rewarding activity (for example, playing pool). In the treatment of heavy drinking of alcohol, changing the situational cues (for example, watching TV) that prompt the drinking may decrease the frequency of drinking (Deardorff et al., 1975). In treating neurotic depression and anxiety, changing a person's assumptions about expected sequences through cognitive therapy is often helpful (Beck, 1971; Beck et al., 1979). For example, a patient may assume the following sequence: "If I am not liked by everyone, then I must be no good." This assumption may be changed through therapy to something like: "If some people don't like me, I still like myself, and that will help some people to like me."

Many first-order psychotherapeutic interpretations, which do not delve much into the past or future, are aimed at pointing out and hopefully interrupting pathological sequences. For example, "When you get angry, you then get anxious." Or "When you overeat, you then get depressed and subsequently overeat even more." It can be seen that such interpretations aim to interrupt a vicious cycle. Likewise, the technique of paradoxical intention is aimed at interrupting a vicious cycle (Frankl, 1978; Watzlawick, 1978). For example, "When you overeat, I want you to try your best to feel bad and unworthy so that you feel you deserve to have more food." Presumably, when the patient realizes he can increase his symptom, he also realizes that he can decrease it. By intending and trying to feel bad, the feeling is brought under the patient's control, and the sequence eating–depression may be interrupted.

At the social level of treatment, sequences of interaction can be structured in order to reduce uncertainty or they can be rearranged in order to modify power struggles. The reduction of uncertainty about future outcomes mitigates anxiety (Masserman, 1972). This can be helpful for many problems associated with anxiety, but making the interpersonal environment predictable and consistent is particularly useful for schizophrenic patients. Achieving closure in communications, unraveling double binds, and instilling expectable rhythms in family life gives sequential structure to the environment which may help the schizophrenic compensate for his tracking difficulties (see Chapters 4 and 7).

With regard to changing power struggles between people, Haley (1977) points out that one of the best ways to do this is to change the sequence of interactions. For example, a mother may involve her son in an attempt to control her husband. By being in between the mother and father, the son is "triangulated" (Bowen, 1976). If the son can be removed from the interaction, the balance of power between the mother and father may shift toward greater equality with less roundabout communication. That is, the sequence of mother → son → father is changed to mother → father.

In this regard, many therapeutic maneuvers in family therapy involve either a direct change of sequences or a reinterpretation of sequences. Contractual tradeoffs, where one person agrees to do something if the other person agrees to do something else, involve joint plans for changing the nature of the sequential interaction. Also the reinterpretation of sequences often consists of reframing an outcome in a different light (Watzlawick, 1978). For example, a wife may report that she stops talking whenever she sees her husband furrow his brow, since she thinks he is angry at her. This may be reframed to indicate that the husband's furrowed brow means "interest and concern" rather than "anger."

One of the most common problems in marital discord is blaming the other person for "starting it." Here the sequences of a mutual interaction are "punctuated" differently by each person (Watzlawick, 1976). For example, for the supposed "cause" of a marital fight, a wife may view a husband's sarcastic comment as the starting point, whereas the husband may view the wife's aloofness as the starting point. This endless game can be shown to be pointless if they can see that both contributed to starting the fight, and moreover, by maintaining the fight through the search for a cause, they are now perpetuating it.

Alterations of Rate

Rate problems are manifested by patients going either too fast or too slow. If a patient is going too fast, the problem is usually mania or anxiety. At the biological level, lithium carbonate can be given to a manic patient so that he eventually slows down. Lithium slows biological clocks (Engelmann, 1973; Johnsson et al., 1979; Wehr, Muscettola, and Goodwin, 1980). For the anxious patient, various types of tranquilizers, such as the benzodiazepines, help to slow down a patient. At the psychological level of treatment, relaxation techniques and meditation exercises may help a patient to slow down (Johnson and Spielberger, 1968). Also, as discussed later, hypnotic techniques for slowing down and ''stretching out'' inner time can help slow down a patient, giving a sense of ''all the time in the world.'' Such methods are useful for treating patients who are anxious because ''too much is coming too fast.'' At the social level of treatment, a common technique of crisis intervention is to help patients or families to pace their responses and to temporize issues so that they do not feel that they must handle everything immediately. Also, for patients who are irritating because of their hyperactivity, social confrontation in group or milieu therapy gives them feedback that may help to slow down their interpersonal pace.

If a person is going *too slow,* once having ruled out dementia, the problem is usually depression. For the treatment of depression, at the biological level, the antidepressant drugs, such as imipramine, appear to speed up rate (Edelstein, 1974; Linnoila et al., 1980). There is some evidence that the tricyclic antidepressant drugs accelerate biological rhythms involved in adrenergic turnover in the brain (Wehr and Goodwin, 1979; Wehr and Goodwin, 1981; Kafka, Naber, and Wehr, 1979). Of course, stimulant drugs, such as methylphenidate or the amphetamines, also speed up rate, but these drugs carry the risk of abuse as well as that of precipitating a psychosis.

At the psychological level, procrastination is associated with slowness of responding. Problems underlying procrastination can be treated with psychotherapy. Procrastination often stems from an excessive need to be perfect so that the person is disinclined to act for the fear of failure. This need to be perfect can be treated with cognitive therapy (Beck et al., 1979). At other times, procrastination may stem from an approach–avoidance conflict which needs to be clarified and resolved.

At the social level, slowness in responding may represent passive-aggression in which a person aggresses against others by deliberately being late or tardy. The problem often stems from rebelliousness against authority figures and is sometimes manifested as rebellion against the strictures of time itself, as though the person was combating Father Time. These problems are best treated with group or family therapy, particularly when they infringe on the rights of other people.

Besides the above interventions, there are some special problems of rate that appear to be aided by mechanical ''pacemakers.'' Some cases of stuttering can be effectively treated by having a patient time his speech output to a metronome beat that he unobtrusively hears through a small hearing aid (Brady, 1969). Also, the frequency of psychomotor epileptic attacks or of recurrent pain episodes can be reduced by electrical inhibition of brain areas through the use of feedback control devices (Delgado, 1969, 1979). That is, brain discharges responsible for the unwanted experience are detected and then promptly inhibited by a monitor embedded within the person's scalp. These are exciting discoveries. Along with new ways to control biological rhythms by chemical means, mechanical pacemakers of the brain may offer ways to regulate rate and frequency not yet envisioned.

Alteration of Temporal Perspective

Changing a person's span of awareness into the past or future and getting the person to achieve a better balance between past, present, and future considerations are implicit but important aspects of most forms of psychotherapy. These factors of temporal perspective cannot be readily altered by biological interventions. Yet there are some drugs which do alter temporal perspective. For example, marihuana appears to foster an increased focus on the present, to the relative exclusion of past and future considerations. (Melges et al., 1971). This increased concentration on the present is associated with euphoria, presumably because the person has less worries about the past or future when he is focusing on just the present. Also, intravenous barbiturates are commonly used to gain access to past material that is repressed because of psychological trauma, as with amnesia and other dissociative states. Psychotomimetic drugs, such as LSD or related hallucinogens, have been used to activate childhood memories or to help patients deal with a fearsome future event, such as death. These drug-induced changes in temporal perspective are of limited usefulness, however, since the person's immediate memory is concomitantly impaired so that a proper integration of the material may not be achieved for a lasting effect. Also, the extreme measure of frontal lobotomy, which is a biological intervention that produces indifference toward the future (see Chapter 2), is of limited usefulness since problem-solving abilities are concomitantly impaired.

At the psychological level of treatment, there are different types of psychotherapeutic interventions that alter temporal perspective. As discussed later, a direct way to do this is to use hypnosis to heighten awareness of the present. The patient can be given the hypnotic suggestion that the present is expanded, with the past and future remote. This induces a state of euphoria, presumably liberating the patient from the time-bound control of past and future considerations (Zimbardo, Marshall, and Maslach, 1971). In this regard, one of the major aims of Gestalt therapy is to induce a greater ''present-centeredness''

(Naranjo, 1977). This increased focus on the present appears to reduce anxiety, decrease obsessional worries about the future, and help the patient become more aware of his surroundings. A similar heightened focus on the present is common to most meditative practices (Goleman, 1977).

Psychotherapeutic interpretations essentially relate the past to the present, sometimes the past to the future. Since psychotherapists usually focus more on content than form, they sometimes are not fully aware that their interpretations of content also may be changing the formal relationships between past, present, and future. For example, if a patient comes to therapy complaining of anxiety about current financial problems and the therapist relates this to envy of his brother when he was a child, the patient's temporal frame of reference may be changed. In this regard, Levy (1963) points out that one of the primary functions of an interpretation is to change a person's habitual frame of reference, the ways in which he conceptualizes events. Changing a person's focus on the past, present, or future (or changing the interrelations between past, present, and future) is an expedient way to change his frame of reference. Altering a person's frame of reference, regardless of the "truth" of an interpretation, is often therapeutic in itself, since it helps the patient gain a different perspective as to how to approach his problems.

Time projection into the past or future also helps the patient to gain a wider temporal perspective on his problems. In contrast to interpretations, which call for a reconceptualization of elements of the past, present, and future, time projection techniques are more experiential. That is, the patient relives segments of his past or imagines himself to be in the future as though it were happening in the present. By "making present" the past or future, the patient gives himself a different set of experiences, not just a different concept. Also, time projection techniques allow the individual to see himself in a different time frame. That is, from the present, he sees himself in the past or future, or from the past or future, he sees himself in the present. By getting out of the present per se, he can set up a dialectical relationship through time so that he can observe himself engaging in alternative experiences which are different than the forces currently impinging upon him. It is easier to observe yourself if you can get out of the present (Gergen, 1969). Transcending the present thus enhances the process of self-observation, which is a therapeutic principle inherent in practically all forms of psychotherapy (Meichenbaum, 1977).

Time projection will be discussed more fully later in regard to hypnosis and other types of time projection therapies (Chapters 10 and 12). The latter include grief-resolution therapy for reexperiencing the past (Melges and DeMaso, 1980) and future-oriented psychotherapy for giving experiential substance to the personal future (Melges, 1972).

At the social level of treatment, temporal perspective can be modified by a variety of means. Some of these are implicit, while others are explicit, forms of intervention. Implicit ways that temporal perspective is altered in psychotherapy include socialization and identification processes. For example, in group therapy, interaction with a number of different individuals who have different perspectives often prompts a resocialization process that includes considering different temporal views of one's problems. Identification with the therapist (or other group members) is an implicit yet powerful way of altering temporal perspective. By identifying with another person, an individual often takes on the other's long-term goals (Lazowick, 1955). In the course of development, this is probably how long-term future outlooks are learned (see Chapter 2). Given enough contact and positive regard for the therapist, a similar process often takes place during psychotherapy.

Social interventions for altering temporal perspective usually consist of psychodramas of the past or future in a group setting. The person is projected back to the past in order to rework a traumatic episode, or he is projected into the future so that he can decide how he will handle an upcoming troublesome event. Other people in the group are assigned roles so that they can play the part of real or imaginary persons in the patient's past or future. In this way, the psychodrama, with the guidance of the therapist, helps the patient to deal concretely with issues of his past or future. Also, the person's span of awareness into the past or future is widened.

I should also mention that there are time management techniques for helping people learn how to plan their use of social time—that is, clock and calendar time. These time management programs are well outlined by MacKenzie (1972) and Lakein (1974). The essence of these techniques involves setting clear priorities and providing enough lead time to meet one's priorities while protecting infringements upon one's time from other people and nuisance interruptions. From Chapters 4 and 5, it should be obvious that many psychiatric patients have problems with managing clock and calendar time. In this regard, schizophrenic patients often have to be actively coached about time management. Also, the neurotic problem of excessively trying to meet the expectations of other people often is revealed in terms of chaotic time management. Moreover, in our hurly-burly society, the learning of skills in time management can be considered as a psychosocial treatment pertinent to just about anyone, normal or otherwise.

In summary, a number of treatment interventions can be conveniently conceptualized as different ways of altering sequence, rate, and temporal perspective. Although current techniques for altering such time factors are not as efficient as one would like, future research is likely to develop refinements in these ways of modifying behavior. If mental illness represents different forms of cybernetic dyscontrol, it is likely that treatment strategies aimed at correcting disorders of sequence, rate, and temporal perspective will be appropriate and useful.

THE TIME FRAMEWORK OF PSYCHIATRIC TREATMENT

Time issues are pervasive in psychiatric treatment. They concern when patients come for treatment, why they come, how long they stay in therapy, their readiness for interpretations, and the timing of interpersonal behaviors. In this section, I will outline a general "bird's eye" view of some of these temporal factors.

Patients generally come for psychiatric treatment because they have lost control of their futures or they are out of synchrony with others. Sometimes they are brought by other people because they are a danger to themselves or to others. Whatever the case, their personal timing or interpersonal timing is out of kilter. As outlined in Table 2, most psychiatric problems can be conceptualized in terms of a different type of time disturbance. That is, patients may have time disorientation, temporal disintegration, rate and rhythm problems, problems with temporal perspective, or desynchronized transactions. Some may have a combination of one or more of these time disturbances. As outlined in Chapters 3 and 4, these time disturbances disrupt the processes of futuring and temporal organization, thereby interfering with the patient's capacities for coping. A key therapeutic task is to correct the time disturbances and to help the patient restructure his future images and plans of action. In this regard, Lewis (1972, p. 223) states, "All therapies involve Plans to change the patient's Plans."

Part of the therapeutic plan is the duration of treatment thought to be indicated. Depending on the nature and acuteness of the patient's problem, different lengths of therapy are prescribed. If the problem is an acute organic brain syndrome such as a delirium, then only a brief period of treatment may be necessary. However, an acute manic or schizophreniform reaction may later merge into a relapsing illness that may require life-long monitoring. Likewise, an acute adjustment disorder may be treated briefly with crisis intervention and may never recur, but it also may forebode a chronic vulnerability that will necessitate longer periods of psychotherapy.

Psychotherapy can be either brief, short term, or long term. Definitions of these time periods of therapy are usually arbitrary (Davanloo, 1978). For purposes here, brief psychotherapy will refer to less than 12 sessions, short term to 12–40 sessions, and long term to anything beyond 40 sessions. The rationale for prescribing brief, short-term, or long-term psychotherapy has not been fully worked out. Often the time course of therapy depends on the theoretical orientation of the therapist. Kasdin and Wilson (1978) point out the need to consider cost-effectiveness, including the number of treatments required, as an outcome measure for evaluating different forms of therapy. There should be a premium on more efficient forms of therapy, given the massive needs of society that are not being met. Research indicates that, for most patients, there are diminishing returns when psychotherapy lasts longer than 14–21 sessions (Meltzoff and Kornreich, 1970), but further research is needed that takes into consideration the severity of illness, the type of therapy, therapist–patient compatibility and so on. Increasing the frequency of visits above once a week does not apparently improve outcome (Meltzoff and Kornreich, 1970).

Setting a time limit on the number of sessions right from the start appears to quicken the pace of therapy and facilitates "getting down to business," as compared with an open-ended unspecified number of sessions. In setting a time limit, issues of termination, such as separation from the therapist, come up earlier and can be used therapeutically (Mann, 1973). Time-limited psychotherapy tends to discourage chronic dependency of the patient on the therapist, whereas no time limit may foster the development of chronic dependency. On the other hand, some psychoanalysts hypothesize that the leisure of no time limit in classical psychoanalysis is necessary for the reactivation of a sense of timelessness similar to that of one's childhood (Nannum, 1972). The psychoanalytic treatment setting gives a dual message about time: there is unlimited time in terms of the duration of treatment, yet there is strict adherence to the time limits of the analytic hour for which the analyst is paid for his time. The former fosters a regressive timelessness, and the latter promotes a reality orientation about time, a contrast which may be therapeutic in itself.

Psychoanalysis is a searching and illuminating process that often takes at least three years, with four to five sessions per week. This requires a commitment beyond the means of most people in society. Yet some of Freud's analyses lasted for as little as three months (Marmor, 1979). Research is needed to find out which kinds of patients, such as those with high degrees of defensiveness and resistance, need longer periods of therapy.

Some therapists pay a great deal of attention to the time factors within a given session (Horney, 1939). For example, lateness for an appointment, particularly if recurrent, may represent resistance or anger at the therapist. Similarly, waiting until the last moment of the session to bring up a highly charged issue may represent resistance.

The duration of an individual psychotherapeutic session usually lasts 55 minutes, but research has shown that 30-minute sessions may be just as effective (Meltzoff and Kornreich, 1970). Because of the greater complexity of issues and a greater number of people involved, many family and group therapists allow 1½–2 hours for an average session. Of course, patients who are being given support, usually in association with use of medication, often can be seen for 10–15-minute sessions per week or month.

The prescribed time course of therapy is obviously linked to the purposes of psychotherapy. The restoration of equilibrium, as with crisis intervention, requires less total time than a major overhaul of one's personality, as with psychoanalysis. Although there is much controversy about the general purposes of psychotherapy, there does appear to be some consensus, at least among researchers such as Strupp (1970) and Frank (1974), about the following general goals of psychotherapy:

1   To raise hope and combat demoralization
2   To restore self-control
3   To modify unrealistic expectations of self, others, and the environment
4   To foster harmonious interactions with others

Both futuring and temporal organization are directed toward accomplishing these general goals. As described in later chapters, futuring helps raise hope and modify unrealistic expectations. Temporal organization helps restore self-control and enhances the timing of interpersonal interactions (see Chapter 12).

Diverse techniques are used to accomplish these general goals. Whether a given technique is superior to another is difficult to prove by systematic studies of psychotherapy. Whatever the technique or theoretical orientation used, it appears that the characteristics of the therapist (that is, what he is like as a person) are highly important for a good outcome in psychotherapy (Strupp, 1978). Therapeutic traits that stand out are empathy, compassion, genuineness, and nonpossessive warmth. Therapists with these traits appear to have the patient's interests at heart. In fostering the patient's own strivings, they engender "virtuous cycles" so that the patient can eventually make it on his own when given a little guidance. Much of psychotherapy can be looked upon as the therapist being a supportive "coach" who guides the patient's reconstruction of goals and serves as a monitor of feedback and feedforward about how well the patient is directing himself toward his evolving goals.

Finally, out of the host of measures that can be used to test whether improvement has taken place, there is a global impression of timing that is used at least implicitly by most therapists for judging improvement: synchrony with other people. That is, patients who have improved in treatment show a gracefulness in the time flow of their interactions with others, including the therapist. They are aware, responsive, sensitive to nuances, and emotionally in tune with both present and anticipated situations. In a word, they "flow" with ongoing changes over time at the right time. In clinical conferences for evaluating a patient's progress, there are frequent references to this synchrony of timing, such as whether or not the patient is "appropriate," "on cue," "with it," or "in synch." Eventually, this synchrony of a patient's interpersonal behavior may be able to be captured in systematic measures of videotape recordings. This might help outcome studies by emphasizing human behavior as a form in motion rather than something that can be measured as static states. The importance of such temporal kinetics was highlighted by Kelly (1955), and has been confirmed by research of nonverbal communication (Harper, Wiens, and Matarazzo, 1978).

THE PAST, PRESENT, AND FUTURE IN PSYCHOTHERAPY

Different forms of psychotherapy vary according to the attention given to the past, present, or future. Different assumptions about how to bring about changes in behavior are reflected in these different temporal emphases.

The past is emphasized by psychoanalysis. One of the main assumptions of psychoanalysis is that, through helping the person to become aware of past events, such as early childhood experiences, the person will be able to decipher past influences from his present interactions. There are many other therapies that are based on this psychoanalytic assumption. For example, the "script analysis" of transactional analysis attempts to show the patient how he was programmed by his parents during childhood. Also, a therapy such as primal scream appears to be an attempt to uproot feelings associated with early experiences. The release of held-back emotions associated with past events is thought to disempower the influence of the past on the present.

The present is highlighted by Gestalt therapy (Naranjo, 1977). In order to become completely aware of one's feelings and sensations, the person is taught to immerse himself in the here-and-now. Perls (1969) emphasized that the present is "the centre of balance" between the past and future, and to shift too far into the past or into the future is to become an unbalanced personality. When a person loses present awareness, he no longer possesses the medium through which to integrate the various polarities of his personality. To become whole, Gestalt therapy expands awareness of the present, since to live in past memories or future expectations is to deny oneself of the vital contact with reality that comes from being in the present. With "present-centeredness," the past and future remain accessible as the person maintains his balance in the present.

Emphasis on the here-and-now also takes place in behavioral modification and in most forms of group and family therapy. In behavior modification, the therapist does not emphasize the past causes of the behavior but focuses on what factors are currently maintaining the behavior. The key questions revolve around how the maladaptive behavior is being reinforced and what can be done to reinforce alternative and more desirable forms of behavior. In group therapy, one of the most potent therapeutic factors is feedback from others about how one is "coming across" in the here-and-now (Yalom, 1970). Although aspects of the past and future may be dealt with in group therapy, they usually are not as important as the interpersonal confrontation and learning that takes place in the present with a group. In most forms of family therapy, there also is a predominant focus on present interactions in an attempt to streamline communications and transactions (Satir, 1967).

Compared to the emphasis given to the past and present in various forms of psychotherapy, the future has been relatively neglected. This is somewhat surprising in light of the important role of anticipations and expectations in governing human behavior (see Chapter 3). Yet existentialist therapists place great emphasis on the realtionship of the present to the future (Yalom, 1980). Commitment, choice, and responsibility for one's actions and feelings are key features of the existentialistic emphasis on the future. Besides existentialism, there are other forms of psychotherapy that have paid attention to the future. These include Adler's (1929) emphasis on strivings and purposes as integrative factors for the personality; Kelly's (1955) constructive alternativism for helping patients to realign sets of anticipations; and the Gouldings' (1979) "redecision" work where patients are encouraged to take a stand against their parental programming in order to make their futures different. Also, as detailed in Chapter 12, there is future-oriented psychotherapy which uses time-projection techniques in order for patients to choose and rehearse a realistic future self-image (Melges, 1972).

Of course, the predominant temporal foci of various forms of psychotherapy, as outlined above, represent matters of emphasis. In actual practice, it is rare for a psychotherapist, whatever his theoretical orientation, to focus exclusively on just the past, the present, or the future. An optimal psychotherapeutic approach usually attempts to integrate past, present, and future. This integration is most explicit in the various forms of "cognitive therapy," which are aimed at helping patients revise their past assumptions and future expectations (Beck, 1971; Meichenbaum, 1977; Beck et al., 1979). A gamut of psychotherapeutic interventions, ranging from emotional catharsis to clarification of unconscious factors, have at least the implicit aim of freeing the patient from his past and opening his future. What happens to the patient in the future, however, is usually left unstructured; the person may be given insight about how the past affects the present, but rarely is one time projected into the future to see how insights might be applied to upcoming situations. This neglected step in psychotherapy is discussed in Chapter 12.

THE USE OF HYPNOTIC TIME DISTORTIONS IN PSYCHOTHERAPY

Hypnosis can be used to alter sequence, rate (duration), and temporal perspective. When used in conjunction with other forms of therapy, these hypnotic time distortions can facilitate psychotherapy. In this section, the therapeutic use of these hypnotic time distortions will be outlined.

Before dealing with the time interventions, some of the temporal characteristics of hypnotic induction will be discussed. Persons who are highly susceptible to hypnosis are capable of an intense degree of imaginative involvement in situations (Hilgard, 1970). It is as if they can quickly lose contact with the present and enter another realm of reality as though it were present. There are systematic tests of this susceptibility to hypnosis (Hilgard, 1965; Spiegel and Spiegel, 1978), but clinically it can be detected by simply asking the person if he cries in movies, gets lost in a novel, forgets about his body in a sports event, and so on. In general, a person who is highly hypnotizable can achieve greater degrees of time distortion, yet these marked degrees usually are not necessary for most uses of hypnotic time distortions in therapy. A light trance with a mild time distortion is often sufficient.

It is interesting that hypnotic induction techniques customarily employ a deliberate focus on the time flow of events. These include the repetition of monotonous sounds, the rhythm of a metronome, attention to breathing, and so on. Also, many hypnotists gain control over the subject's expectancies by employing what can be called "the prediction of the inevitable." That is, inevitable sequences of bodily sensations are predicted by the hypnotist. For example, "Make a tight fist; now relax it completely; sooner or later you will notice a tingling in your fingers." The tingling of the fingers is an inevitable response, once a person's attention is drawn to it. When the hypnotist draws the person's attention to the tingling in advance of its occurrence, it seems as though the hypnotist has powers of prophecy. He can predict what will happen to the person's own body. In this way, the hypnotist appears to have control over the patient's responses by carefully timing his comments just as the person's inevitable natural responses are emerging. Milton Erickson was a master of this technique (Erickson and Rossi, 1979). By commenting on what the patient was about to experience slightly ahead of the patient's awareness of certain sensations, Erickson appeared to gain control over the patient's intentions by being "one step ahead of them."

There are other similar induction techniques that attempt to set up a positive feedback and feedforward cycle through time. For example, "When you relax, you will feel more sleepy, and when you feel more sleepy, you will feel more relaxed." Setting up "an illusion of alternatives" also induces a progressive cycle that will occur sooner or later as a matter of time (Watzlawick, 1978). For example, "You will want to close your eyes either *now* or *later,* and then you will be entering a trance." This makes use of the fact that sooner or later the person will want to close or blink his eyes.

In using hypnotic time distortions, it is advisable that they should not be employed with psychotic individuals whose temporal disintegration might be further aggravated by the time distortions. In general, hypnotic time interventions are indicated as an adjunct to treating neurotic or personality disorders where it might be useful to "imprint" a desired change by highlighting it in the mind via a time distortion. Below I will discuss separately hypnotic alterations in sequence, rate, and temporal perspective, but in actual practice, combinations of these time interventions may be employed during a given hypnotic session.

Alterations of Sequence in Hypnosis

Hypnotically induced changes in sequence are well known in the form of posthypnotic suggestions. Here, the hypnotized subject is told that after he awakes from hypnosis, he will emit a certain response when a specific cue occurs. For example, he will take off his shoe when somebody opens the door. This will occur quite out of his awareness. These posthypnotic suggestions for a change in sequence can be used therapeutically. For example, for a person who wants to quit smoking, he is told that whenever he reaches for a cigarette, he will feel nauseated, and whenever he avoids smoking, he will get a feeling of well-being. In my experience, unless the patient is highly hypnotizable, these alterations in sequences are best rehearsed in imagination during hypnosis if they are to be effective in changing if–then contingencies in real life.

Under hypnosis, imagined outcomes can be rearranged so that they become temporally juxtaposed to a behavior or attitude, using the principle of covert reinforcement (Cautela, 1970). Covert reinforcement means that an inner image, rather than an external reward or punishment, is used for reinforcement. For example, a man wanted to be more warm toward his wife; under hypnosis, he was asked to imagine himself being warm with his wife and immediately after this to experience the thrill of making a good tennis shot, something he found exhilarating. In this way, events ordinarily separated in time were juxtaposed temporally so that the image of making a good tennis shot "rewarded" the image of being warm. Negative consequences also can be used in this way. For example, a kleptomaniac, who ordinarily felt "charged up and thrilled" when she was not caught for her thievery, was asked under hypnosis to see herself stealing and immediately thereafter to experience her hands covered with feces, something she found abhorrent. In this way, consequences can be rearranged in the mind so that patients can modify their behaviors according to their conscious choices. Although hypnosis is not altogether necessary for covert reinforcement, it appears to have the advantage of inducing a "ribbon of concentration" that imbues the transformed consequences with a sense of reality, even though they might seem absurd in the waking state (Spiegel and Spiegel, 1978).

Alterations of Rate in Hypnosis

Alterations of internal rate and the sense of duration go together (see Chapter 2). To recapitulate, a speeding of internal rate makes clock time, by comparison, seem to be "dragging," whereas a slowing of internal rate makes clock time seem to be "flying by." Under hypnosis, the suggestion that time is speeded up (so that a minute seems like a second) should give rise to responses that are faster than clock time, whereas the suggestion that time has slowed down (so that a second seems like a minute) should give rise to responses that are slower than clock time. These hypnotic alterations of rate have been experimentally demonstrated in an operant task that required subjects to press a lever at a certain rate (Zimbardo et al., 1973). That is, the hypnotic suggestion that time was speeded up or slowed down was objectively manifested in the subjects' speed of responding. These hypnotic time distortions were significantly greater than those of role-playing and awake control subjects. Moreover, the hypnotically induced time distortions persisted even when the hypnotized subjects were given feedback about their erroneous objective performance. These findings indicate that hypnotic time distortions are "real" phenomena in which subjects actually experience an alteration in the passage of time.

Clinically, Erickson has used the hypnotic acceleration of subjective time for therapeutic purposes (Cooper and Erickson, 1959). For example, under hypnosis the patient is told that, within a span of 20 seconds, he will be able to review a vast number of past experiences related to his problem and, by the end of the 20-second period, he will arrive at a solution. During such a procedure, most subjects report a panoramic array of experiences that, during the waking state, might have taken hours to review. Or to put it another way, rather than experiencing, say, 20 events in 20 seconds, the hypnotized subject might experience 200 events within the same 20-second time. Cooper and

Erickson (1959) believe that this technique can accelerate therapy by uncovering a host of relevant associations more quickly than usual.

Hypnosis also can be used to slow down time for treatment purposes. The patient is told that inner time will gradually become slowed down and stretched out. Initially, the hypnotist counts aloud at a rate of one per second and then gradually lengthens the intervals between counts until there is about one count per every four breaths (that is, one count approximately every 30 seconds). As this is being done, the patient is given the suggestion that he will have "much more inner time" and that his mind will become "peacefully empty." In my experience, this usually induces a state of profound relaxation. It is particularly useful for anxious patients who feel that "too much is coming too fast."

I also use the slowing of inner time as an adjunct to other therapeutic interventions, such as for highlighting certain images or as a prelude to time projection. The rationale for the highlighting of images is as follows: If more subjective time can be given to a desired image, then the person seems to concentrate on it more and gives it more value, and the image appears to linger longer in the mind than during normal consciousness. Also, the altered state of consciousness induced by the slowing of inner time appears to be conducive to the projection of one's self into the past or future as though these times were taking place in the present. Perhaps this stems from giving the past or future a sense of duration, thereby making it seem more real than a fleeting memory or fantasy. The clinical use of these hypnotic time distortions in future-oriented psychotherapy is discussed further in Chapter 12.

There is need for much more experimental work on hypnotic alterations of rate, even though there have been systematic attempts to study the phenomenon (Cooper and Erickson, 1959; Weitzenhoffer, 1964; Zimbardo et al., 1973). Some intensive studies of highly hypnotizable subjects have produced remarkable effects. For example, Fogel and Hoffer (1962) gave a normal subject the posthypnotic suggestion that a metronome was beating at one per second. Unbeknown to the subject, the experimenters then altered the rate of the metronome. When the metronome was sped up to three beats per second, the person became gay and lively; at eight beats per second, she became manic. When the metronome was returned to one beat per second, her behavior again became normal. Yet when it was further slowed to 40 beats per minute, she became sluggish and depressed. When the metronome was stopped, she became immobile and catatonic. These findings have been essentially replicated by Aaronson (1966, 1968) in his intensive study of five hypnotizable subjects, using one subject as a simulator control. That is, a speeding of rate induced hypomania, a slowing of rate induced either tranquility or depression, and stoppage of time gave rise to a feeling of unreality that was occasionally associated with schizophreniclike postures. These changes in the clinical picture also were reflected in changes in MMPI scales. Further experimental work in this important area is needed.

Given the above changes, one might wonder whether it is safe to use hypnotic alterations of rate for therapeutic purposes. In this regard, I have used the "slowing of inner time," in the manner described above, in over 300 neurotic patients with no adverse effects. As noted, the usual response is profound relaxation, not depression. This hypnotic procedure differs from the above experiments in that the subject knows that psychological time is being deliberately slowed down during the hypnotic state, whereas in the experiments the subjects were given the posthypnotic suggestion that a metronome was beating according to clock time, and then the rate of the metronome was altered. Thus in the latter case, changing the rate of the metronome was like changing "world time," thereby altering the perception of reality.

Alterations of Temporal Perspective in Hypnosis

The form of temporal perspective can be changed through hypnosis. A focus on the past, present, or future can be highlighted. Also, different relationships among one's past, present, and future can be created. Hypnosis appears to facilitate the formation of these alternative foci and relationships since hypnotized subjects more readily accept nonordinary experiences.

The hypnotic expansion of the present appears to induce euphoria. Zimbardo et al. (1973) found that, compared to nonhypnotized subjects, the hypnotic suggestion to allow "the present to expand and the past and future to become distanced and insignificant" produced a more frequent use of the present tense in spontaneous language, more laughing at funny events, a preoccupation with sensory experience, and less concern with social appearances. The euphoria was interpreted to arise from "liberating behavior from time-bound control" since the hypnotic subjects seemed unaffected by past traditions or future worries.

Aaronson (1968) also found that the hypnotic expansion of the present induced euphoria. By contrast, the hypnotic obliteration of the present (for example, "there is no present") often produced a schizophreniclike state in normal subjects. A similar psychotic picture was produced by the simultaneous ablation of past and future, suggesting that the present has little meaning unless it is related to the past and future. Expansion of the past produced either happiness or sadness, depending on whether subjects viewed their past positively or negatively. Expansion of the future produced a state of joy in which the person felt he had ample time to do what he wanted to do. The expansion of both the future and present produced a mystical euphoria with an intense interest in happenings around oneself. From these findings, it would appear that either an expanded present or the simultaneous expansion of the present and future could be used for the treatment of anxiety and depression.

Besides expanding or contracting the past, present, or future, hypnosis can be used for time projection into the past or future. Hypnosis appears to make these episodes of "time traveling" seem real, at least to a degree. Hypnotic age regression into the past can be used for a number of therapeutic purposes, such as recovering repressed material, reawakening positive aspects of childhood, restoring a sense of continuity with one's past, and so forth. Usually a patient has to be highly hypnotizable for complete age regression to occur, but incomplete forms of age regression can be useful in therapy. What is most important is that the patient reconstructs elements of his past.

Whether or not a person is completely age-regressed can be checked in a number of ways. The most obvious is to compare the subject's report of, say, his birthday at age four with details remembered by a relative who was there. In a truly age-regressed individual, the degree of recall and reexperiencing of minute details of the past is remarkable. For example, one patient reexperienced receiving a gift of a music box at age four; she could hear the tune and saw the face of the elderly German man who had made it for her. These details were confirmed by other sources of information. Another way to check if age regression has taken place is to ask the patient after he has awakened whether he noted any change in his body during the hypnotic process. A person who is age-regressed commonly will report that his body became smaller, like that of a child. Many subjects report that their feet were just dangling over the chair, not touching the floor. Still another way of checking is to ask the subject, while hypnotized, about current events. Many age-regressed subjects respond by reporting current events appropriate to the age to which they are regressed, and they are often childishly inarticulate in discussing these events. Moreover, they often have no knowledge of the real present, as though what is future to them in their regressed state has not yet occurred (Spiegel, Fishman, and Shor, 1945). For example, when asked who is President, a subject may say "Truman," and even when given cues about the current President, the subject will look puzzled. This ablation of whole periods of time is an interesting phenomenon which could be used therapeutically.

Under hypnosis, a person also can be age-progressed into the future. Of course, there is no suggestion that this will enable the person to foretell exactly what might happen in the future, but it can be a way of discovering a patient's expectations. For example, a mother of three children was extremely fearful of having a hysterectomy one month hence for a low-grade carcinoma of the cervix. When she was age-progressed to the operation and the hospital stay, everything was fine, but when taken ahead to when she went home, she entered her house (in her imagination) and cried out, "All the furniture is gone!" This signified her fear of losing her procreative powers and her role as a mother. Although she was intellectually aware of this threat before the hypnosis, the experience under hypnosis vivified the conflict for her. This facilitated subsequent psychotherapy around these issues.

Sensitivity to the patient's readiness for time traveling is crucial. In actual practice, a great deal of psychotherapy can take place while preparing a patient for age regression or progression, particularly around issues as to whether the patient really wants to change. Many patients believe that the material that they will uncover during these procedures will be so over-powering that they will have to give up their symptoms or change their customary behavior immediately thereafter. They often resist the prospect of such a rapid change, since their symptoms have become familiar aspects of their identities and often serve as ways of controlling others. Dealing with this resistance to change from the familiar is therapeutic in itself, regardless of whether the hypnotic age regression or progression is carried out.

When the procedure is actually carried out, I have found that it is best first to slow down inner time, in the manner described above, so that the patient enters a relaxed altered state of consciousness. Then depending on whether age regression or progression is being used, the hypnotist either counts the years going backward or forward. It is important to go slowly and to time the years appropriately to the patient's ability to recapture different segments of time. Initially, there should be an emphasis on positive experiences before dealing with traumatic issues. When using hypnotic age regression, it is important that the therapist have a specific purpose in mind, such as obtaining experiences relevant to helping the patient make a redecision (see Chapter 12).

There are other forms of time projection that are facilitated by hypnosis. Rather than suggesting a gradual change in one's age, as with age regression or progression, the person can travel more quickly to segments of the past or future. Using a tape recorder analogy, rapid time projection into the future can be called "fast forward," whereas rapid reversal of time into the past can be called "fast backward." With these fast-forward and fast-backward tech-niques, compared to age regression or progression, the person usually retains a greater hold on the present as he travels into the past or future. Obtaining differences between one's present views and views taken from the past or future can be therapeutic in changing a patient's frame of reference. The dissociation of time periods can set up a dialectical relationship between the present self and the future self, or between the present self and the past self. This is similar to the dissociation between the body and self under hypnosis that is useful for having the self "take care of" the body, as with the treatment of cigarette smoking and other physical problems (Spiegel and Spiegel, 1978). That is, in separating various temporal views of the self, the future self can guide or take care of the present self, or the present self can declare its differences from the past self. In this way, what is ordinarily experienced as an amalgam of self-images is strung out in time into different temporal views of the self.

Also, time distancing from traumatic events can be experienced through time projection techniques. For example, a college student was flagellating herself for having failed a recent examination, thinking that her hopes for a career as a lawyer were ruined. When time-projected into the future six months ahead, she looked back at her present dilemma as "only a drop in a bucket, only one test among many," and she gained a more balanced perspective on her current problem. Time distancing makes use of the old adage "time heals" by helping patients to experience inner time separating the self from an event.

By way of concluding this section, it is important to repeat that hypnotic time distortions should be used cautiously, if at all, in persons with a history of psychosis. In particular, patients with current tracking difficulties or temporal indistinction should not be asked to engage in hypnotic time projection, since the time traveling might further confuse them. That is, these time-traveling techniques might overtax the psychotic patient's impaired ability to index memories as past, perceptions as present, and expectations as future (see Chapter 7). Yet with neurotic and personality disorders who can index past, present, and future, the separation of events in time appears to facilitate a later new integration which can be therapeutic. Thus, time traveling may be harmful to the psychotic patient, whereas it is often helpful to neurotic and personality disorders. The use of hypnotic time distortions, such as changes in sequence, rate, and temporal perspective, in conjunction with future-oriented psychotherapy is further described in Chapter 12.

SUMMARY AND CONCLUSIONS

The aim of this chapter was to introduce various ways that time can be used in psychiatric treatment. The major points can be summarized as follows:

1 Alterations of sequence, rate, and temporal perspective can be used for the treatment of psychiatric disorders.
2 These time interventions can take place at the biological, psychological, or social levels of interaction.

3 Issues of time structure and timing are pervasive in many forms of psychiatric treatment.

4 Various schools of psychotherapy differ according to predominant foci on the past, present, or future.

5 Hypnotic alterations of sequence, rate, and temporal perspective can be used to facilitate psychotherapy.

PART THREE

Psychosis:
Loss of Control
of the Future

During an acute psychosis, there is marked loss of control over the future. The person has lost the ability to direct himself toward goals. The lack of goal-directed behavior and thinking is perhaps the most striking clinical clue that a patient may be psychotic. Objectively, it can be observed in the disorganization of the patient's speech and actions. Subjectively, when asked about his future, the psychotic patient often reports that the future seems uncanny and mystifying, and he feels that he himself has little control over what might happen to him in the future.

Part III of this book will deal with the loss of control over the future in acute psychosis. Two central themes will be explored:

1 Loss of control over the future during an acute psychosis is related to difficulties in sequential thinking.
2 Attempts to regain control over the future through over-projections into the future generate paranoid thinking, which then augments feelings of loss of control.

Chapter 7, which deals with the first theme, provides a model for understanding the progressive symptoms of an acute psychosis in terms of increasing difficulties with sequential thinking. This is an extension of the proposal made in Chapter 4 that difficulties with keeping track of sequences are fundamental to the formal thought disorder of active schizophrenia. The focus of Chapter 7, however, is not on diagnosis but rather on the progression of psychotic symptoms. In terms of the cybernetic concepts presented in Chapters 3 and 4, I propose that impaired sequential thinking during an acute psychosis disrupts the temporal organization of plans of action, and this, in turn, induces incoordination of the person's futuring and emotions. In short, during an acute psychosis, since the patient has difficulty with sequentially organizing his plans of action toward goals, he loses control over his future.

There are two different reactions to this loss of control over the future: either withdrawal from activities and pursuits or attempts to regain control. The attempts to regain control by making over-projections into the future often give rise to paranoid thinking. These over-projections into the future are termed *over-futuring*. In essence, this means that the paranoid person develops an overly elaborate set of future images with regard to suspicions about other people's plans in relation to himself.

Chapter 8 explores the role of over-futuring in all types of paranoid thinking. Over-futuring can occur as a reaction to a threat of loss of self-control in an attempt to regain control over the future. It can occur without there being difficulties with sequential thinking, as in various paranoid disorders such as acute paranoid disorder, paranoid states, and paranoid personalities.

However, its escalation is particularly aggravated when there are difficulties with sequential thinking, as in paranoid schizophrenia. Even though over-futuring can be conceptualized as a style of coping with anticipated threats, it often increases the sense of threat and loss of control over the future since the person comes to believe that his future is controlled by others.

Thus in discussing the loss of control over the future during an acute psychosis, I will first deal with the temporal disorganization of plans of action and then with over-futuring. The combination of temporal disorganization and over-futuring, as in paranoid schizophrenia, is particularly conducive to loss of anticipatory control.

CHAPTER SEVEN

Temporal Disintegration and Psychotic Symptoms

My body is an hour glass and my mind is like sand pouring through it.

Quote from a schizophrenic patient

The above patient felt that the "world had become timeless." She knew that the "clocks still march onward," but she was in "a different realm" where "everything is happening at once." Along with this, she had lost her "grip" on who she was and felt "pushed and pulled" by "strange forces and voices" that made her do things against her will. Prior to the onset of these terrifying symptoms of loss of self-control, she had experienced a "mystical awareness" in which she felt she could "see beyond" ordinary reality. But later her sense of "psychic powers" and revelations dissipated as she entered the "abyss of timelessness."

The progression of psychotic symptoms in this patient, beginning with a mystical awareness and followed by lack of control over one's thinking, fragmentation of identity, and finally feelings of control by outside forces, is quite common during the course of an acute psychosis (Conrad, 1958; Chapman, 1966; Bowers, 1974; Docherty et al., 1978). In this chapter, I will explore how this progression of psychotic symptoms might be related to the disintegration of the experience of time.

TEMPORAL DISINTEGRATION AND PSYCHOTIC DYSCONTROL

The basic postulates to be explored are as follows:

1 *The disintegration of sequential thinking is associated with loss of control over the future during an acute psychosis.*

2 *Progressive degrees of the temporal disintegration of sequences are associated with increasingly severe psychotic symptoms.*

In essence, it is proposed that when time becomes disorganized so does the person. It should be noted that psychological time can become disorganized during a psychosis without there being the time disorientation typical of organic brain disease (see Chapter 4). In a study of acute mental illness that excluded patients with organic brain disease, psychotic patients had significantly greater distortions of time sense than nonpsychotic patients (Melges and Fougerousse, 1966). This study prompted further investigations, to be summarized below, on the role of temporal disintegration in the emergence of psychotic symptoms.

Temporal disintegration refers to the breakdown of sequential thinking. There is an incoordination of making serial adjustments to reach a goal (Melges et al., 1970a, 1970b). Subjectively, temporal disintegration is experienced as difficulty in indexing memories as past, perceptions as present, and expectations as future. Cognitive and subjective report measures of temporal disintegration are given in Appendix A.

The term *psychosis* refers to defective reality testing. Simply stated, defective reality testing means that the person has difficulty in telling the real from the unreal. An important aspect of reality testing is the capacity to test predictions or hunches in terms of actual occurrences. This necessitates adequate sequential thinking. From these considerations, our research group proposed that *temporal disintegration impairs reality testing*.

In terms of cybernetic concepts (see Chapter 3), we proposed that temporal disintegration impairs reality testing since the person would have difficulty comparing what is happening (feedback) with what is likely to happen (feedforward) and what is intended (goal-directedness). In this way, the dysfunction in sequential thinking would give rise to regulatory dyscontrol (Melges et al., 1970b).

Thus it is proposed that when sequential thinking becomes impaired, the person may lose his capacity for anticipatory control. Adequate sequential thinking is necessary for the temporal organization of plans of action, since a plan is a hierarchy of sequences (see Chapter 3). When a person's planning functions become impaired, his futuring and emotions also become disorganized. Goal-directed behavior becomes chaotic since there is a disharmony between the person's future images, plans of action, and emotions. The deranged sequential thinking makes it difficult for the person to make serial adjustments and corrections in order to reach goals. He loses control over his future.

Moreover, the difficulty with sequential thinking would make it difficult for the person to distinguish the *now* from the *then*. When an experience in the here-and-now appears to have nothing before or after it, it may seem isolated from the continuum of time and hence seem timeless.

Our research group found that timelessness is a common alteration of consciousness during the severe stages of an acute psychosis. In this regard, our further clinical and experimental work, which is summarized below, indicated that the more pronounced forms of temporal disintegration were associated with more florid types of psychotic symptoms. Some of the key relationships between progressive degrees of temporal disintegration and increasingly severe psychotic symptoms are listed in Table 3. I will deal with each of these relationships in separate sections of this chapter. Table 3 provides an overview of the findings that represent a blend of clinical and experimental approaches. For now, suffice it to say the table proposes that progressive degrees of temporal disintegration are related to increases in defective reality testing.

INVESTIGATIVE APPROACH

In examining these relationships, I should be careful to point out that our findings consist of correlated relationships that change together through time. This does not mean that our research has established that temporal disintegration is the necessary and sufficient cause of psychotic symptoms. Nevertheless, as described below, we have attempted to examine the role of temporal disintegration as at least a contributing cause of psychotic symptoms by manipulation experiments in which we induced temporal disintegration in normal volunteers in order to test whether psychotic symptoms would emerge.

In this regard, it is possible to look at temporal disintegration as either a manifestation or mechanism of psychotic illness. For example, an underlying

Table 3   Progression of Temporal Disintegration and Psychotic Symptoms

Degrees of Temporal Disintegration	Associated Psychotic Symptoms
Prolongation of the present	Psychedelic experiences
Tracking difficulties	Loosening of associations
Temporal discontinuity	Depersonalization
Temporal indistinction	Delusional ideation
	Paranoid connectivity
	Inner–outer confusion

biochemical cause could be manifested at the psychological level of inquiry by giving rise to both temporal disintegration and psychotic symptoms. However, the heuristic approach taken here, as outlined in the Prologue, is that once a time distortion takes place, whatever its underlying cause, it alters the organization of consciousness at the psychological level. Thus in line with this cybernetic approach, temporal disintegration can be considered as a contributing and aggravating factor in psychotic symptoms, although there may be other underlying causes.

Our investigative approach entailed going back and forth between clinical and experimental studies. Besides the comparisons of groups of patients, we focused on intensive studies of individuals over time to test whether there was a dynamic interrelationship between changes in temporal disintegration and certain measurable psychotic symptoms. This method of correlating within-subject changes over time is outlined in the previously published research reports and in Appendix B. The essential question of the method is, What changes with what? The method is a form of "intensive" design that uses each subject as his own control as he is studied over time (Chassan, 1979). It is only through studying relationships between changes over time within an individual (or a system) that the possible influence of one change upon another can be determined; this cannot be determined by group comparisons (Melges, 1972). But this method of studying concomitant variation is not just an individual design, since the aggregate changes can be averaged across individuals studied. Moreover, using the same method, findings from longitudinal studies of psychiatric patients can be compared with experimental studies using normal volunteers.

If our research group found a substantial change correlation between temporal disintegration and a psychotic symptom through studying psychiatric patients longitudinally, we then proceeded to test whether the psychotic symptom would emerge in normal volunteers if we induced temporal disintegration in them. For these manipulation experiments, the way we induced temporal disintegration was to use tetrahydrocannabinol (THC), usually in high doses in the range of hashish. It is well known that one of the most prominent effects of THC is the alteration of time sense (Bromberg, 1934; Tinklenberg et al., 1972; 1976). All the THC experiments summarized below used double-blind controls with placebo and, in some experiments, comparable intoxicating doses of alcohol for comparison purposes. The major intent of these THC experiments was not to compare drug effects but, rather, to test whether the induction of temporal disintegration would be associated with the emergence of certain psychotic symptoms.

Our measures consisted largely of systematic subjective reports and cognitive tasks (see Appendix A). One reason for this was to increase the clinical utility of our findings. That is, it was our hope that the questions and tasks could be used by clinicians in their examinations of patients.

The same measures of temporal disintegration and of psychotic symptoms were used in both the clinical and experimental THC studies. Thus although a clinical psychosis may differ from a hashish psychosis, the findings reported in this chapter are in terms of identical or similar measures. A number of investigators have pointed to the similarity of a hashish psychosis to clinical acute psychoses (Ames, 1958; Thacore and Shukla, 1976; Tennant and Groesbeck, 1972; Isbell et al., 1967). This should *not* be taken to mean, however, that THC in its usual form as a marihuana cigarette (which is a much lower dose than hashish) produces a psychosis.

Although it is well known that at low "recreational" doses of THC, the usual effects are euphoric, high doses of THC produce psychotomimetic effects that are similar to that of LSD-25, except that there are less perceptual distortions with THC (Melges et al., 1974). These effects can be terrifying, particularly if the subject loses awareness that he has taken a drug and the effects will be time limited. In addition, during the early stages of a clinical psychosis, as explained below, there often is a euphoric exhilaration similar to the initial effects of low doses of THC; at later stages, this initial euphoria gives way to uncanny experiences and feelings of loss of control.

Thus our experimental approach entailed using high doses of THC as a rough model of psychosis. Although we focused on progressive psychotic symptoms and not on broad diagnostic categories, we were essentially interested in processes relevant to the active stages of acute schizophrenia, particularly in the role of incoherent thinking and a formal thought disorder in relation to other psychotic symptoms. At the time that our research was conducted, however, we felt that the diagnostic criteria for schizophrenia were too imprecise for investigative purposes. Although there are different theories about the genesis of the schizophrenic thought disorder, our bias was that there is a primary deficit in processing information in immediate memory (see Chapter 4). As discussed later, sophisticated techniques have been developed that demonstrate this deficit in processing information in immediate memory in acute schizophrenics (Saccuzzo and Braff, 1981) as well as during THC intoxication (Braff et al., 1981). This lends support for using THC as a model of the psychotic processeses we were studying. Such a deficit in immediate memory could be the underlying cause of the temporal disintegration of sequences during active schizophrenia and during THC intoxication. That is, if a person has problems with immediate memory, he is apt to have difficulties with tracking sequences. It is hoped that these more sophisticated techniques will expand and refine the relationships between temporal disintegration and progressive stages of psychosis described below in terms of clinical questions and measures that can be used in psychiatric examinations (also see Chapter 5).

As discussed later, the proposed relationships between temporal disintegration and progressive stages of psychosis provides a clinically useful model for dealing with acute psychotic patients. Let us now turn to the proposed progressive stages.

PROLONGATION OF THE PRESENT AND PSYCHEDELIC EXPERIENCES

The first stage of temporal disintegration is characterized by the prolongation of the present and psychedelic experiences (Table 3). It is proposed that when mental sequences become mildly disconnected, present experiences seem to last longer since they are relatively isolated from past and future events. That is, they seem to "stand alone." Rather than the future continually becoming present and then fading into the past as in normal consciousness, the disconnection of sequences makes the present seem relatively isolated from the past and future. Moreover, the inability to sustain a continuous train of thought prompts the person to attend to a variety of present stimuli that ordinarily would be excluded from consciousness. As a result, for a given amount of clock time, the person is aware of many more events than usual and his thoughts seem to race. It is proposed that this incipient breakdown in sequential thinking and the racing of thoughts give rise to the prolongation of the present, which, as explained below, may account for psychedelic experiences.

The term *psychedelic* means "mind-manifestation." Psychedelic experiences often take on the form of revelations and heightened sensations. Psychedelic experiences are common during the early, prodromal stages of the development of an acute psychosis (Bowers and Freedman, 1966). The person feels exhilarated with a "new creativity." This is an altered state of consciousness that is awesome and mystical. It is similar to the emergence of primary process thinking, as in dreaming (see Chapter 2).

Norma McDonald (1960) described this early phase of her psychosis as a state of unusual "wakefulness" in which "the brilliance of light on a window sill or the color of blue in the sky would be so important it would make me cry." Unusual visual imagery has been highlighted by Chapman (1966) as common during the early phases of schizophrenia. It also is common during the initial stages of THC intoxication. For example, one subject during THC reported he was having a flood of visual images, "like spontaneous El Greco scenes." Another THC subject described his experience as "multiple reality with a strobe-light effect'' in which there were ''jarring bursts of sensations that seemed timeless.''

These psychedelic experiences appear to be related to an early stage of temporal disintegration in which the experience of the present is prolonged. That is, the present seems ''stretched out'' and seems to last longer than usual. This apparent lengthening of inner duration and a heightened focus on the present per se have been found during acute mental illness as well as during the initial stages of THC intoxication (Melges and Fougerousse, 1966; Melges et al., 1971). The racing of thoughts appears to contribute to the feeling of more inner time, since there is a greater frequency of inner events compared to those noticed in the external environment (Tinklenberg et al., 1972). This makes clock time seem to be passing by slowly by comparison; inner time is faster compared to outer time. Considerable research has shown that a greater frequency of internal events is associated with the illusion that outside (clock) time is passing by slowly (Fraisse, 1963; Frankenhauser, 1959; Ornstein, 1969). This illusion is particularly prominent when there is a lack of organization of the inner events. An incipient dissociation of sequences may contribute to this lack of organization so that present experiences seem somewhat isolated from the continuum of past and future experiences. A heightened focus on the present, with the relative exclusion of past and especially future references, is characteristic of acute psychotic illness as well as THC intoxication (Melges and Fougerousse, 1966; Melges et al., 1971).

The racing of thoughts and images may contribute to the increased frequency of unusual ''connections'' and ''revelations'' during the early stages of an acute psychosis. That is, with an accelerated internal tempo, there are more frequent opportunities for events to become linked in the mind compared to when the mind is going at its normal rate. An oscillation in the rate of internal events also could produce a chain of ''connections'' during thought racing that would then linger in the mind when thinking processes intermittently slowed down, as with poverty of thought. In addition, the heightened focus on the present per se may make certain events ''stand out'' in the mind, since they would be isolated from the contexts of past or future considerations. The increased focus on the present may make experiences seem vivid and fresh, as though never experienced before. The present focus may enhance one's awareness of current sensations (Melges et al., 1971). In these ways, the prolongation of the present may produce the psychedelic experiences of unusual connections and heightened sensations during the early phases of an acute psychosis.

In this regard, Aldous Huxley (1963, p. 21) emphasized temporal changes as central to his experience with the psychotomimetic drug mescaline: ''My actual experience had been . . . . of an indefinite duration or alternatively of a perpetual present made up of one continually changing apocalypse.'' Other psychedelic drugs, such as LSD, also produce similar marked alterations in the sense of time (Aronson, Silverstein, and Klee, 1959; Kenna and Sedman, 1964).

TRACKING DIFFICULTIES AND LOOSENING OF ASSOCIATIONS

As a psychosis progresses, the person has increasing difficulties with keeping track of sequences. These difficulties with tracking information over time are usually experienced as frequent lapses in the person's train of thought or as blocking. These tracking difficulties are manifested in the person's speech as ''loosening of associations'' (Melges et al., 1970a), which is a prominent feature of the formal thought disorder of schizophrenia (Bleuler, 1911; see Chapter 4). The content of the person's speech appears loosely tied together, irrelevant, and lacks goal-directedness. Since the person frequently forgets what he just said or what he intends to say, his thoughts wander haphazardly from subject to subject. Because he is unable to keep a goal in mind and to coordinate sequences of thought relevant to the goal, the train of his associations appear to be loose and lack organization toward a goal. Thus it is proposed that the inability to track sequences accounts for loosening of associations.

Tracking difficulties not only are prominent during the active phases of schizophrenia but also are common during THC intoxication (Melges et al., 1970a; Weil, Zinberg, and Nelson, 1968; Casswell and Marks, 1973). For example, a schizophrenic patient reported: ''I can't keep a train of thought. . . . Thoughts slip away before I can quite grasp them.'' Similarly, a THC subject reported: ''I can't keep hold of my thoughts. . . . I can't dial the words or memories I want at the right time.'' These difficulties with tracking information over time have been demonstrated by systematic cognitive tests as well as subjective report measures (see Appendix A). Increasing doses of THC produced increasingly severe impairments of tracking information over time.

Tracking difficulties interfere with the person's ability to comprehend and sustain a conversation. To quote a schizophrenic patient: ''When people talk to me, I can't follow what they're saying. . . . I get all mixed up, especially when they don't talk simply . . . or when several people are trying to tell me something.'' Similarly, a THC subject reported: ''I don't think you're understanding me or getting what I'm saying—possibly because I don't think *I* get what I'm saying or what you're saying. . . . There seems to be a time-gap between my hearing a question and understanding it, so by the time I'm ready to respond you seem to be off on something else. . . . Because of this, I'd rather just go into myself and not try to make conversation.''

These dysjunctions in comprehending the flow of conversation have been found to disrupt comparisons between the self and others and contribute to paranoid ideas (Melges, 1976). For example, a THC subject with marked tracking difficulties likened his experience to being on an elevator whose doors would intermittently open and shut, giving him only ''glimpses'' of what other people were saying and doing. He would then try to ''fill in the gaps'' and ''piece together the glimpses, like making a puzzle.'' In doing this, he came up with a host of suspicions about interwoven events beyond his immediate mental grasp. A schizophrenic patient reported that she was only getting ''chunks'' of what other people were up to, and when she would lose her train of thought, she felt ''somebody seems to steal my thoughts away.'' In this way, tracking difficulties, as a disturbance in the *form* of thinking, can give rise to unusual thought *content,* such as paranoid ideas.

Tracking difficulties appear to be related to intermittent dysfunctions of immediate or ''working'' memory (Melges et al., 1970a). Immediate memory pertains to the initial registration and ''holding in mind'' of input, and differs from short-term and long-term memory (see Chapter 2). Immediate memory has been found to be deficient in schizophrenia (Braff, Callaway, and Naylor, 1979; see Chapter 4). However, deficiencies in immediate memory do not appear to be the whole story, since tracking difficulties are usually manifested in terms of an inability to coordinate information serially so that it is not brought to mind at the right time. In other words, the information often can be recalled accurately but it is mistimed (Melges et al., 1970a). In a later section, I will explore some of the possible brain mechanisms that may account for tracking difficulties.

TEMPORAL DISCONTINUITY AND DEPERSONALIZATION

As difficulties with keeping track of sequences become worse, the person may begin to experience the past, present, and future as discontinuous and segregated. This temporal discontinuity is reflected in statements that the past, present, and future seem like ''separate islands of experience with little relation to each other.'' Along with this feeling of discontinuity of time, there is often a pervasive feeling of loss of self-direction and an incapacity to plan toward goals. Temporal discontinuity and impaired goal-directedness have been found to be related to the experience of depersonalization in a number of clinical and THC investigations (Melges et al., 1970b; Melges et al., 1974; Melges and Freeman, 1977; Freeman and Melges, 1977).

The findings indicate that, as the timeline of the past, present, and future becomes discontinuous and fragmented, the self comes to feel strange and unfamiliar—that is, depersonalized. That is, without past and future frames of reference through which a person becomes familiar with himself, the person's experience of the self seems unfamiliar. There is a lack of feeling of self-sameness over time, which Erikson (1968) has emphasized as being important for the sense of identity (see Chapter 2).

The fragmentation of the sense of self is common during the acute stages of schizophrenia (Bowers, 1974). Patients often express their profound deper-sonalization as the self "going to pieces." During high doses of THC, a similar fragmentation of the self takes place. To quote one THC subject: "My self is broken in time."

We also have found that severe degrees of temporal disintegration are associated with diffusion of the body image (Freeman and Melges, 1977). The body image is an important aspect of the self concept. Depersonalized patients often report that the self is "separate" from the body. In particular, we found that the outer boundaries of the body felt "fluid and changing" in association with temporal disintegration. If the body image is taken to represent personal space, the findings indicate that the diffusion of personal space is related to the disintegration of personal time.

In our studies, the correlations between changes in temporal disintegration and depersonalization were quite substantial, being as high as .87 and .92 in the THC experiments (see Appendix B). This indicates a dynamic relationship between these processes. Moreover, the THC induction of temporal disintegration slightly preceded the emergence of depersonalization; thereafter, the two processes covaried until the effect of the drug wore off. Higher degrees of temporal disintegration produced higher degrees of depersonalization.

Thus it appears that temporal disintegration, particularly the discontinuity of past, present, and future, is related to the emergence of depersonalization. This should not be taken to mean, however, that temporal disintegration is the only factor involved in depersonalization. The latter can occur in milder forms in neurotic individuals, particularly as a defense against emotional contact, and even in normal individuals in face of an impasse that blocks valued goals (Sedman, 1970; Dixon, 1963; Noyes and Kletti, 1976). Nevertheless, the more severe forms of depersonalization, as when the self feels that it is "going to pieces," is most commonly seen in an acute psychosis.

TEMPORAL INDISTINCTION AND FLORID PSYCHOTIC SYMPTOMS

As the fragmentation of sequences becomes even more pronounced, the person begins to have difficulty in distinguishing the past and future from the present. This telescoping of past, present, and future is called temporal indistinction. This extreme degree of temporal disintegration has been found to be related to florid symptoms of psychosis, such as delusions, paranoid connectivity, and the confusion of inner and outer events (Melges et al., 1974; Melges and Freeman, 1977).

The basic process that appears to underlie these florid symptoms of psychosis is that the person has difficulty in distinguishing the *now* from the *then*. That is, the past and future collapse into the present which is experienced as a "timeless now" where memories and expectations appear to be as real as present perceptions. This telescoping of past, present, and future is usually an ineffable experience that is hard to describe in words. Acutely schizophrenic patients commonly describe it as "everything happening at once." A THC subject described this state retrospectively as follows: "Words, images, and concepts from many times of my life tumbled as in a kaleidoscope."

Delusional Ideation

The emergence of unsystematized delusions of influence by outside forces, paranoid suspicions, and grandiosity has been found to covary with temporal disintegration, particularly temporal indistinction (Melges et al., 1974). Paranoid delusional patients have been found to have significantly greater time distortions than other acute forms of mental illness (Melges and Fougerousse, 1966). Difficulties with sequential thinking impair reality testing, since the person has problems in distinguishing his hunches and predictions from actual occurrences (Melges, 1976). But more important, with an extreme confusion of sequences, the person's sense of reality may be altered. The sequences may fuse and coalesce to be experienced as uncanny coincidences. Uncanny coincidences are common experiences during the development of delusory ideas. Past memories and future expectations appear to intersect with present perceptions as uncanny "connections" that are hard to dismiss on the basis of just chance occurrences. These uncanny coincidences may take the form of deja vu and precognitive experiences. The uncanny coincidences often form the nidus for further delusional elaborations.

Paranoid Connectivity

Uncanny coincidences may merge into the experience of a vast web of connections related to the self. This paranoid connectivity is often described as a "conspiracy," "plot," or "masterminded scheme." This feeling of a global-interconnected conspiracy directed at the self has been found to be related to the temporal indistinction of past, present, and future (Melges et al., 1974). What appears to happen is that many events of the past and future, ordinarily separated and spread out in geophysical time, seem to become interconnected in psychological time. Sequences of the past and future coalesce into a timeless now.

The experience of paranoid connectivity is both awesome and terrifying. Because the past and future are intermingled and transposed, the person often feels that he is clairvoyant. In particular, he feels that he can foretell the future, yet the experience of the future as fixed, rather than open, robs him of freedom of choice. To quote a paranoid schizophrenic patient: "My prophecies are truths that trap me." Similarly, a THC subject who had marked temporal disintegration felt that everything had been "planned ahead" to "trap" him: "Those people out there [outside the window] are plants. . . . So many coincidences. . . . Everything is connected. . . . I know what's going to happen before it happens. . . . The future seems memorized, like it's coming 'at' me, like I'm part of a script, and I don't have any choice."

The experience of the future as "rigged" is common during paranoid connectivity in clinical and drug-induced psychoses. This poses a severe threat to loss of self-control, which, in turn, often prompts suspicions of control from other people, thereby augmenting the paranoid ideas (see Chapter 8). Moreover, with temporal indistinction, the person's predictions of others' motives may be experienced as actualities, since he has problems in distinguishing the future from the present (Melges and Freeman, 1975).

Inner–Outer Confusion

The interpenetration of past, present, and future and the fusion of sequences have been found to be a prominent process in the confusion of inner events with those occurring outside the person (Melges and Freeman, 1977). That is, when the past (memories) and the future (expectations) became indistinguishable from the present (perceptions), there appeared to be a confusion between inner events (memories and expectations) and outer events (present perceptions).

The measures of symptoms of inner–outer confusion were derived from the works of Schneider (1959) and Mellor (1972). These symptoms included the degree of auditory hallucinations, experiences of alien control by outside forces, thought diffusion, uncanny coincidences, and feelings that one's body was being moved or touched by strange forces. Besides tracking difficulties and temporal discontinuity, temporal indistinction appeared to play a major role in inner–outer confusion. It appeared that the strange forces and sensations which seemed to be coming outside the person were inner events (memories and expectations) confused with present-time outer perceptions. It was as though memories and expectations, dislodged from the continuum of inner time, revisited the person and seemed to be coming from realms outside the self. In short, events lost in time were dislocated in space.

Experiences of inner–outer confusion are typical florid symptoms of an acute psychosis. Examples include: "Outside forces put impulses into me. . . . My inner thoughts are broadcast to other people even when I don't speak aloud. . . . I hear voices outside my head arguing or talking about me." Further examples are given in Appendix A. In acute psychiatric patients, higher degrees of temporal disorganization, particularly temporal indistinction, were related to greater frequency of these symptoms of inner–outer confusion (Melges and Freeman, 1977).

With regard to hallucinations, Moreau (1845, p. 168) described the transposition of inner and outer events during his experiments with hashish: "And what is more extraordinary, certain combinations of thought are transformed into sensory impressions—that is to say, are endowed with the property of acting physically upon our senses in the manner of exterior stimuli." Along this line, Horowitz (1975) has proposed a cognitive model of hallucinations which suggests that images not embedded as linear sequences may become "lit up" in the mind, making them more vivid so that they might be labeled as external present perceptions.

In summary, it appears that progressive degrees of temporal disintegration are related to increasingly severe psychotic symptoms. The most extreme form of temporal disintegration, temporal indistinction, appears to be involved in florid psychotic symptoms, such as delusional ideation, paranoid connectivity, and inner–outer confusion. The findings thus far are consistent with the postulate that aberrations of time are involved in the defective reality testing seen in acute psychoses.

For a pictorial overview of the alterations of consciousness associated with the progressive degrees of temporal disintegration, as outlined in Table 3, an analogy to the fragmentation of a motion picture may help illustrate this process. The stream of normal consciousness is like a movie, in which each frame of a film merges with the next to give the impression of a continuum with smooth transitions of content. With the prolongation of the present, the person becomes more focused on the present as though it were magnified. As tracking difficulties emerge, he is still focused on the magnified present, but this seems to be haphazardly separated from past and future frames of the film, which sporadically jump into his present awareness. As the fragmentation of sequences becomes more severe, temporal discontinuity ensues in which the magnified present seems disconnected with past and future sequences, which seem remote and discontinuous with the present. Finally, with temporal indistinction, past and future frames of the film collapse into the present so that there is a superimposition of images that flick in and out with no temporal relation to one another. Since there is no progressive continuum of past, present, and future, or—in the words of Henri Bergson (1947, p. 278)—no "continuous progress of the past which gnaws into the future," the experience seems timeless.

POSSIBLE BRAIN MECHANISMS

Thus far, I have dealt with temporal disintegration at the psychological level of inquiry. In this section, I will explore some possible brain dysfunctions that might underlie temporal disintegration.

One possibility is that the temporal disintegration of sequential thinking may stem from an intermittent disorder of immediate memory in the left cerebral hemisphere. The left cerebral hemisphere is primarily involved in the analysis of sequences, such as language (see Chapter 2). Recent evidence suggests that information processing in the left cerebral hemisphere is impaired in schizophrenia (for review, see Wexler, 1980). Also, THC has been found to predominantly impair left hemispheric functions (Heath et al., 1980). In addition, disorders of immediate memory have been highlighted as the central cognitive deficit in schizophrenia (see Chapter 4). In this regard, research indicates that, in both schizophrenia and THC intoxication, there is impaired transfer of information from immediate memory to short-term memory (Saccuzzo and Braff, 1981; Braff et al., 1981). Defective processing of information in immediate memory, particularly in the left cerebral hemisphere, may account for difficulties with tracking sequences over time.

From a clinical standpoint, since tracking difficulties and loosening of associations appear intermittently in schizophrenia (that is, occurring off and on for a few minutes during an hour), it is likely that whatever dysfunction is taking place in the brain, it is intermittent. A likely candidate for an intermittent disorder is some kind of seizure. In this regard, it is possible that a minor seizure in the limbic system might intermittently interrupt immediate memory functions of the left cerebral hemisphere.

Along this line, Chapman (1966) has described the similarity of schizophrenic blocking and psychomotor epileptic attacks, which involve the temporal lobe and limbic system. There are other symptoms of psychomotor epilepsy that resemble those of acute schizophrenia (Bear and Fedio, 1977; Monroe, 1978). These include not only hallucinations but also peculiar time distortions such as uncanny coincidences, deja vu, and time telescoping. It is of interest, moreover, that lesions of the hippocampal formation in the limbic system can produce psychotic, dreamlike states (Scoville and Milner, 1957; Gascon and Gilles, 1973). The hippocampus, besides being involved in emotional experience, plays a major role in immediate memory and the tracking of sequences (Douglas, 1967; Turner, 1969). On the basic of longitudinal studies of identical twins discordant for schizophrenia, Mednick (1971) proposed that the twin who eventually becomes schizophrenic has higher degrees of birth trauma, thereby depriving the hippocampus and related structures of oxygen and making that twin more vulnerable to the schizophrenic cognitive deficit. It is also relevant that psychotomimetic drugs, such as LSD, psilocybin, and THC, are primarily distributed in the limbic system and produce seizures in these areas deep within the brain (Adey, Bell, and Dennis, 1962; Miller, 1979; McIsac et al., 1971; Heath, 1972; Heath et al., 1980).

Of course, there are other relevant hypotheses. Another possibility is that since tracking difficulties represent an incoordination of sequences, this incoordination may be related to cerebellar or vestibular dysfunctions. There is some evidence for impaired vestibular and cerebellar dysfunctions in schizophrenia (Levy, Holzman, and Proctor, 1978). In this regard, years ago, Stransky (1904) described the mental incoordination seen in schizophrenia as "psychic ataxia."

THERAPEUTIC IMPLICATIONS

The proposed relationships between temporal disintegration and progressive stages of psychotic symptoms, as outlined in Table 3, provide the clinician with a model for approaching the acutely psychotic patient. That is, since changes in temporal disintegration appear to be dynamically related to changes in psychotic symptoms, treatment methods for correcting temporal disintegration are likely to be helpful for the therapy of psychotic symptoms. In my clinical experience, I have found that empathizing with the patient's cognitive difficulties in tracking sequences enhances a therapeutic alliance with the patient and helps him understand that his uncanny experiences of loss of control may not be due to outside alien forces but rather may be coming from his jumbled thought sequences. Although this is a clinical extrapolation that may not be fully justified in terms of the change correlation data, it nevertheless gives the patient a way of understanding his unusual experiences and often helps forestall further delusional elaborations and attributions. It also helps enlist cooperation in treatment.

In addition, I have found that knowledge of the stages of an acute psychosis, as outlined in Table 3, helps to educate patients and their families about the early signs of a relapse so that they can get treatment before florid psychotic symptoms reappear. I educate them to be on the alert for changes in their sense of time, thought racing, and troubles with keeping a train of thought. When these symptoms occur, they are to call their psychiatrist. In this way, especially with cooperative and intelligent patients, I have been able to taper and discontinue antipsychotic medications and yet prevent full-blown relapses by reinstituting relatively low doses of antipsychotic medicines during the prodromal stages. The merit of this educative approach is that troublesome side effects of the antipsychotic medications, hopefully including tardive dyskinesia, are reduced.

Thus my therapeutic approach for treating acutely psychotic patients is to consider temporal disintegration as a key process in need of treatment. I will therefore propose some general guidelines for treating temporal disintegration at the biological, psychological, and social levels of intervention. It is hoped that more definitive forms of treating temporal disintegration will be developed in the future, since not only will this provide further tests of our thesis, but it also may provide better ways of helping psychotic patients with their extremely disabling and terrifying symptoms.

At the biological level of intervention, it may prove worthwhile to search for neurochemical methods for enhancing the timing of sequences and immediate memory. In this regard, there is evidence that the phenothiazines, which have already proven to be effective in treating acute psychotic symptoms, improve immediate memory and timing functions (Callaway, 1970; Fischer, 1967; Angle, 1973; Stone et al., 1969; Spohn et al., 1977; Zahn, Carpenter, and McGlashan, 1978). Of course, the phenothiazines also have other effects, and more research is needed on their possible role of enhancing the timing of sequences. In the future, there may be drugs that specifically enhance immediate memory and the coordination of sequences, without having the adverse side effects of the phenothiazines and related drugs. One possibility is that fragments of the ACTH molecule appear to improve immediate memory (DeWied, 1976). Since such short peptide chains are natural substances within the body, they may have fewer side effects.

In acutely psychotic patients, the antipsychotic drugs appear to improve the temporal disintegration of sequences within about one week (Melges and Freeman, 1977). Also, these drugs appear to improve judgments of 30-second durations (Melges and Fougerousse, 1966). On the other hand, these drugs apparently impair the estimation of very short durations of around one second (Goldstone, Nurnberg, and Lhamon, 1979). Thus further research is needed to clarify whether the antipsychotic drugs act differently on sequential processing and the estimation of various durations.

With regard to biological approaches for treating temporal disintegration, another neurochemical possibility is the further development of implanted electrical "pacemakers" deep within the brain, which could detect and correct intermittent seizure discharges. Such pacemakers have already shown promise for treating intractable pain and epilepsy (Delgado, 1969, 1979). This, of course, is a wave of the future that needs careful evaluation.

At the psychological level of treatment, it is important for the therapist to realize that the psychotic patient often is experiencing an alteration in the temporal form of consciousness. It is as though he is in a different "time warp." Acknowledging the different temporal form of his existence, particularly his difficulty with keeping track of sequences, helps build rapport. In order to help him register and keep track of sequences, the therapist should slow down his responses, parse his phrases, and punctuate his questions and replies with gestures so as to facilitate the clarity of the communications (McGhie, Chapman, and Lawson, 1965). In this regard, it is well known that when schizophrenics are given enough time, their performance on a variety of tasks improves (King, 1950; Usdanksy and Chapman, 1960). Besides slowing and punctuating his statements, the therapist should help the patient to mark sequences and to put them in temporal perspective (Seeman, 1976). Along this line, a useful technique is to help the patient distinguish the present from the past or future. This helps the patient to restore what Minkowski (1927, 1931, 1933) called the "I–here–now" position so that he can distinguish the *now* from the *then*. This aids reality testing by helping the patient to integrate, yet keep distinct, past, present, and future. To quote Arieti (1974, p. 575): "Whereas the world of psychosis has only one temporal dimension—the present—the world of reality has three: past, present, and future." Helping the psychotic patient to sort out memories and expectations from his "timeless now" thus aids reality testing.

At the social level of intervention, it is helpful to make the patient's interpersonal milieu as predictable as possible. This includes helping the patient's family to learn how to reach point-for-point closure in their communications, to refrain from interruptions and several people talking at once, and to avoid giving "double messages" that convey conflicts between verbal and nonverbal communications. In this regard, research has shown that schizophrenics have inconsistent and incoherent ways of anticipating events, particularly the reactions of other people (Bannister and Fransella, 1966; Adams-Webber, 1979). It is possible that their chaotic ways of anticipating and construing the reactions of others may be secondary to tracking difficulties. Whatever the case, making their interpersonal environment as predictable as possible will at least help prevent the aggravation of tracking difficulties that occurs when social feedback is chaotic and confusing.

Thus in light of the cybernetic concepts presented in Chapter 3, I propose that the restoration of sequential thinking helps in the treatment of psychosis by enhancing the temporal organization of plans of action. When the psychotic patient can plan sequences toward goals, he is then able to regain control over his personal future through the sequential organization of his future images, plans of actions, and emotions.

SUMMARY AND CONCLUSIONS

Two basic postulates were explored in this chapter:

1 The disintegration of sequential thinking is associated with loss of control over the future during an acute psychosis.
2 Progressive degrees of the temporal disintegration of sequences are associated with increasingly severe psychotic symptoms.

The temporal disintegration of sequences, it is proposed, prompts the person to lose control over his personal future since he is unable to plan ahead and make serial adjustments to reach goals. That is, during an acute psychosis, the relationships between plans of action, future images, and emotions are incoordinated and sequentially disorganized. Moreover, the temporal disintegration of sequence impairs reality testing since it is difficult to test hunches or predictions in terms of actual occurrences if the person has trouble distinguishing the *now* from the *then*. As time becomes disorganized so does the person.

Increasing degrees of temporal disintegration provide a model for understanding increasingly severe psychotic symptoms. These relationships are presented in terms of four progressive stages of an acute psychosis:

1 During the prodromal stages of an acute psychosis, the prolongation of the present is related to psychedelic experiences.
2 Difficulties with tracking sequences are related to loosening of associations.

3 The discontinuity of past, present, and future is related to depersonalization.

4 The indistinction and telescoping of past, present, and future are related to florid psychotic symptoms, such as delusional ideation, paranoid connectivity, and inner–outer confusion. Events that are lost in time become dislocated in space.

The therapeutic implications of this model are that the correction of temporal disintegration may be a key process for the treatment of acute psychosis. There are already biological, psychological, and social interventions that enhance the timing and organization of sequences and appear beneficial to the acutely psychotic patient. As a further test of this model, it is hoped that more refined methods for correcting temporal disintegration will be developed for the treatment of acute psychotic symptoms.

CHAPTER EIGHT

Over-Futuring
and Paranoid Thinking

I know of no rule which holds so true as that we are always paid for our suspicions by finding what we suspect.

HENRY DAVID THOREAU, *Journal*, 1837–1847

In this chapter, we propose that over-futuring is a core process in paranoid thinking. Over-futuring refers to over-projections into the future that are unchecked by present-time feedback from others. In an effort to regain and attain control over his personal future, the paranoid person over-projects into the future and comes to believe in these over-projections to such a degree that he discounts or misconstrues feedback from others.

Over-futuring can give rise to psychotic loss of control over the future. The person's view of reality may become so dominated by over-projections into the future that past and present realities are neglected. This can occur without the impairment of sequential thinking outlined in Chapter 7. However, as explained later, the combination of over-futuring and the temporal disorganization of plans of action, as in paranoid schizophrenia, is particularly conducive to paranoid spirals and loss of control over the future.

In this chapter, we propose that paranoid spirals occur when there is a threat to loss of control of the personal future and the person attempts to regain control through over-futuring. As outlined in Chapter 4, the person vulnerable to paranoid spirals has a tendency to over-focus on the future. When threatened with loss of self-control, he tends to focus even more on the future. Although futuring usually is a process conducive to coping (see Chapter 3), excessive futuring can become maladaptive in paranoid processes.

This chapter was written in collaboration with Arthur M. Freeman, III, M.D., Professor of Psychiatry, University of Alabama Medical School in Birmingham.

Before we elaborate this thesis further, a brief clinical vignette may help to illustrate what we mean by over-futuring:

A 33-year-old truck driver, who had no previous psychiatric contacts, was apprehended by the police after he had maintained a daylong vigil on top of a hill by shooting at cars passing by below. On admission to a psychiatric hospital, this man had no tracking difficulties or hallucinations. History from his wife revealed that, about one month before, he had tried to recoup some financial losses by collecting insurance on some trucks that were destroyed by fire after making a "shady deal with some strangers." At the time of hospitalization, he believed that there was a specially organized "Mafia" that was plotting against him. Their plans were to threaten him subtly and then eventually kill him. He believed that they were doing this because they knew his "secret" and, by threatening to reveal his secret, they were trying to extort the insurance monies due to him about three months hence. The way that they would threaten him was to follow his truck with "certain cars, mainly Chevys and Fords." Wherever he drove, his suspicions seemed confirmed since there were "Chevys and Fords behind me, ahead of me, or crossing in front of me." His wife's disbelief in this scheme prompted him to think that she might be "in" with them. Nevertheless, he was able to convince his 13-year-old daughter that there was a plot against him by taking her along with him in his truck. The daughter said, "He was right; no matter where we went, there were Chevys or Fords following us or ahead of us; if they weren't there just at the time he thought, they'd trick us and show up later." As he became increasingly threatened, he became more and more suspicious about their plans. He believed that they were using him as an "example" in order to keep "other guys in line" in the future. His suspicions about "what they were up to" in the future heightened his sense of threat. Finally, he felt he had to take action to resist his supposed attackers: he took his gun, perched himself on top of a hill, and shot at every Chevy and Ford within eyesight.

This case is a good example of over-futuring. The threat to his personal future was that his secret would be found out. To prevent this, he became suspicious of what others might do. But his suspicions increased his sense of threat. Moreover, feedback in the present was misconstrued to fit his future projections: if the Chevys or Fords were there, this confirmed his suspicions—a rather likely event, given the ubiquity of Chevys and Fords—if they were not there now, it was a trick and they were bound to show up later.

This case history shows some of the common processes involved in paranoid thinking. The purpose of this chapter is to present and review a general model of paranoid processes (Melges and Freeman, 1975). As teachers at a Stanford-affiliated hospital which had the only locked wards for a large district, we were faced with the need to develop a comprehensive teaching approach to the management of the more than 500 acutely paranoid patients of diverse types admitted each year to these wards.

OVER-FUTURING AND THE PARANOID THREAT–PREDICTION SPIRAL

Our central thesis is that *paranoid thinking stems from an interaction of threats and predictions: The threats prompt predictions and suspicions that often increase the threats that initially prompted the suspicions.* We propose that such a vicious cycle is involved in the formation of paranoid thinking in diverse types of psychiatric disorders. As explained later, the nature of the threat is usually loss of control over the self or over significant others. The threat prompts predictions and suspicions of control from others. That is, others are suspected of plans intended to control or dominate the self. This heightens the person's sense of threat to loss of control over himself. In attempting to prevent control from others by predicting it, the feeling of being threatened increases. The attempts to solve the problem by projecting into the future about the intentions of others may eventually become the problem.

In many paranoid reactions, there is no attempt to obtain feedback from other people about present-time happenings. Rather there is mainly a series of projections into the future, which give rise to a threat–prediction or future–future interaction. In terms of some of the cybernetic concepts of this book, there is excessive feedforward unchecked by present-time feedback. That is, anticipations prompt other anticipations that, in turn, "feed into" the initiating anticipations, leading to a vicious cycle. In this way, a person's world view may become dominated by misconstrued anticipations that are divorced from ongoing reality.

In terms of the concepts of futuring and temporal organization (see Chapter 3), our central thesis can be stated as follows: Paranoid thinking is likely to occur when there is *over-futuring,* especially when coupled with a lack of temporal organization. The combination of over-futuring and temporal disorganization is particularly common in paranoid schizophrenia, as will be discussed later.

DEFINITIONS

Paranoid and Paranoid Delusions

Our use of the term *paranoid* refers to the person's unfounded belief that he is being persecuted. This equivalence of the terms *paranoid* and *persecutory* is in line with the definitions of paranoid disorders in the *Diagnostic and Statistical Manual of Mental Disorders* (DSM-III) of the American Psychiatric Association (1980). Our purpose in this chapter is not to differentiate the various paranoid syndromes, but to point out processes that are common to various types of paranoid disorders. It should be well recognized that paranoid thinking occurs in a wide variety of mental disturbances other than paranoid schizophrenia, such as manic-depressive illness, personality disorders, metabolic and toxic states, and psychotomimetic drug experiences (Swanson, Bohnert, and Smith, 1970; Manschreck and Petri, 1978).

A person can be paranoid, in the sense of being overly suspicious, without being delusional. A delusion is an unshared outlandish belief that is held with great subjective certainty and is resistant to modification by logical argument or subsequent experience (Jaspers, 1968). Thus a delusion is a false belief that is difficult to falsify. When a person has a paranoid delusion, it means that he has an unshakable conviction that other people are conspiring to do him harm or to control him.

A paranoid delusion can be systematized, as when its content remains fixed and unchangeable, or unsystematized, as when its content varies over time yet still contains the general theme of being persecuted. Our use of the term *delusional ideation* refers to unsystematized delusions. Finally, as described in Chapter 7, the term *paranoid connectivity* refers to the experience of a vast web of interconnected events directed against the self. A host of uncanny coincidences and feelings of precognition often occur during paranoid connectivity (Melges et al., 1974).

Control and Vicious Cycles

As discussed in Chapter 3, the term *cybernetics*, derived from the Greek word for steersman, is closely linked to the concept of control: Control is achieved through reducing discrepancies between inputs and a reference condition or goal (Powers, 1973). That is, through the detection of errors (feedback), deviations from the goal are counteracted. Lack of control often takes the form of vicious cycles, technically called *deviation amplifications* in which one deviation amplifies another (Maruyama, 1963; Wender, 1968).

As a simple term for these deviation amplifications, the word *spiral* was introduced in Chapters 3 and 4. A downward spiral is a vicious cycle whereby a person becomes increasingly emotionally upset.

Downward spirals commonly stem from the following processes:

1 Lack of goals, or goals being obscured by faulty thinking and conflict
2 Inability to detect and correct for deviations from goals
3 Excessive feedforward unchecked by present-time feedback

It is this latter process of over-projection into the future that we propose as common to the genesis of all types of paranoid thinking. Of course, the paranoid spiral can be augmented by the first two processes listed above, as when a person has a formal thought disorder with temporal disintegration. But, as detailed below, it is the paranoid penchant for trying to gain rigid control over the self and others that predisposes the person to excessive projections into the future about intentions of others in relation to the self. That is, the paranoid person over-futures.

A CYBERNETIC MODEL OF PARANOID PROCESSES

Interpersonal Control and Initial Conditions

In interpersonal behavior, the concept of control has at least three interacting domains: control over self, control over others, and control from others. We propose that the person likely to develop a paranoid reaction is one whose overriding goals are (1) to maintain control over himself and over other people and (2) to prevent control from others. Although such goals are valued to some degree by most people, a rigid and all-inclusive control over the self and others, plus the fear of being dominated by others, characterizes what Shapiro (1965) calls the "paranoid style." These preoccupying goals are the initial conditions that fashion an over-focus on the future and set the stage for the cybernetic paranoid processes we will describe.

In this chapter, we will not deal with developmental factors that bring about these preoccupying concerns with control over the future, such as the sensitivity of the self to slights and threats from peers during early adolescence (Sullivan, 1953) and the need to affirm one's significance in the eyes of others (Schwartz, 1963). We should also point out that in experimental studies normal subjects under conditions of threat and uncertainty demonstrate a need to predict and control (Pervin, 1963). In this sense, then, most individuals are predisposed to some extent to paranoid ideation under conditions of threat.

Formation and Maintenance of Paranoid Delusions

In light of the initial conditions of the person's extreme need to maintain rigid personal and interpersonal control, our thesis can be reframed as follows: *Paranoid delusions stem from the threat of loss of personal control over the self or others and the attempts to prevent this loss of control by predicting and counteracting control from others.* The essential cybernetic processes of this thesis are outlined in Figure 1.

During the *formation* of paranoid ideation, there is a threat of loss of personal control *over* the self or others; this prompts predictions and suspi-

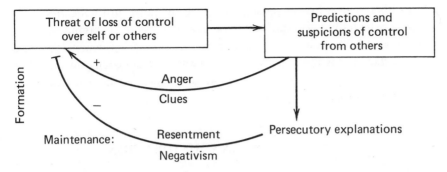

Figure 1 Proposed cybernetic processes involved in the formation and maintenance of paranoid reactions. Plus (+) sign indicates deviation-amplification processes; minus (−) sign, deviation-counteraction processes. (Reprinted with permission from F. T. Melges and A. M. Freeman, Persecutory delusions: A cybernetic model. *American Journal of Psychiatry* 132:1038–1044, 1975.)

cions of control *from* others. The latter arouses anger since personal plans of maintaining interpersonal control are perceived as being potentially interrupted (Melges and Harris, 1970). The aroused anger carries with it the expectation of retaliation from others, increases the threat of loss of personal control, and prompts further predictions and suspicions of control from others. Suspicions abound about others' motives in relation to the self. Since the suspicions are biased predictions in the sense that the person needs to confirm them so that he will feel he is right and thereby in control, they are likely to lead to the finding of clues (that is, indicators of portentous events yet to come) that others are motivated to control him. Through these feedforward processes, the person eventually comes to feel highly threatened about the loss of self-control and highly suspicious about being controlled by others.

This downward spiral may become such a vicious cycle that the person grows panicky and does lose control. One way to halt the cycle, however, is for the person to make an assumption that other people are indeed controlling him and have indeed been persecuting him. These persecutory explanations provide a present-time new focus—the goal of resisting others' influence. The individual's previous anger about future possibilities is transformed to resentment about what has supposedly happened. His persecutory explanations and his resentment provide him with a way of reducing his threat of loss of personal control by negativistic behavior aimed at counteracting control from others (see the bottom of Figure 1).

Thus for the *maintenance* of paranoid delusions, in order to decrease the threat of loss of self-control and to prevent control by others, the individual presumes that he is being persecuted (or has been persecuted), and he adopts a mode of resisting others' influence. In this way, he reestablishes some sense of self-control by being against others. Since being against others is a goal and modus operandi that eventually becomes essential to his identity in that it reduces his threat of loss of personal control, his persecutory ideation is not only a false belief but also difficult to falsify. This is how paranoid delusions are maintained. In addition, through protesting others' influence and consequently antagonizing them, a person with a paranoid delusion often provokes actual rejection or control from others, which further substantiates his persecutory explanations.

STAGES OF PARANOID IDEATION

We offer these proposed cybernetic processes as general postulates for the formation and maintenance of all types of paranoid delusions, although the nature of the threatened loss and the ways of attempting to prevent it may be different for the various paranoid syndromes. In Table 4, progressive stages of paranoid ideation are outlined in terms of escalating threat–prevention interactions and their outcomes. The essential stages are premonition, pursuit, projection, and presumption and protest.

In Table 4, it can be seen that the major outcomes of an earlier threat–prevention interaction may compound the initial threat and prompt further attempts at prevention and prediction that, in turn, escalate the sense of threat. That is, the outcomes of an earlier stage may become the threat of the next stage.

Because the stages are derived from clinical observations and retrospective histories of paranoid patients, they are heuristic at this point. A given person may not progress through all stages. For example, suspiciousness may bring about adaptive consequences, such as the interruption of clandestine plans of a political cabal; this is healthy skepticism. On the other hand, a patient with a

Table 4   Stages of Paranoid Ideation and Threat–Prevention Interactions

Stage	Threat	Attempts at Prevention	Outcomes
Premonition	Loss of control over self or others	Predictions of others' plans in order to prevent control from others	Suspiciousness and anger
Pursuit	Being found suspicious and angry	Pretenses to hide suspicions, anger, and sense of threat to prevent retaliation	Feeling pursued and self-conscious
Projection	Feeling pursued and self-conscious	Projection into the future to outplot supposed pursuers	Feelings of influence and passivity
Presumption and protest	Feelings of influence and passivity	Presumption of plot, and decision to resist others' influence	Persecutory explanations and negativism

Adapted with permission from Melges, F.T. & A.M. Freeman, Persecutory delusions: A cybernetic model. American Journal of Psychiatry, *132:1038–1044, 1975.*

thought process disorder, in which the distinction between present and future threats becomes blurred, may progress rapidly to feelings of influence, bypassing earlier stages (see Chapter 7).

Premonition Stage

As the initiating event for paranoid ideation, we emphasize not a loss but rather the *threat* of a loss. The threat prompts suspiciousness and anger, since the person thinks he can do something to prevent the loss from occurring. If the loss is acknowledged as already having taken place, the individual will experience depression and may give up rather than experiencing anger and suspiciousness (Melges and Bowlby, 1969; Melges and Harris, 1970). Because of the potentially paranoid person's overriding concerns with maintaining control, the initial threat is usually a loss of control over the self, loss of control over significant others, or both.

The threat of loss of control *over the self* can take many forms. These include incipient memory impairment with organic brain disease, the emergence of automatisms or reduplicative experiences with temporal lobe epilepsy, the arousal of unwelcome sexual or aggressive impulses, unpredictable startle reactions during drug intoxication or withdrawal, the emergence of illusions or hallucinations, a developmental crisis that the person experiences as an impasse, and the inability to direct one's thinking. The loss of control over one's thinking is particularly important during the early phases of paranoid schizophrenia.

A threat to loss of self-control makes the person feel vulnerable to control from others, and he begins to predict others' plans in order to prevent being controlled. The more he predicts control from others, the more threatened he becomes; suspiciousness and anger mount, and he is beset with the premonition that something strange is going on.

The premonitory feeling that "something strange is going on," often called delusional mood or *trema* (Conrad, 1968), also can occur with the threat of loss of control *over others*. This is particularly likely to occur when there is a threat of separation from a significant other person with whom the patient has had a close and dependent relationship. Jealousy that escalates to suspicions of infidelity, and finally paranoid ideation typifies the ramifications that may be initiated by the threat of loss of control over a significant other (Vauhkonen, 1968). We have observed such paranoid reactions in overt homosexuals, particularly when the dominant member of the pair becomes threatened by signs of indifference from his or her partner.

In this regard, for a person who needs almost total control over himself or over others, the indifferent reactions of others to the self are often interpreted by the person as clues signifying that he does not have control of the others' view of himself or is insignificant and inferior in others' eyes (Schwartz, 1963). Such clues heighten his sense of threat, and the emotional arousal accompanying the finding of clues reinforces their apparent validity and prompts further searching for clues (see Figure 1).

Pursuit Stage

Whereas the premonition stage involves the person searching others for their intentions, the pursuit stage involves the expectation that others are searching the person for what he feels, knows, or might do. His initial threat is now compounded by the threat that others will retaliate if they discover his suspicions and anger. As one patient stated, "If they knew what I know about what they're up to, they'd kill me." To prevent the retaliation, the person begins to pretend that he is not suspicious, angry, or threatened; yet the more he pretends, the more self-conscious he becomes about others discovering his vulnerabilities. He believes that if others find out how vulnerable or how phony he is, they will be even more likely to control him. Here the person is hiding secrets and his inner turmoil from others (Artiss, 1966), and he is afraid he will be found out; he feels pursued by others. Ideas of reference, such as "being followed" or "being watched," are common during this stage.

Projection Stage

At this stage, since the person feels self-conscious and pursued by others, he is likely to attempt to outguess and outplot his supposed pursuers. Rather than the self looking at others, his focus is now on reacting to others looking at the self (Laing, Phillipson, and Lee, 1966). Rather than being self-directed toward his own internal goals, he feels directed by what he anticipates to be the schemes of others in relation to himself. As he loses self-direction, he begins to feel increasingly passive and under the influence of others (Table 4).

By this time, his initial threat of loss of personal control is considerably compounded by threats of being found out or controlled by others. In order to prevent being trapped by his supposed pursuers, he projects into the future what he thinks their plans of action will be. The more he projects into the future, the more he becomes entrapped by his own predictions. The ruminative vicious cycle common to this stage can be paraphrased as follows: "If I do this, they will do that; and if they don't do that, it's because they are pretending (much like I am) in order to catch me off guard later on." In this way, his predictions appear confirmed no matter what happens, and his seemingly correct predictions ensnare him further in what seems to be a preordained web of events determined by others.

We emphasize projection in time (especially into the future) as well as in space (from self to other and then back to the self). That is, on the basis of his threat of loss of personal control, the person predicts in time what he expects others might do in relation to himself. This use of the term *projection* is in accord with its derivation from the Latin *projicere*, meaning to throw forward and ahead as well as outward. Its use in this way incorporates the expulsive and essentially spatial use of the term by Freud (1911) with the expectancy and essentially temporal types of projection emphasized by Sullivan (1953) and Laing and associates (1966).

In capsule form, during the projection stage, that which the person projects onto others and the future is projected back at him. In this regard, many acutely paranoid patients state that the future seems to be coming "at" them rather than them going into the future.

Presumption and Protest Stage

Feelings of influence and predestination heighten the threat of loss of control over the self to such a degree that panic about being controlled by others supervenes. The person has become acutely disorganized, and his identity disintegrates because he now lacks internal reference conditions and personal goals (see Chapter 7). In order to prevent his disorganization from continuing, the individual must find some kind of focus or goal about which he can reorganize his personal identity. Since he has been preoccupied with how others are reacting to him and influencing him, he is likely to seize an external focus to explain his predicament. In his panicked state, he can no longer tolerate the uncertainties of prediction and testing: he presumes that there is indeed a conspiracy directed against him, and this presumption provides him with the new goal of protesting others' influence (Table 4).

The presumption of a plot, which Cameron (1963) called "sudden paranoid crystallization," is often accompanied by a sense of relief, since the person feels he now knows what is going on and has a new plan of action—his decision to protest others' influence. A "paranoid pseudocommunity" (Cameron, 1963) is gradually specified and systematized as a conspiratorial group to which the person relates in a reactionary way by protesting its influence. His anger about future possibilities turns to resentment about what has happened and is happening. By becoming reorganized around the goal of resisting others, he reestablishes some sense of self-control: by supposedly preventing and counteracting control from others, he reduces his threat of loss of self-control. The reduction of threat reinforces his modus operandi of resisting others. As a result, his persecutory explanations become impervious to logic and persuasion from others. Attempts to dissuade him that there is no conspiracy against him are paradoxically threatening, for they challenge his newfound identity of being against others. In this manner, persecutory delusions are perpetuated.

TEMPORAL DISINTEGRATION AND LOSS OF CONTROL

As outlined in Chapter 7, the temporal disintegration of sequences can lead to loss of control and paranoid ideas. The impaired sequential thinking disrupts the temporal organization of plans of action and is particularly prominent in paranoid schizophrenia (Chapter 4). Of course, the pervasive problems with sequence, rate, and temporal perspective in organic brain disease can also give rise to loss of control and paranoid ideas. In addition, the racing of thoughts as in mania and amphetamine psychoses may speed up the threat–prediction cycle so that relatively there are more interactions per unit of clock time than there are when mental processes are at a normal rate. Yet the confusion of sequences is particularly likely to enhance the threat–prediction interactions during the formation of paranoid ideation (see top of Figure 1). That is, a confusion of sequences may make it difficult for the person to distinguish a future threat or prediction from present occurrences.

Moreover, impaired sequential thinking is itself a threat to loss of self-control. The inability to direct one's thinking sequentially toward goals, commonly seen in acute schizophrenia as well as in hashish and LSD intoxication, poses a considerable threat to loss of volitional control over the self and thereby may prompt predictions and suspicions of control from others. The unpredictable and intermittent occurrence of these difficulties with tracking information over time, such as losing one's train of thought or blocking, may be attributed to outside forces interfering with self-direction. In addition, tracking difficulties have been found to be highly correlated with misconstrued interpersonal perceptions and paranoid ideation (Melges, 1976). Chapman (1966) highlighted the importance of blocking, which he described as being similar to psychomotor epileptic attacks, as an early symptom of schizophrenia that patients often experience as alien control and later attempt to explain in terms of being persecuted.

If a person has difficulty keeping track of what he just said or what he intends to say, loosening of associations is apt to occur, since his thoughts wander in many different directions (Melges et al., 1970). The resultant thought content, although bizarre, is not necessarily delusory or persecutory in the sense of an unwarranted conviction that one is at the center of an interconnected conspiracy directed against and influencing him. Experimental evidence suggests that the attribution of such a global scheme may stem from the telescoping and indistinction of past, present, and future, so that memories, perceptions, and expectations, which are ordinarily separated by geophysical time, seem to be interconnected in psychological time (Melges et al., 1974). Such temporal confusion might blur the distinction between inside events (memories and expectations) and outside events (perceptions). As described in Chapter 7, this process gives rise to "paranoid connectivity." In short, that which is lost in time may also seem lost in space, and internally generated threats and predictions may seem to be coming from the outside. Uncanny experiences of influence and feelings of being predestined may emerge in this way (see Chapter 7).

The blurring of temporal boundaries would also enhance the interaction between threats and predictions (see the top of Figure 1), since predictions would be endowed with a sense of reality similar to present-time or past occurrences. That is, rather than thinking, "They might attempt to control me," the temporally confused individual would be more likely to think, "They are [or have been] controlling me."

RECONSIDERATIONS: FREUD AND SULLIVAN

Concerns with being controlled or dominated by others are frequent in the clinical descriptions of paranoid patients in the writings of both Freud (1911) and Sullivan (1953). Feelings of being influenced by outside forces and becoming emasculated were central features in Schreber's memoirs (1955), which Freud used as the expository case for his thesis about paranoid delusions. Fears of "being taken advantage of" and of being "exploited" by others were highlighted by Sullivan. These themes of domination and submission resonate with our cybernetic model. Since the proposals of Freud and Sullivan are often used in teaching about the development of paranoid delusions, a brief comparison of their models with ours is in order.

Freud (1911, p. 485) hypothesized that persecutory delusions developed from the denial, reversal, and projection of homosexual strivings: "I (a man) love him" became transformed, through contradictions and reversals mediated by primary process thinking, into "I do not love him—I hate him," which was then transformed by unconscious projection processes into "He hates (persecutes) me, which will justify me in hating him." How and why such contradictions and reversals came about rested heavily on Freud's (1915) categorical declaration that primary process thinking allows for logical contradictions and transmutations, in contrast to the sequential linear thinking characteristic of secondary process (see Chapter 2). Our thesis about temporal disorganization, in which nonlinear thinking is prominent, offers one way of operationally explaining Freud's proposed reversals from love to hate and from subject to object (that is, they are mediated by a confusion of temporal sequences). Indeed, Freud (1915, p. 184) emphasized that timelessness was a fundamental characteristic of primary process thinking. In this regard, the question can be raised whether temporal disorganization accounts for other primary process phenomena, such as the allowance of mutually contradictory ideas, reversals to the opposite, and displacements of affects and impulses to other sources (Melges et al., 1974).

Schreber also demonstrated temporal confusion. In translating Schreber's memoirs, MacAlpine and Hunter (1955, p. 27) stated that they left Schreber's frequent changes in tense unchanged because they revealed his confusion about past and present, which occurred even during the recuperative phase of his illness at the time of his writing. Moreover, Schreber himself noted that the early phase of his illness was accompanied by experiences of profound timelessness, "as if single nights had the duration of centuries" (1955, p. 71). Furthermore, Niederland's (1974) reanalysis of the Schreber case indicated that Schreber's experiences of "divine miracles" (for example, feelings of being physically contorted and transformed) probably represented revived memories of actual childhood experiences; Schreber was subjected, as a boy, to extreme physical contortions in accord with his father's orthopedic child-rearing practices that were directed toward domination of the will of the child. How these past childhood experiences later came to be experienced as present reality in adulthood could be explained by a telescoping of past, present, and future.

As in the case of Schreber, the nature of the delusory thought content is often explainable on the basis of the person's past history. How and why such thought content emerges at a particular time involves questions of process. In our model, we propose that no particular thought content by itself can precipitate paranoid formation unless it poses a threat to loss of control over the self or over others. Although Freud emphasized the specific role of latent homosexual strivings in the formation of paranoid delusions, such thought content (for example, Schreber's fears of becoming emasculated and exploited homosexually) could be placed in the larger context of threats of being dominated or controlled.

The evidence for the specific role of homosexual thought content in paranoid delusions is controversial (Arthur, 1964; Schwartz, 1963; Kline, 1972). When it does occur, it may reflect more general concerns such as loss of personal identity (Schwartz, 1963). Also, the occurrence of paranoid ideation in overt homosexuals is difficult to reconcile with classical Freudian theory that emphasizes the role of repressed homosexual strivings (Klaf, 1961). Nevertheless, in accord with our model, the emergence of homosexual thought content may be threatening to a person who believes himself to be heterosexual and who lives in a predominantly heterosexual society that shuns homosexuality. We propose then that the more general initiating event is the threat of loss of control over the self or others, of which the emergence of homosexual thought content is a special case.

A second major feature of Freud's (1911, p. 457) thesis about paranoid delusional formation is often neglected—that the delusional explanations are attempts at recovery or restitution of the self in relation to others. This is in accord with our cybernetic model, particularly the maintenance stage, in which the person's persecutory explanations provide a way of regaining personal control through protesting the influence of others.

Themes of domination and submission are also common in Sullivan's writings (1953) about paranoid formation. His ideas are difficult to systematize but can be paraphrased as follows: the potentially paranoid person feels inferior to others, and he conceals these inferiority feelings from himself and others by dissociating them. A paranoid transformation takes place when such a person feels he is "being taken advantage of" in the sense of being humiliated by others and led to reveal his concealed weaknesses. The previously dissociated aspects of his personality are then reawakened as uncanny "not-me" experiences. To protect his self-system, he further disowns these not-me experiences by blaming others for his plight: certain others become the personification of his disowned not-me experiences. By transferring blame to others, he downgrades them so that he will not feel further humiliated—that is, it is possible for him to believe that others are just as bad or worse than he is. This face-saving maneuver is similar to recent theories about the reduction of cognitive dissonance in paranoid transformations (Berkowitz, 1960), in which an idealized self-image is maintained through derogating others and setting them in contrast with the self. These formulations can be readily recast into our cybernetic model, which centers around attempts to reduce the threat of loss of self-control by preventing control from others.

Sullivan (1953, p. 359) averred that projection was a universal normal anticipatory process usually adaptive for foresight about self–other transactions. In contrast to Freud, Sullivan did not emphasize projection of latent homosexual wishes as the central mechanism for paranoid transformation. He proposed that only when projection became distorted by face-saving maneuvers did it become pathologically involved in inappropriate self–other anticipations and a paranoid transfer of blame onto others. This emphasis on misconstrued interpersonal anticipations is in line with our model.

IMPLICATIONS FOR TREATMENT

In terms of the general model depicted in Figure 1, optimal treatment would entail diminishing the interaction between threats and predictions. If therapy can mitigate the threat–prevention interactions listed in Table 4 for the various stages of persecutory ideation, the outcomes of each stage, testable by observer ratings or subjective reports, should lessen in frequency or intensity. In this way, along with the systematic collection of longitudinal data, the model and its stages can be tested by tailoring treatment according to each proposed stage.

The treatment of paranoid reactions is easier said than done. With an acutely paranoid patient, it is difficult to minimize the patient's fear of being controlled when he himself is so out of control that he poses a danger to himself and others. This is a crisis situation that must be handled expediently by making sure that the patient's worst fears—complete loss of self-control with harm to himself and others—do not materialize. This may require hospitalization and medication. Although most acutely paranoid patients vigorously protest such measures, at a later time many are grateful that they were not allowed to completely lose self-control.

Even in this crisis situation, attempts can be made to preserve the patient's feelings of self-control. Initially, the therapist and his assistants should minimize the threat of dominating the patient by not standing over him and by giving him plenty of room. At the same time, enough assistants should be in the background in order to neutralize the possibility of attack or escape. A sufficient number of people are necessary for all to feel supported and remain calm in order to diffuse the patient's angry outbursts and accusations. Within certain constraints, the patient can also be given some options. For example, "You'd feel more in control if you could calm down; to calm down, you can either be given some medicine or go in a room by yourself. Which would you prefer?"

Once an acute paranoid patient has calmed down or if from the beginning the patient is capable of some degree of rational discourse, the primary task of the therapist is to begin building a nonthreatening relationship with the patient. This is difficult to do, since the bellicose and suspicious nature of paranoid patients often threatens the therapist and arouses hostility, even in experienced therapists. The following guidelines often help in establishing this all-important nonthreatening relationship:

1   Empathize with the threat as the patient is (or has been) experiencing it. For example, "If those things were happening to me, I would feel threatened, too."

2   Avoid a fact-finding scrutiny about the patient's allegations of a plot against him. In this regard, an interrogation of the patient's bizarre ideas is the most common error made with paranoid patients, since they soon surmise that their beliefs, which are very real to them, are being challenged or subtly ridiculed.

3   Join the patient in testing reality about present happenings, and take the focus off the past and especially the future. For example, if the patient says, "I think they're waiting outside to get me," the therapist gets up and asks the patient to walk outside the office with him to see if "they" are there now. In this regard, brief walks with a paranoid patient are often more therapeutic than the stereotype of the psychiatrist sitting with the patient in his office.

4   Do not assume that everything the patient says, even if bizarre, is delusional. Some real surprises can occur in this regard. For example, one woman claimed that she was a spy and that her hotel room had been recently ransacked. Since she had several foreign airplane tickets, we checked her story, and it turned out to be true. Her other paranoid delusions could not have been worked with if we had not accepted this reality. The same principle applies to reality-based perceptions that the patient has about certain people or situations (Arieti, 1962).

5   Discriminately reinforce the patient's strengths and nondelusional thinking. In this context, discriminate reinforcement means rewarding the patient (for example, with nods, empathic statements, and so on) for correct thinking while remaining passive and noncommital when the patient emits delusional thinking. This helps extinguish the focus on the delusional ideas and also avoids the pitfall of marshalling counter-arguments against the delusions, which usually just escalates their intensity.

6   Avoid gimmicks and wild interpretations. This should be obvious, but unfortunately we have witnessed that some therapists and mental health workers have attempted double-chair Gestalt work, Jungian dream interpretation, and uncovering of latent homosexual wishes with acutely paranoid patients. These procedures are contraindicated, since they often diminish the patient's sense of self-control.

7   When making interpretations or statements to the patient, couch them so as to enhance the patient's sense of self-control and to lessen his tendency to predict control from others. For example, "By deciding to ignore them, you have restored your own power."

The above guidelines not only help build a nonthreatening relationship with the patient but also diffuse the patient's threatening feeling of loss of self-control. Once the patient feels that his sense of threat is understood by a nonthreatening person, the way is opened for the therapist to guide him in modifying his predictions and suspicions about control from others. It is beyond the scope of this chapter to deal with the many ramifications of treating paranoid patients, but since this topic has received insufficient attention in the literature, we will develop further some therapeutic implications of our model that have seemed to work well. Establishing a nonthreatening relationship with the patient, as described above, is basic not only for treatment but also for getting the patient to share information relevant to discovering factors underlying his sense of threat.

Right from the start, one of the most useful distinctions is whether the primary threat is loss of control over the self or over others. The threat to loss of control over the self can stem from a host of metabolic and organic factors, including the surreptitious taking of stimulants such as amphetamines (Manschreck and Petri, 1978; Ellinwood, 1968). Whenever possible, these toxic and chemical factors should be corrected. More common, the threat of loss of control over the self stems from a thought process disorder, typified by temporal disintegration in paranoid schizophrenia. In such instances, pharmacotherapy should be used to restore the patient's control over his thinking. The dosage of antipsychotic medication can be monitored according to the degree and frequency of tracking difficulties (see Chapters 5 and 7). Once these have been brought into control, it is important not to overmedicate the patient, since extrapyramidal and sedative side effects of antipsychotic drugs may in themselves be experienced as alien control.

It is also important to realize that persecutory thought *content* can be present without a thinking *process* disorder (McPherson, 1969). For example, a patient can have marked paranoid delusions and yet have no tracking difficulties. In fact, some paranoid disorders, such as paranoid personalities and paranoid states, may show unusual abilities in keeping track of information relevant to their over-futuring and the supposed schemes of others. Moreover, even when the persecutory thought content was initiated by deranged thinking it may persist after the thought process disorder has been adequately treated with medication. Attempting to eradicate the persecutory explanations or content by increasing drug dosage to sedative levels may aggravate the degree of paranoid content, since most paranoid patients at this stage need to be in cognitive control, not only for their self-esteem but also for their participation in psychotherapy.

If the history reveals that the primary problem is loss of control over a significant other person, rather than loss of control over the self, antipsychotic medications are usually not necessary although the judicious use of antianxiety drugs may help calm the patient for his or her participation in psychotherapy. When the primary issue is loss of control over another person, the therapist should realize that the current problem may be a reactivation of past conflicts, much like a neurotic conflict centering around motives for revenge. For example, a 54-year-old woman with no formal thought disorder was extremely apprehensive that ''somebody was going to kill her.'' She had an eerie feeling that somebody would retaliate if they knew how angry she was at her father-in-law, who reminded her of her own brutalizing father whom she had always wanted to ''get even with.''

More common, the loss of control over a significant other person is with a loved one. In the past, the loved one usually has been the submissive partner and the patient has been dominant. When the loved one becomes more assertive or finds a new attachment, the patient experiences a loss of control over the other person. This often prompts the patient to engage in further attempts to over-control the other person, usually manifested as a vigilant search for clues about infidelity in order to justify jealous accusations. In such instances, the therapist should assist the patient in clarifying issues with this other person. If a reunion or rapprochement cannot be effected, then the therapist should help the patient transform the threat of a loss to the acknowledgment of the loss. When the patient grieves the loss, his suspiciousness usually diminishes. At the same time, the patient should be helped to discover other plans and goals that do not involve this significant other person.

Whether the primary problem is loss of control over the self or over others, psychotherapeutic statements should be aimed at empathizing with the threat of loss of personal control while helping patients to test reality in terms of here-and-now transactions with other people rather than by predicting their supposed intentions. The general aim of such statements should be to help the patient gain control over himself rather than to prevent control from others by predicting their plans. In this regard, some useful statements geared to the stages of paranoid ideation (Table 4) are briefly exemplified below:

1 *Premonition stage.* ''I can understand how upsetting that might be.'' ''We never know what people really mean or intend to do in the future, so we are just hurting ourselves by letting our imaginations run wild.''

2 *Pursuit stage.* ''It's hard to reveal inner feelings and secrets to people you don't trust.'' ''Perhaps you can talk about your suspicions and anger here in this office, to me alone, since it's hard to master something that is hidden.'' ''Sometimes we try to hide things even from ourselves, and that makes us feel like we're not being ourselves.''

3 *Projection stage.* ''It must feel terrible to have your every move watched or interfered with.'' ''Perhaps by trying to outguess them, you are letting them make you worry too much . . . or letting yourself get too tied up by your thoughts about them.'' ''By letting yourself get upset by them, perhaps you're giving them too much power.''

4 *Presumption and protest stage.* ''What would happen if you just ignored them and went about your own business?'' ''Who is 'they'? Is there one person that we can focus on?—You know the old adage 'divide and conquer.' '' ''How could we check out if the phones are bugged?''

"When you just said that you think I'm in league with them, that hurt my feelings. Is that what you want?"

When a patient has reached the late stage of presumption and protest, the psychotherapist should realize that the patient's persecutory explanations are serving to reduce the threat of loss of personal control; to contradict them verbally is to pit belief against belief and to entail the risk of augmenting the patient's protest of others' influence. A more useful approach is to identify in the past the specific circumstances that initiated the threat–prediction inter-actions; in the process of historically reviewing the progression of paranoid ideation, including reality-based "insights" about certain situations (Arieti, 1962), the patient may gradually reconstruct his current beliefs and here-and-now readiness to protest. In addition, sometimes a direct approach in which the therapist (or a companion lay therapist) joins the patient in actively testing specific instances, such as delusions about phones being bugged, increases the patient's reality testing and lessens some of his presumptions (Jackson, 1963). Therapy for this late stage is often difficult, yet some patients are helped considerably when they are gently guided to find or rediscover personal long-range goals that do not involve their current paranoid preoccupations with certain other persons. After a patient's paranoid ideation has subsided and he has regained self-direction, supportive therapy should be aimed at helping him lessen his need for rigid control over himself or over others.

In summary, the model we have proposed suggests different treatment strategies for the formative and maintenance stages of paranoid delusions. The ultimate test of the model will be in its effectiveness in guiding treatment for the various stages of paranoid ideation.

SUMMARY AND CONCLUSIONS

Paranoid thinking can give rise to behavior that endangers the self as well as society. In order to understand and suggest ways of treating paranoid think-ing, we have proposed that the following cybernetic processes are involved:

1 During the *formation* of paranoid ideas, threats to loss of control over the self or others prompt suspicions of control from others, that, in turn, augment the initiating threat of loss of control. When this threat–suspicion interaction consists of projections into the future, unchecked by present-time feedback, a paranoid vicious cycle is initiated by *over-futuring*. This vicious cycle usually goes through the following stages:

(a) Premonitions about control from others, resulting in suspiciousness and anger

(b) Feeling pursued by others because of expecting their retaliation for one's suspiciousness and anger, which the person often attempts to hide

(c) Projection into the future in an attempt to outplot supposed pursuers, but ending up feeling manipulated by them because of overconcern with their plans.

2 The *maintenance* stage of paranoid delusions starts when the person is so threatened by the loss of self-control that, as a way to maintain at least a semblance of control, he presumes that others are indeed against him and he must resist them in order to survive. His persecutory explanations and his decision to resist others' influence provide him with a ready plan of action that serves to reduce his threat of loss of self-control. He learns that by resisting others, his sense of threat is reduced. This reinforces his persecutory ideas, which eventually become vital for his personal identity. This is how persecutory delusions are perpetuated.

Along with correcting metabolic factors and temporal disintegration, which can aggravate the above paranoid processes, therapy of paranoid patients should be aimed at interrupting the vicious cycle stemming from the interaction of threats to loss of self-control with suspicions about control from others.

PART FOUR

Depression:
Blocks to the Future

In depression, the future seems blocked. The severely depressed patient may give up trying to pursue anything in the future. Part IV will explore two common blocks to the future: hopelessness and grief. With hopelessness, a person's plans of action are deemed to be ineffective for reaching future images (goals). In unresolved grief, a person's images and plans remain fixed to the past, making the future seem empty and devoid of meaning.

These blocks to the future—hopelessness and unresolved grief—are common in severe depressive disorders. As outlined in Chapter 4, there are two time features that are common in severe depressive disorders: (1) slowing of mental processes and (2) hopelessness to the point of giving up future pursuits. These two time factors often interact to give rise to a depressive spiral as follows: The mental slowing may induce the person to feel hopeless about the efficacy of his plans of action, and the hopelessness may prompt him to give up and slow down even further. This is different from the normal sadness and disappointment that is to be expected with everyday losses. That is, in contrast to a severe depressive disorder, normal sadness is not characterized by marked mental slowing or the feeling that one's future is globally bleak.

The block to the future and the slowing of a severe depressive disorder are usually easily differentiated from the psychotic loss of control seen in acute schizophrenia. As previously outlined (Chapters 4, 5, and 7), in psychotic loss of control the images of the future are fragmented and confused with past memories. In acute schizophrenia, thought sequences are jumbled and the rate of thinking may shift intermittently from thought racing to thought blocking. By contrast, in a severe depressive disorder, even though the patient may have difficulty in concentrating because of his slowed thinking, he is usually able to keep track of sequences and to distinguish past, present, and future.

In addition, the psychomotor slowing and hopelessness of a severe depressive disorder can be distinguished readily from the neurotic dread of the future. As introduced in Chapter 4 and more fully developed in Chapter 11, one of the prominent characteristics of neurotic anxiety is uncertainty about the personal future. This uncertainty of images and plans is different from the hopeless giving up of a severe depressive disorder. That is, the neurotically anxious patient is still striving; he has not given up hope even though he has many conflicts and uncertainties as he enters his future.

Of course, the syndrome of "neurotic depression" (now called dysthymic disorder) does not have the psychomotor slowing and the marked hopelessness of a severe depressive disorder. Neurotically depressed patients are perhaps better labeled as suffering from chronic low self-esteem (Chapter 11). That is, they are uncertain about the value of the self in relation to others, and their sense of identity is unstable since it depends heavily on their meeting the expectations of other people. In short, the neurotically depressed person is uncertain about himself rather than being hopeless.

In contrast to the uncertainty and dread of the future seen in neurosis, the hopelessness of a severe depressive disorder is characterized by a dysjunction between future images and plans of action. The patient believes that his plans of action are insufficient for meeting future goals. The reasons for this may be an incapacity for carrying out plans of action, perfectionistic or unrealistic goals, or both.

The dysjunction between plans and future images (goals) in a depressive disorder can have diverse biopsychosocial causes. At the biological level, in the depressed phase of manic-depressive illness, there is a slowing of mental processes that appears to be induced by a shift in circadian rhythms (see Chapter 4). The psychomotor slowing is accompanied by a lack of energy and zest, making the patient feel incapable of carrying out his plans. A similar slowing can stem from other types of metabolic derangements, such as hypothyroidism. At the psychological level, the loss of a close person or a cherished goal is a common triggering event for the onset of a depressive disorder. How the patient construes or distorts his future in view of the loss is an important psychological determinant of depressive disorders. At the social level, lack of a support group and expected rewards also can contribute to depressive disorders as can the inability to deal assertively with one's anger in order to sustain healthy relationships with others. All these biopsychosocial causes of depressive disorders can give rise to the dysjunction of plans and future images that is characteristic of the hopelessness of severe depressive disorders.

Part IV of this book will focus on the following general themes:

1 Hopelessness reflects a dysjunction between future images and plans of action.
2 Whatever its triggering cause, once hopelessness sets in, it becomes a vicious cycle (spiral) since it forecloses consideration of alternatives.
3 The interruption of spirals of hopelessness is highly important for the treatment of depressive disorders.

In Chapter 9, I will focus on underlying expectations that predispose a person to becoming severely depressed and hopeless. The hopelessness of depression will be contrasted with a different type of hopelessness seen in sociopathy. General approaches for treating these different spirals of hopelessness will be outlined.

Chapter 10 will deal with methods for identifying and treating unresolved grief. Unresolved grief gives rise to a depressive spiral of hopelessness since the person's images, plans, and emotions are fixed in the past rather than being directed toward the future.

CHAPTER NINE

Spirals of
Hopelessness

The future looks cold and bleak, and I seem frozen in time.

Statement of a depressed patient

The loss of hope can be paralyzing in a severe depression. The future seems blocked and devoid of meaning and pleasure. Time seems to drag endlessly. Time seems monotonous and empty. There is little zest for living.

In this chapter, I will deal mainly with spirals of hopelessness that occur in severe depression. Also, I will contrast depressive hopelessness with the avoidance of hope seen in antisocial personalities. Although hopelessness is most prominent in depressive disorders, it also can occur as an end-state in many forms of psychiatric and physical illnesses. The prodigious struggles of man against illness can end in hopelessness. The poet Virginia Woolf (1970, p. 3) showed this. Shortly before killing herself by walking into the sea, she wrote: "I am certain that I have gone too far this time to come back again. . . . I am always hearing voices, and I know I shan't get over it now. . . . so I am doing what seems to be the best thing to do."

Hopelessness is at the core of most completed acts of suicide. Once hopelessness blocks the future, the risk of suicide is high. Hopelessness prompts the person to give up striving. It also foreshortens and constricts future time perspective, thereby closing off consideration of other alternatives for coping with one's problems. This giving up and foreclosure of the future is different from the paranoid attempt to regain control over the future by over-futuring, as discussed in Chapter 8. Hopelessness also is different from the neurotic dread of the future in which the future seems uncertain and

---

Thanks are due to Sir John Bowlby for his help in generating some of the early formulations of this chapter (Melges and Bowlby, 1969).

perhaps foreboding at times but still there are glimmers of hope toward which the person strives (Chapter 11). In severe depression, hopelessness is like a dark cloud that draws a curtain on the future.

My central thesis is that *spirals of hopelessness occur when (1) the person believes that his plans of action are no longer effective for meeting goals and (2) a constriction of future time perspective forecloses considerations of alternative plans and goals*. That is, even though the person believes that his plans of action are incapable of reaching his goals, he nevertheless remains committed to a rather narrow range of future images and relationships, and as these come to seem hopeless, he does not switch to other alternatives but gives up striving. In essence, hopelessness, by constricting future time perspective, breeds further hopelessness.

Before dealing with this thesis as it applies to hopelessness in depressive disorders, I will first define hope and hopelessness in light of cybernetic concepts and then outline some common predispositions to depressive hopelessness.

HOPE AND HOPELESSNESS

As used here, hope is an overall positive attitude toward the personal future. It differs from expectancies and anticipations, which refer to specific events forthcoming in the future. As commonly used, hope is the belief that although events may look uncertain or foreboding at the moment, positive opportunities will eventually arise. A person who has hope believes that, in the process of attempting to link his plans with his goals, not only will he have reasonable success, but also he will be able to participate in unforeseen and exciting opportunities that will arise in the near and distant future (Scher, 1971). Thus, with hope, the personal future is not certain and fixed but is viewed as being open, unfrozen, and full of opportunities.

Sustaining hope has been found to be important for coping with imprisonment (Frankl, 1974), with physical illness (Schmale, 1958), and with a variety of crises (Coehlo, Hamburg, and Adams, 1974; Stotland, 1969). There is some evidence to suggest that the progression of a terminal illness may be slowed if hope is aroused (Holden, 1978; Cousins, 1976). Raising hope is central to all forms of psychotherapy (Frank, 1974) and is thought to be the guiding "integrative field" of the ego for structuring goal-directed activity (French, 1952, 1970). Although cognitive appraisals of the future contribute to hope, it is mainly an overall emotional attitude that goes beyond the considerations of logical inferences about the future. Hope can be sustaining even when there are insufficient facts to sustain it.

Hopelessness, the opposite of hope, reflects an overall negative outlook on the personal future with a constriction of opportunities. Hopelessness is associated with poor coping, the aggravation of physical illness, and even death insufficiently explained by organic factors (Stotland, 1969). Hopelessness is common during many forms of severe mental illness, but it is most prominent during severe depressions (Beck, 1967). Although hopelessness is a global, subjective feeling, it can be systematically measured and has been validated as a meaningful construct in a variety of clinical settings (Beck et al., 1974). Typical statements of hopelessness are, "My future seems dark to me;" "I might as well give up because I can't make things better for myself;" "All I can see ahead of me is unpleasantness rather than pleasantness."

With hopelessness, there is the feeling that it is most improbable that plans will bring about goals, or that goals are even meaningful to strive for. As outlined in Chapter 3, plans of action refer to hierarchically organized sequences of intended action. Goals are preferred future images; they are the desired outcomes of intended action. Normally, plans of action and goals usually go hand in hand. When a given plan proves effective in reaching a goal, that plan of action is more likely to be called upon later, when the individual is striving for the same or a similar goal. Conversely, if the plan proves ineffective, the plan is less likely to be adopted again. Or with repeated frustrations and failures, the goal itself may be abandoned. Within this cybernetic framework, the kinds of goals a person sets for himself are seen to interact with the plans he adopts to achieve those goals (Melges and Bowlby, 1969).

When a person believes that his plans are likely to reach his goals, he is likely to have hope and high morale. This is particularly true if he perceives linkages between his short-term plans and goals and his long-term plans and goals. In this regard, Lewin (1942, p. 59) stated, "To develop and to maintain high goals and, at the same time, to keep the plan of the next action realistically within the limits of what is possible, seems to be one of the basic objectives for and a criterion of high morale."

With hopelessness, the linkages between plans and goals become disconnected. The dysjunction between plans and goals can take different forms of hopelessness depending on how the person habitually anticipates that outcomes will occur. These beliefs commonly center around the following general expectations:

1 To what degree is skill or chance expected to influence future outcomes?
2 Whether loyalty to others or exploitation of other people will bring about desired outcomes?

3 Whether important outcomes will take place in the short-term or long-term future?

The above general expectations determine, in large measure, how a person approaches the future as he structures his plans in relation to the kinds of goals he sets for himself. As discussed below, these general expectations often set the stage for the occurrence of hopelessness in depression. That is, the person prone to becoming depressed and hopeless often is oriented toward skill, loyalty, and the long-term future (Melges and Bowlby, 1969). This is in contrast to the orientation toward chance, exploitation, and the near future in antisocial personalities.

PREDISPOSITIONS TO DEPRESSIVE HOPELESSNESS: THE NARROW FUTURE

It is here proposed that a person predisposed to becoming hopeless and depressed usually has a narrow view of his personal future. By narrow, I do not mean that future time perspective is foreshortened, but rather it is limited in breadth, like an elongated and narrow tunnel. The person's future is channelized toward just a few relationships with significant other people or toward just a few important goals in life. When he loses a close person or when he fails at one of his goals, his narrow future seems blocked, and since he is not accustomed to seeing options beyond his narrow future, he may become hopeless.

There are, of course, genetic predispositions to depressive disorder, as with manic-depressive illness. As outlined in Chapter 4, this may be a genetic predisposition to certain phase shifts in circadian rhythms that induce a slowing of mental rate. The latter can make a person feel that he is incapable of carrying out his plans of action, thereby inducing hopelessness. As discussed later, this also induces a spiral of hopelessness. It should be noted, however, that a person with manic-depressive illness does not necessarily have a narrow view of his personal future, but when he does, it can aggravate his predisposition to depressive hopelessness. But in this section I will deal mainly with psychological predispositions to a narrow future.

From a psychological standpoint, I propose that the narrow future stems from the person's predominant beliefs in (1) the efficacy of skilled action, (2) loyalty to other people, and (3) the value of long-term goals (Melges and Bowlby, 1969). In this sense, persons who are predisposed to depressive hopelessness are often viewed as ''solid citizens'' who are dedicated workers, nonmanipulative with others, and conscientiously committed to long-term goals. Such traits are valued in a future-oriented society such as exists in the middle class of America today (Kluckhohn and Strodtbeck, 1961). When the hopelessness of depression overtakes such an individual, friends and families often are puzzled how such a "good person" could become hopeless.

The belief in the efficacy of skilled action is called the "internal control of reinforcement" (Rotter, 1966). This means that the person believes that, whatever happens to him, outcomes are determined largely by his own skilled action rather than by chance or luck. Moreover, he is responsible for his destiny; others are not to blame. Furthermore, this belief that future rewards are contingent on one's skilled behavior is associated with high-achievement motivation. They set high standards for themselves and often are compulsively perfectionistic. This pertains not only to achievement goals but also to their affiliations with other people. If something goes wrong with their interpersonal relationships, they tend to hold themselves responsible, rather than to blame others, and tend to think if only they had done something, things would be better. Their sense of competence and self-esteem depends largely on their capacity to make events happen (White, 1963). While this feeling of self-efficacy is important for self-esteem for most people (Bandura, 1977), it is a rigid and an inflexible belief in those persons vulnerable to depressive hopelessness. The depressive-prone individual gives little credence to chance or fate for determining his destiny. When negative events happen to him, he holds himself responsible for not executing an appropriate plan of action.

The person vulnerable to depressive hopelessness also tends to be loyal and trusting toward others. He believes that he can make relationships work well by being dedicated and committed. Moreover, he often is exclusively attached to a "dominant other" who becomes the be-all and end-all of his or her existence (Arieti and Bemporad, 1978). He commonly has few other important relationships than this dominant other person. He lives predominantly to meet the expectations of this other person. Moreover, since he is loyal, he expects this other person to be loyal toward him. He cannot brook manipulation or mistrust from this other person. This exclusive attachment to a dominant other person may be rooted in earlier losses of a parental figure, particularly during late childhood and adolescence, thereby prompting the person to highlight the importance of forming a trusting and loyal relationship with another person (Melges and Bowlby, 1969).

In addition to his beliefs in skill and loyalty, the person vulnerable to depressive hopelessness tends to believe in the value of long-term goals. He focuses largely on working toward long-term goals while neglecting outcomes in the present and near future. Moreover, he often is exclusively driven toward accomplishing a "dominant goal" (Arieti and Bemporad, 1978). He pins his sense of worth on accomplishing this goal. He has few other goals of value. This emphasis on accomplishing a dominant goal is currently more frequent in males. For his self-worth, the person believes he must become president of his company, be nominated for a Nobel Prize, make a million dollars, and so forth. When it looks like he will fall short of his dominant goal, he feels his whole life is a failure.

These rigid and inflexible beliefs in skill, loyalty, and long-term goals produce a narrow view of the personal future. The person vulnerable to depressive hopelessness believes that whatever skills he has, they must work or all else will fail. He believes that since he is loyal to others, other people should be loyal to him; if they are not, he becomes utterly disillusioned about his expectations of loyalty and help from others. His belief in the long-term future is usually limited to just a few goals in which he is highly invested; if it looks like one of these goals is unreachable, he sees few, if any, alternatives and the future looks bleak.

In this regard, the person prone to becoming depressed often has "rigid cognitive schemas" that limit his capacity to see alternatives and predispose him to bleak expectations about the future (Beck et al., 1979; Kovacs and Beck, 1978). These rigid cognitive schemas distort his views of the future. Common beliefs in this regard are as follows: "If I am not perfect, then I will be a total failure." "If this person is disloyal to me, it means that I am unworthy and will never again have a close relationship." "If I cannot reach this particular goal, then there's no use trying for anything else." It can be seen that many of these rigid cognitive schemas can be boiled down to a limited view of contingencies; that is, rather than thinking, "If A does not work out, then I'll do B, C, D, or E," the depressive-prone individual thinks, "If A fails, then everything else also will fail."

SPIRALS OF HOPELESSNESS IN DEPRESSIVE DISORDERS

It is here proposed that a narrow view of the personal future predisposes a person to hopelessness when some aspect of that future is lost. That is, the narrow future makes him vulnerable to having his hopes dashed, and since he foresees few alternatives, he becomes disillusioned about his future. He has placed "too many eggs in one basket," so to speak. When life events disrupt his beliefs in skill, loyalty, and the value of long-term goals, he is at a loss as to how to reenter his future.

Hopelessness is a common feature of severe depression (Beck, 1967). Also, the more severe the depression was rated, the greater was the feeling of hopelessness, and hopelessness was the factor most highly correlated with the depth of a depression as well as the likelihood of suicide. Grinker et al. (1961)

also found that hopelessness was a central factor in depression and was related to feelings of unworthiness, helplessness, indecisiveness, inability to act, and guilt about not maintaining duties. Changes toward a more negative view of the future have been found to be dynamically related to changes toward lower self-esteem (Melges et al., 1971). In addition, depressed patients, compared with other diagnostic groups, report having "no purpose in life," and yet they remain preoccupied with the future and show little interest in the present (Melges and Fougerousse, 1966). A preoccupation with a purposeless future produces a sense of futility.

In terms of the cybernetic concepts outlined in Chapter 3, I propose that *spirals of hopelessness occur when the person believes that his plans of action are no longer effective for meeting his goals, yet he still clings to his goals.* His goals may consist of maintaining an important relationship with another person or an important long-term achievement. The dysjunction between the person's goals and plans initiates spirals of hopelessness.

The gap between these goals and plans of action is common to the plurality of models of depression reviewed by Akiskal and McKinney (1975). Writers of different theoretical schools use different terms to describe this gap, but they point to the same phenomenon. For example, Bibring (1953), a psycho-analyst, posits "as the basic mechanism of depression, the ego's shocking awareness of its helplessness in regard to its aspirations . . . such that the depressed person . . . has lost his incentives and gives up, not the goals, but pursuing them, since this proves to be useless." A. Lazarus (1968), a behaviorist, holds that "depression may be regarded as a function of inade-quate or insufficient reinforcers . . . some significant reinforcer has been withdrawn." In other words, the plans of action are no longer expected to be reinforced by reaching goals or through sustaining a relationship.

It is proposed that this dysjunction between plans and goals is common to the hopelessness of all types of depression, including mild (dysthymic) and severe (psychotic) depressions as well as unipolar and bipolar (manic-depressive) types of depression. In the case of depression occurring in a person with manic-depressive illness, it is probable that an inherited predis-position triggers a neurochemical dysfunction in the brain, such as a phase shift in biorhythms (Wehr, Muscettola, and Goodwin, 1980), which slows down the person's overall rate of functioning, making him feel that he no longer has the energy to carry out his plans (see Chapter 4). Whatever the triggering event, once there is the dysjunction of plans from goals, hopeless-ness sets in and may become a downward spiral when the person remains attached to his goals.

Since the person clings to his future images, such as his former relation-ships and goals, long after he knows it is impossible to reach or sustain them, the gap between his plans and his future images widens and he becomes increasingly hopeless. As the hopelessness deepens, he often gives up trying to execute his plans and becomes inactive. This further widens the gap between his plans of action and the goals to which he remains attached. Furthermore, the depressed patient often misconstrues events of the present and near future to fit his bleak expectations about the distant future.

The precipitating stress for the hopelessness of depression is commonly a loss of some kind (Akiskal and McKinney, 1975). Usually it is a loss of skill, a loyal relationship, or the long-term future. The loss of efficacy in skilled action can be caused by a number of factors, such as mental slowing during the depressed phase of manic-depressive illness, skills becoming outmoded by technological advances or impaired by metabolic derangements, physical illness, lack of youthful energy, or beginning organic brain disease. Also, interpersonal skills can be challenged by moving to an unfamiliar environment, such as when one retires. In addition, a person's sense of skilled efficacy can be challenged by being trapped in a situation that demands accomplishing a continuing goal for which he is inadequately prepared. A common example of this is the new mother who feels she must take excellent care of her infant even though she feels helpless as to how to do it. She desperately wants to be a good mother but feels that her plans of action are inadequate to meet this task. She often interprets the infant's crying as evidence of her lack of skills. This may result in a postpartum depression (Melges, 1968).

Perhaps the most common precipitating stress that triggers hopelessness in depression is the loss of a significant other person (Stenbeck, 1965; Bowlby, 1980; see Chapter 10). As previously mentioned, the loss is usually that of a "dominant other" with whom the patient has had a loyal and dependent relationship. The loss makes the future seem empty. A shared plan of action is interrupted by the loss, making the continuing goal of affiliating with this other person seem hopeless. The person feels denied of a host of anticipated reinforcements. The loss may not be overt, as with death, separation, or infidelity, but can be subtle, such as the relationship not meeting up to mutual expectations of support, trust, and loyalty. Because the patient expects loyalty in return for his own loyalty, when he loses the other person or if the relationship becomes strained, he often feels betrayed. Yet since the patient has been so attached to this other person, it is difficult for him to give up the goal of somehow maintaining the relationship. He clings to this goal even though it seems hopeless.

Finally, the loss can be of the long-term future itself. This can occur when the person realizes that he will never reach his dominant goal in life. It also can occur when a patient is given the diagnosis of a terminal illness, such as untreatable cancer. When a person is customarily oriented toward the long-term future, the prospect of losing it often robs the present and near future of zest and meaning, making life seem even more hopeless.

Why does the depressed person cling so tenaciously to his goals long after it seems unlikely that he will reach them? Why does he not just give up and switch to realizable goals or other relationships? This often stems from his basic perfectionism, sense of duty, and loyalty that has narrowed his personal future. Also, part of the answer may lie in the finding that skill-oriented behavior is quite resistant to extinction (James and Rotter, 1958; Rotter, 1966). That is, a person who has been previously rewarded for skilled behavior will persist in that behavior long after rewards are not forthcoming. This is in contrast to a chance situation, such as gambling at a slot machine, where the rewards are viewed as being outside of one's personal control (Melges and Bowlby, 1969). Another way of stating this is that when rewards are viewed as being governed by external chance circumstances, the person is more likely to adjust his behavior according to recent and present outcomes, whereas when rewards are believed to be contingent or internally generated skills, the person is likely to persist in striving to reach future goals while discounting feedback from present outcomes. In this regard, depressed patients have been found to neglect the present and remain preoccupied with future goals, even when the latter appear futile (Melges and Fougerousse, 1966; Wyrick and Wyrick, 1977).

As the depressed patient's current plans of action become increasingly alienated from his distant goals, it seems as though time's arrow into the future is broken. Associated with this is the feeling that the passage of time seems inexorably slow and devoid of meaning and pleasure (Melges and Fougerousse, 1966; Wyrick and Wyrick, 1977; Scher, 1971; Straus, 1947). In addition, hopelessness may prompt the person to give up striving, and this may induce further slowing of mental rate. The mental slowing, in turn, may induce further hopelessness, since the person views himself to be sluggish and inefficient, no longer skilled in carrying out his plans of action.

As the spiral of hopelessness worsens, the depressed person comes to feel increasingly doubtful about the efficacy of his skills, more unworthy of expecting loyalty and help from others, and increasingly negative about reaching valued long-term future goals. As the hopelessness worsens, future time perspective foreshortens and there is an increase in ideas of suicide (Melges and Weisz, 1971). Of all the factors involved in depression, hopelessness has been found to be most highly correlated with suicide (Yufit et al., 1970; Wetzel, 1976). When future time perspective in the depressed person becomes not only narrow but also foreshortened, the risk of suicide is at its highest, particularly when it seems to be the only alternative way to escape from suffering and disillusionment.

In this regard, negative emotions, such as depression and anxiety, are significantly correlated with a foreshortening of future time perspective (Melges and Fougerousse, 1966; Teahan, 1958; Wohlford, 1966; see also Chapters 2 and 3). In depressed patients, changes toward greater unpleasant emotions were highly correlated with changes toward a loss of internal control of reinforcement, a foreshortening of future time perspective, and increases in suicidal ideation (Melges and Weisz, 1971). This suggests that the occurrence of hopelessness and negative emotions may induce a foreshortening of future time perspective, thereby aggravating the hopelessness by closing off consideration of alternatives.

Thus, by way of conclusion, I propose that the dysjunction between future images and plans of action in depressive hopelessness is commonly triggered by two factors: mental slowing and/or the loss of an important person or achievement. These factors are associated with two related spirals of hopelessness:

1   The mental slowing, by impairing skilled action, induces hopelessness about the future, which may prompt the person to give up striving, thereby inducing further mental slowing. As a result, the person's inactivity robs him of opportunities and rewards that would otherwise become available. This spiral is common in the depressed phase of manic-depressive illness, but it also can occur in endogenous depressions (now called melancholia) which often is complicated by psychomotor slowing.

2   The loss of an important person or goal, because of the individual's narrow view of his personal future, makes the future seem hopeless, and the hopelessness, in turn, may foreshorten future time perspective so that the person even further excludes alternatives from consideration. His constricted and narrow view of his future makes the pain of the loss seem all consuming, and he sees no way out. This spiral of hopelessness is common during unresolved grief.

These spirals of hopelessness may combine to give rise to another spiral: a negative view of the self, others, and the future. Beck (1967) has highlighted this triad of negative views as common to all types of depression. In my experience, however, the main interaction is between negative views of the self and negative views of the future; other people usually are not viewed negatively in the sense of blaming them, as with paranoid disorders, yet the depressed person may feel so hopeless that he believes other people cannot be of help to him. The interaction between negative views of the self and negative views of the future has been documented as psychiatric patients were studied longitudinally: changes toward hopelessness were highly correlated with changes toward lower self-esteem (Melges et al., 1971).

Before discussing how to dissect and treat these spirals of hopelessness in depression, I will first contrast depressive hopelessness with another form of hopelessness seen in antisocial personalities. In making this contrast, I realize that, for heuristic purposes, I am making sharp distinctions that do not pertain to each and every case and in some cases there may be an overlap of the proposed dynamics.

HOPELESSNESS IN ANTISOCIAL PERSONALITIES

The hopelessness of antisocial personalities (sociopaths) often is not recognized. Because of the sociopath's impulsive hedonism and reckless seeking of pleasure in risky situations, it is easy to miss his particular kind of hopelessness. In contrast to the depressed person who becomes disillusioned about his long-term future, the sociopath, beginning in childhood, has never had much hope for the long-term future. The sociopath is in a chronic state of hopelessness about the long-term future. As a consequence of this foreshortened future time perspective, the sociopath is geared primarily to getting immediate gratification in the present and near future (Melges and Bowlby, 1969). When this present-orientation meets with repeated frustrations, he then experiences hopelessness, particularly when he feels forced to consider long-term consequences which he habitually views as futile and hopeless.

An antisocial personality is an individual who repeatedly violates the norms of society. Crime, illicit drug taking, and promiscuity are common in this disorder. Formerly, antisocial personalities were called sociopaths, and I will use the latter term to refer to the same condition in this chapter. Sociopathic behavior often begins before age 15 and is usually manifested in a variety of delinquent acts. I will therefore review studies of future time perspective in delinquents as relevant to antisocial personality, while realizing that an antisocial personality does not become fully crystallized until after age 18. Also, it should be pointed out that antisocial acts can stem from other mental disorders, such as schizophrenia, mania, and mental retardation. These other disorders are to be excluded when considering factors involved in the personality constellation of sociopaths.

In terms of general expectations about how outcomes will take place, the sociopath believes primarily in (1) chance rather than skill, (2) exploitation of other people rather than expecting help from forming trusting and loyal relationships, and (3) the present and short-term future rather than the long-term future. These beliefs can augment one another, giving rise to the sociopathic spiral of hopelessness. That is, his risky and impulsive behavior aimed at exploiting others often breeds hostility from others; this aggravates his distrust of long-term commitments and further prompts him to seek whatever rewards he can find in the present through impulsive acts that exploit others.

Impulsivity is the hallmark of sociopathic behavior. There is considerable evidence that impulsive behavior is spurred by an inability to delay gratification and a neglect of long-term consequences (for review, see Melges and Bowlby, 1969; also Chapters 2 and 3). In Halleck's (1967) words, the sociopath is "a basically ahistoric individual for whom the the past and the future are meaningless and for whom only the existing moment is important." This focus on the existing moment makes them vulnerable to drug taking, alcoholism, thievery, and "making it" within a violence-prone gang that offers immediate support for risk taking. To quote one delinquent in this regard: "People will mess over me anyway, so I just take what I can get now. . . . I can make it now with these other dudes. . . . Why wait for it?"

Predisposing Factors to Antisocial Hopelessness

What might account for the sociopath's predominant beliefs in chance, disloyalty, and the present? Although there is some evidence that genetic factors and attention deficits during childhood contribute to this order, the bulk of research suggests that early environmental factors, particularly family disorganization marked by illegitimacy, divorce, and separation, play a major role (Melges and Bowlby, 1969). It is as if the sociopath has been so repeatedly disappointed in the past that he is afraid to hope for anything in the future. Since his early life has been so full of chance and changes over which he had little control, he expects the future to be the same. Since in the past he has been repeatedly hurt whenever he trusted others for loyalty and help, he now distrusts others in order to rob them of the power to hurt and to exploit them before they exploit him. Since committing himself to a long-term future goal or relationship has rarely worked out in the past, or has been poorly modeled by his parental figures, it seems foolish to invest in a distant future that will not materialize.

Precipitating or Aggravating Factors

Because of the sociopath's basic orientation toward the present, it is difficult to find a systematic or psychodynamic explanation for why he commits certain acts at a given time. Sometimes the explanation which is most accurate is that an opportunity presented itself, and the sociopath seized the moment. In this regard, gang violence amongst delinquents has been likened to a "pick-up game" of basketball in a neighborhood park—that is, somebody starts the action and others just join in (Cloward and Ohlin, 1960). Unless they are motivated by revenge, acts of violence commonly eclipse the past and future, and are most likely to occur when taking personal action in the present appears to offer immediate rewards or relief from tension (Melges and Harris, 1970). By contrast, the capacity to resist temptations of the moment, whether aggressive or sexual in nature, has been shown to be related to a greater concern for the future and to a tendency to endow the future with a sense of reality (Levine and Spivack, 1959; Cottle and Klineberg, 1974).

Paradoxically, sociopathic sprees of impulsive behavior often occur when the sociopath feels forced to consider long-term consequences. That is, when his present-oriented, exploitative behavior meets with repeated frustrations and control from authority figures, forcing him to at least look at long-range consequences of his behavior, he then may become doubly hopeless— hopeless about the present as well as the future. Since he distrusts the long-range future, he accentuates his basic modus operandi of seeking rewards by exploiting others in the present. A well-known example of this is the increase in derelict and unruly behavior in a prisoner who realizes that he will soon be released. He becomes anxious about his hopes for release, since it means that he has to count on the actions of others, which is against his basic beliefs. Since he fears hoping for the future, he regresses to his former present-oriented impulsive behavior.

In conclusion, different types of hopelessness are proposed to be central to the psychopathology of depression and sociopathy. The depressed patient, while deeply concerned about his future, has lost the hope he once had because he has come to believe that his plans will no longer achieve his long-range goals and maintain his relationships. Also, because he has a narrow and limited future outlook, when his plans become blocked, he foresees few, if any, alternative opportunities. By contrast, the sociopath has long since given up hope of striving for continuing and long-term goals and, instead, habitually seeks goals and opportunities available in the present.

I have seen this contrast between depressive hopelessness and antisocial present-centeredness take place in a single person in cases of multiple personality. For example, Jane 1 (the predominant personality) had a narrow view of her personal future. She was highly invested in skilled action as a computer programmer and dutiful mother. She was extremely loyal to her adoptive parents, her husband, and her children. She was very committed to getting her Ph.D. in mathematics. By contrast, her alternate personality, whom she called Jane 2, was excited by chance and risky situations in the sleezy bars she would frequent, was exploitative and manipulative of others, and delighted in impulsive, promiscuous behavior aimed at present gratifications. Jane 2 never looked into the future; she saw only the present; the here-and-now was to be seized for every mischievous pleasure possible, without regard to future consequences. Jane 2 ridiculed Jane 1 for her long-term commitment to a narrow range of duties and obligations. On the other hand, when Jane 1 would learn of the escapades of Jane 2, she felt guilty and ashamed that someone living in her own body could be so irresponsible, particularly with regard to her children. Thus two different kinds of temporal perspective—a rigid future outlook and a completely present-orientation—appeared to give rise to different personalities in the same person.

THE TREATMENT OF DEPRESSIVE HOPELESSNESS

The treatment of spirals of hopelessness entails altering the negative expectations that are augmenting one another and foreclosing the future. The treatment strategies should take into account the predisposing beliefs about the future that have made the person vulnerable to hopelessness. Empathy with the person's basic beliefs about the future helps combat demoralization and helps overcome resistance to change (Frank, 1974). Most therapists, who are usually future oriented, have little difficulty in empathizing with the basic future-orientation of depressed patients, yet they often are at odds with the present-orientation of antisocial personalities (Lager and Zwerling, 1980).

According to the model presented here, the general treatment strategies for hopelessness in depression and sociopathy are opposite. The treatment of the hopelessness of depression entails (1) increasing chance and risk taking rather than just relying on the performance of skills, (2) inducing an attitude of taking care of one's self and getting self-satisfaction rather than just being dependently loyal on a dominant other, and (3) highlighting rewards in the present and near future rather than the distant future. By contrast, the treatment of the hopelessness of antisocial personalities entails (1) the building of skills rather than risk taking, (2) the formation of loyal bonds to foster identification rather than manipulation of others, and (3) the extension of awareness into the distant future rather than just focusing on the present and near future.

It is beyond the scope of this chapter to deal extensively with specific treatment measures that will foster the above general strategies. Nevertheless, some guidelines for treating depressive hopelessness will be outlined.

Hopelessness is the most dangerous sign of severe depression since it is highly correlated with the risk of suicide. Therefore, it requires vigorous treatment. This may require hospitalization until the hopelessness and risk of suicide subside. Of course, for a person with mild or neurotic depression (better termed chronic low self-esteem), hospitalization is usually not necessary. Future-oriented psychotherapeutic strategies for dealing with neurotic depression are discussed in Chapter 12.

For the treatment of the hopelessness of severe or moderate depressions, a biopsychosocial approach is useful. If the patient is markedly slowed down (psychomotor retardation), it is usually necessary to use biological treatments, such as antidepressant medications or even electroshock therapy, in order to restore him to a normal rate of functioning (see Chapters 4 and 5). In using antidepressant medicines, it is useful to follow the degree of early morning lethargy typically seen in a severe depression. When this morning lethargy decreases, it is an indicator that the antidepressant medication is working and that the patient's normal rate of functioning will soon return. This slowness has to be treated since it contributes to the patient's hopelessness by limiting his capacity to think of future options and to have the energy to pursue them.

While the patient is still slowed down, the therapist should be active, nurturant, and reassuring. He should actively tell the patient that although the future may *seem* hopeless, he has a 90–95% chance of getting better. Meanwhile, about three weeks will be necessary for the antidepressant medications to take effect. In order to help the patient tolerate this delay, it is appropriate to appeal to his basic character in the past of being able to "tough things out" and "hang in there."

When the patient is still hopeless about his future, it is appropriate for the therapist to assume the role of a surrogate "dominant other" who is nurturant and will take care of things until the patient "gets back on his feet again." The patient is actively encouraged to engage in daily activities, however minute, from which he will gain some sense of being able to act and get self-satisfaction. Nihilistic delusions about the future, such as, "I will always be depressed" or "My family is better off without me," have to be repeatedly challenged and questioned. If the patient has had a previous depression from which he recovered, this should be repeatedly reviewed in order to remind the patient that since he got better in the past, it is likely that he will do so in the future.

Most depressed patients feel guilty about being depressed and not meeting responsibilities. This has to be vigorously challenged: "What good is it doing you to feel guilty? Why are you making things worse for yourself? You have an illness—a depression; and it's going to take some time before you're better. If you had a pneumonia, would you blame yourself?" Some patients are guilty about attempting suicide or thinking about it. Helping the patient forgive himself for attempting suicide or thinking about it can often be accomplished through some brief guided imagery. The patient is prompted to take the role of a nurturant parent with regard to himself. For example: "From what you've told me, you have always been a good mother. Close your eyes and think how well you took care of your son. Now, keeping that image of yourself as a caring mother, look back on yourself to a month ago when you were so ill and depressed that you wanted to take your life. Can you mother yourself and forgive yourself?''

Meanwhile, at the social level, the therapist should clearly explain the nature, course, and treatment of the depression to the family. His initial role is that of a teacher who gets the family to rally around the patient for support. This is a great aid to combating hopelessness.

The timing of later psychotherapeutic strategies, including family therapy, is tuned to the patient's improvement of slowing and the emergence of glimpses of hope. As these signs begin to appear, the therapist gradually shifts his role from that of a nurturant take-charge physician to that of a supportive guide who helps the patient find his own directions.

Thus when the depressed patient's psychomotor slowing begins to improve, he is more ready to become an active participant in psychotherapy. It is at this juncture that the therapist can begin to help the patient modify his rigid expectations about the future that have made him vulnerable to becoming hopeless. This includes (1) encouraging risk taking and helping him to become more spontaneous, (2) giving him permission to seek a wider array of relationships with other people rather than being excessively loyal to a dominant other, and (3) helping him to take note of and register rewards in the present and near future rather than focusing on the distant future.

The enhancement of risk taking and spontaneity is greatly aided by a milieu setting that reinforces the patient for having fun. Many depressed patients have forgotten how to play. They are skill-oriented work-aholics. To change this orientation, massive social support is needed so that whims, humor, and playful daring are rewarded. Risk taking also can be reinforced during group or family therapy.

Helping the patient change his loyal dependency on a dominant other often requires extensive psychotherapy. The patient often has lived his life trying to gain the approval of a dominant other. He favors the security from such an external relationship over the self-satisfaction that would come from meeting internal expectations of himself. The shift toward self-satisfaction can be made through psychoanalytically oriented therapy (Arieti and Bemporad, 1978). Also, the patient's rigid beliefs about his need to be loyal and dependent can be challenged with cognitive therapy (Beck et al., 1979). For example, the therapist can show the illogicality of such assumptions as, ''I am worthless without him'' or ''I can't live without her.'' With patients with unresolved grief after the loss of a dominant other, grief-resolution therapy, followed by future-oriented psychotherapy, is a useful way to begin the process of letting go of a loyal relationship and forming internalized choices for the self that are projected into the future (Chapters 10 and 12).

Helping the depressed patient to focus more on the present and near future, rather than the distant future, requires a cognitive-behavioral approach. Whenever the patient discounts a compliment or disavows the importance of a present accomplishment, the therapist (or staff) points out to him how he is robbing himself of pleasure. On the other hand, when he does register compliments and accomplishments, he is reinforced and helped to savor them. In addition, assertiveness training for helping patients to deal with interpersonal issues in the here-and-now, rather than protecting a long-term relationship by not saying anything, can aid the overcoming of a rigid belief in the narrow future. Moreover, helping patients to overcome perfectionistic standards about lofty long-term goals often allows them to become more aware of present satisfactions. In this regard, the following paradoxical statement sometimes initiates a change in attitude: "If you're trying to be perfect, then you are not perfect."

In summary, the primary task for treating the hopelessness of depression is to *unfreeze the future*. After giving biological treatments for overcoming psychomotor slowing, psychosocial therapies should be designed to interrupt the spiral of hopelessness by inducing positive expectations about risk taking, taking care of the self, and present rewards. By making the patient aware of the wealth of options that can bring pleasure and satisfaction in the present and near future, the patient begins to realize that his plans of action can become meaningfully connected with his future images. By restructuring the expectations underlying hope, hopelessness is combated.

SUMMARY AND CONCLUSIONS

The major points of this chapter can be summarized as follows:

1   In severe depression, hopelessness is a common block to the future.
2   The person predisposed to becoming depressed and hopeless often has a narrow view of his future that is channelized toward beliefs in skill, loyalty to a dominant other person, and/or pursuit of a dominant long-term goal. When events disrupt his narrow future, he foresees few alternatives for himself.
3   In depression, spirals of hopelessness occur when the person believes that his plans of action are no longer effective for meeting his goals (affiliations or achievements), yet he still remains attached to his goals. This gives rise to a dysjunction between the person's plans and goals.

4   There are two related spirals of hopelessness that commonly occur in depression:

   (a)   Mental slowing, induced by changes in biological rhythms, impairs the efficacy of a person's plans of action, prompting him to feel hopeless about reaching goals. The hopelessness, in turn, may prompt the person to give up striving, thereby slowing him down even further. This spiral is common in the depressed phase of manic-depressive illness.

   (b)   The loss of an important person or of a valued goal induces hopelessness, which, in turn, foreshortens future time perspective, thereby closing off consideration of alternatives and prompting further hopelessness.

5   The treatment of spirals of hopelessness in depression entails a biopsychosocial approach aimed at:

   (a)   Increasing mental rate and associated activities to make more rewards available in the present.

   (b)   Unfreezing the future so that the person does not feel he has lost everything.

6   The hopelessness of depression is different from the hopelessness of antisocial personalities who have never had much hope and maintain a present-orientation.

CHAPTER TEN

Grief-Resolution Therapy: Reliving, Revising, and Revisiting

Loss of a loved person is one of the most intensely painful experiences any human being can suffer.

JOHN BOWLBY (1980, p. 7)

Grief clouds the future. When a family member or close friend dies, not only is that person lost, but also the hopes tied to that person are lost. The future then seems bleak and empty.

As described in Chapter 9, a person whose hopes have been highly vested in a relationship with a "dominant other" is particularly vulnerable to hopelessness when he or she loses this other person. Since the future seems hopeless without the dominant other, the bereaved person has difficulty in accepting the reality of the loss and yearns to find the lost person in the present and the future. This yearning commonly takes the form of visual images of the deceased (Bowlby, 1980). These visual images often are intrusive and disrupt adaptive modes of projecting into the future. In this way, anticipatory control becomes impaired (Chapter 3). That is, the patient's futuring is disrupted by visual images of the deceased and wishes to reunite with the lost person. Also, since the images of the future are unrealistic, they serve as maladaptive templates for the temporal organization of plans of action. During unresolved grief, temporal organization frequently is manifested by restless aimlessness

This chapter was written in collaboration with David R. DeMaso, M.D., Fellow in Child Psychiatry, Children's Hospital Medical Center and Judge Baker Guidance Center, Boston, Mass.

(Lindemann, 1944). In short, the person's images, plans, and emotions are fixed to the past rather than serving as guides to the future.

The purpose of this chapter is to outline and illustrate a systematic method for identifying and treating unresolved grief so that a person's sense of control over the personal future is restored. This method was originally developed by Melges and DeMaso (1980) as a focal form of treatment that can be used within the context of other therapies. The treatment method makes use of present-time guided imagery for the facilitation of normal grieving processes through the imaginary removal of obstacles, such as binds with the deceased and blocks to emotional expression, that previously have inhibited the detachment necessary for finding new images and plans of action.

The emphasis will be on unresolved grief reactions subsequent to the death of a close relative or friend. The question of whether or when to treat grief has become controversial. Freud (1917) asserted that the normal processes of grieving should not be interfered with, and there is a widespread belief that "time alone heals." Yet recent studies (Schoenberg et al., 1975; Parkes, 1972; Maddison and Viola, 1972) have shown that the time taken for healing is much longer than formerly thought, sometimes taking two to four years. During this time, a vast number of the bereaved have been found to be highly vulnerable to physical and mental deterioration (Greenblatt, 1978). Treatment programs, such as widow-to-widow support groups, have been successful in dealing with this public health problem (Silverman, 1976). Although our method of treatment is designed for clinicians dealing with classical unresolved grief reactions, it may also have some usefulness in facilitating the grief–hope process in those suffering from "normal" grief.

GRIEF: NORMAL OR ABNORMAL

Grief is easy to detect clinically, but whether grief is unresolved and pathological is difficult to define operationally. Clinically, just asking the person how he feels about the deceased individual usually prompts the reactions of grief. There are two common responses: explosive weeping or attempts to avoid the subject. Often these go hand in hand (for example, "I know I'm crying about my husband, but I don't want to talk about him"). Among others, the works of Lindemann (1944), Bowlby (1961, 1963, 1973, 1980), and Engel (1961) have outlined the panoply of emotions and defenses that occur in normal grief. The usual stages are (1) shock and disbelief, (2) protest and anguish, and (3) mourning and restitution. The acute phase of grief usually lasts six to eight weeks, but mementos and questions can bring on emotional reactions throughout the first year after death, sometimes years later (Parkes, 1972).

During so-called normal grief, symptoms similar to depression (sadness, insomnia, weight loss, loss of interest, difficulties in concentrating, and so on) are almost universal in the acute phase, and persist intermittently throughout the first year after the loss in about half the bereaved subjects, being present in 74% if the loss was sudden and unexpected for widows under age 45 (Parkes, 1972). Akiskal and McKinney (1975) have reviewed the literature that shows it is difficult to differentiate grief from depressive symptomatology. During grief, phenomena ordinarily indicating the loss of contact with reality can occur. Rees (1975) found that 47% of widows and widowers reported postbereavement hallucinations; 39% reported "the sense of the presence" of the deceased; 13% had auditory hallucinations; and 14% had visual hallucinations. Some of these hallucinations lasted for years after the loss.

Since depression and even sense deceptions occur in so-called normal grief, the definition of unresolved grief cannot depend merely on the enumeration of symptoms and signs. Time and intensity help identify the problem as abnormal but are not conclusive: In abnormal grieving, the person has too little grieving soon after the loss *or* too much grieving too long after the loss, or both. The limits of what is too much or too little, too soon or too late, are hard to define. Also, each person has his own way of grieving, and there are different rates of grieving according to different cultures. The Texas Inventory of Grief (Faschingbauer, Devaul, and Zisook, 1977), which focuses on emotional concern and preoccupation with the deceased, denial of the death, identification responses, and anniversary reactions, is a step forward toward operationally defining the limits of normal and abnormal grief. At the present stage, the clinician should be aware that some patients presenting the classical symptoms and signs of depression may have an unresolved grief reaction even though the loss was years ago.

DETECTION OF OBSTACLES TO GRIEVING IN UNRESOLVED GRIEF

The detection of unresolved grief reactions, from a clinical standpoint, involves finding the dynamics that have inhibited the normal grieving processes. Our approach to detecting unresolved grief reactions which require therapy is to identify depressive disorders that have started shortly after the loss of a significant person whose image still preoccupies the bereaved's mind for longer than a year after the loss. We then begin to look for one or more of the following obstacles to normal grieving that are likely to maintain the grief in an unresolved state:

1 *Persistent yearning for recovery of the lost object.* This has been emphasized by Bowlby (1963, 1980) as a cardinal sign of unresolved grief. In such instances, the bereaved gives evidence of searching for the lost object and often refers to the deceased in the present tense rather than the past tense. Dreams of reunion are common. "Linking objects," such as pictures and mementos of the deceased, are frequently reviewed or touched in order to maintain hopes for reunion (Volkan, 1975). The chronic hope of finding the lost person impairs the process of giving up and building new realistic hopes. For example, one woman who lost her husband three years ago remained preoccupied with clues signifying the return of her husband, such as listening for the sound of his car, the turn of his key in the door, and so on.

2 *Over-identification with the deceased.* The bereaved may have unexplainable somatic symptoms or changes in personality that mimic those of the deceased. For example, a man experienced recurrent chest pain similar to his beloved brother's pain who had died from a myocardial infarction. Another woman patient began to drive recklessly and felt compelled to wear a wig like that of her best girlfriend who committed suicide. Also, persistent and severe anniversary reactions often reflect over-identification with the deceased, particularly when the patient's symptoms mimic the terminal complaints of the deceased (Hilgard and Newman, 1959, 1963).

3 *The wish to cry or rage at the loss coupled with an inability to do so.* Such persons have not allowed themselves the full expression of affect that would enable them to differentiate from and subsequently give up the deceased. Bowlby (1963, 1973) points out that anger and weeping are necessary biologically ingrained responses leading toward the recognition that the loss is final. The inability to cry or rage at the loss frequently stems from the bereaved trying to "not fall apart" at the time of the loss, and at a later time, grieving seems inappropriate. That is, shortly after the loss, the survivor-victim was so preoccupied with funeral preparations, hosting friends and relatives, and maintaining a stoic yet cheerful facade that he or she did not grieve adequately when the time was appropriate. At a later time, after societal sanctions for abreaction are no longer present, the person feels foolish and out of order if he or she gives vent to the welled-up feelings. Sometimes this inhibition of affect is mediated by projective identification with other bereavers, whereby the bereaved guards against his own expression of affect through identifying with and caring for others (Bowlby, 1980). At other times, the initial grieving has been inhibited because the death was stigmatized (for example, suicide) or experienced in part as a relief from pain and suffering (for example, terminal cancer).

4 *Misdirected anger and ambivalence toward the deceased.*   Research suggests that the closer the relationship, the more turbulent and protracted the grief upon loss of the relationship (Schwab et al., 1975). The loss of a close relationship entails the interruption of shared plans of reinforcement, which leads to dashed hopes and anger, since the person feels he deserves to have his hopes and plans continue (Melges and Harris, 1970). The loss is not just of past interactions but also of the expected attachments projected in the future. Anger at the deceased for having deserted the bereaved is perplexing to those who will acknowledge only positive feelings toward the dead person. Former ambivalent feelings, attendant to any close human relationship, become buried under the facade of adoration of the deceased. As a result, the anger is not expressed at the deceased but rather misdirected at the self or others (Freud, 1917; Fenichel, 1945). This blaming of the self or others allows for maintaining the illusion of closeness to the deceased, in the present and future, and inhibits the demarcation of the survivor from the dead person. Excessive self-reproach often reflects anger directed at the self for "not having done enough" or for guilt about being angry at the deceased for having left the person helpless. In this sense, anger directed toward the self is an attempt to control the guilt and expected retaliation from the deceased, as though the latter were still alive.

5 *Interlocking grief reactions.*   A recent loss may awaken the pain of previous losses that were troublesome and conflict laden and thereby never completely handled. The dimly perceived relationship between the losses inhibits the person from fully grieving the current loss for fear the old conflicts will arise again. The person fears he will become overwhelmed with the awareness of superimposed losses. Previous losses, particularly during childhood, appear to predispose a person to pathological mourning (Bowlby, 1980).

6 *Unspoken but powerful contracts with the deceased.*   These invisible loyalties are much like covert "contracts" made during marriage. Some common contracts seen in patients with unresolved grief are as follows: "I will not leave you like you left me" or "I will always obey you and stay by your side."

7 *Unrevealed secrets and unfinished business.*   Some patients cannot accept the death of a loved one for fear that the deceased will then have knowledge of a carefully guarded secret, such as an extramarital love affair, greed for inheritance monies, and so on. Others feel that somehow they must keep the deceased "alive in their bosom" so that they will still have a chance to express love and forgiveness they never did while the deceased was living.

8 *Lack of a support group and alternative options.* With the fragmentation of the modern extended family and the breakdown in socially supporting networks of people, many bereaved persons literally have to start all over again when a spouse dies. The support that they are given is often ritualistic, short lived, and superficial. As a result, they may cling to hopes they once had with their spouses, since the availability of alternative attachments is lacking (Greenblatt, 1978).

9 *Secondary gain or reinforcement from others to remain grief stricken.* Some patients remain in a helpless state after a loss, especially if they learn from the reactions of others that this is a way to escape responsibilities and to obtain continuing succor. Such patients are usually chronically dependent personalities, and treating the unresolved grief alone cannot be expected to change the person's dependency needs. Yet, in some patients, a whole family may be grieving and is using the identified patient as a vicarious object for their own grieving. Family therapy is indicated in such instances as an adjunct to grief-resolution therapy.

In summary, unresolved grief reactions can usually be detected by noting whether a person is time bound to a loss that time alone has not and will not heal. That is, the person's hopes are pinned to the past rather than to the present and future.

ESSENTIAL TECHNIQUES AND PROCESSES OF GRIEF-RESOLUTION THERAPY

Grief-resolution therapy is aimed at helping patients resolve their grief by removing one or more of the above obstacles to mourning. The therapist first identifies the obstacles, then helps the patient remove them by revising scenes in imagination of the loss, and then has the patient revisit and regrieve the loss in present-time imagery with the obstacles removed. The intense work of grieving and giving up is supported by the concurrent building of new images and plans of action.

Table 5 presents an overview of the essentials of grief-resolution therapy. There are three basic techniques: (1) the decision to regrieve, (2) guided imagery, and (3) future-oriented identity reconstruction. These technical stages are related to three fundamental processes: (1) decrease in the defensive avoidance of the reality of the loss, (2) controlled detachment from the lost person, and (3) the building of new images and plans of action.

Each technique and the related process will be given further discussion in separate sections below. The decision to regrieve is important in order to

Table 5   Essentials of Grief-Resolution Therapy

Obstacles	Techniques for Removing Obstacles	Processes
Yearning for lost object Overidentification Blocked affect	1 Decision to regrieve	1 Decrease defensive avoidance

Anger and ambivalence
Interlocking grief
Unspoken contracts
Secrets
Lack of support group
Secondary gain
	2 Guided imagery
	     Relive, revise, revisit
	     Scenes of loss:
	     News
	     Funeral home
	     Funeral
	     Burial
		2 Controlled detachment

	3 Future-oriented identity reconstruction	3 Building new images and plans

reduce the tendency of the patient to defensively exclude information about the reality of the loss. This defensive avoidance has been highlighted by Bowlby (1980) as a key factor in pathological mourning. The guided imagery allows the patient to undergo gradual detachment from the deceased in a manner that enables him to gain control over events which, shortly after the loss, he could not control. The therapist serves as a supportive guide while the patient undergoes controlled detachment from the lost person. The future-oriented identity reconstruction helps the patient to consolidate his own identity vis-à-vis the deceased and to crystallize new future directions. This is particularly important for those patients who view themselves as helpless victims after losing a close person (Horowitz et al., 1980).

Since the guided imagery is the core of the method, emphasis will be placed on this stage of therapy. Guided imagery has been found to be useful in helping patients reconstruct their views of the past, present, or future (Leuner, 1969; Kosbab, 1974; Singer, 1974; Shorr, 1972; Melges, 1972). In grief-resolution therapy, the patient is actively encouraged to visualize scenes of the loss as though they were happening in the here-and-now. This is done in the mind's eye of the patient whose eyelids should be closed. There are essentially three aims of using this present-time guided imagery: (1) Recall of the scenes of the loss, the emotions, and the obstacles to grieving seems to be more complete with present-time imagery than when the events are talked about in the past, (2) the present-time imagery is experienced as more vivid and real than the past (see Chapter 2), and (3) the present-time imagery facilitates the externalization of binds and obstacles with the deceased that can be actively confronted and reworked in imagination.

With regard to the confrontation of binds and conflicts with the deceased, the guided imagery makes use of "dialogues with the dead." This may seem peculiar, yet in our experience the activation of present-time imagery of scenes like viewing the body in the funeral home recreates the sense of ''the presence'' of the deceased. That is, shortly after a person dies, those close to the person usually have the sense that somehow the deceased is present still. This seems to take place regardless of a person's beliefs in an afterlife. The guided imagery recreates this sense of the presence of the deceased so that silent dialogues can take place and be reworked between the patient and the lost person.

A useful way to get the patient to begin dialogues with the deceased is to recreate a scene of the loss (for example, viewing the body in the funeral home) and then have the patient complete sentences such as: ''I will not leave you because . . . I will keep you alive in my bosom because . . .'' This usually reveals some of the obstacles and binds that have been repressed. In order to rework the binds and obstacles, the feeling that the presence of the deceased has somehow responded is encouraged. In this way, the patient's anger or love is thought to be felt and understood, and opportunities for mutual forgiveness can be opened. Feelings of forgiveness and permissions from the deceased to be different and start again are particularly freeing. This use of dialogues with the presence of the deceased can be likened to doing family therapy with the patient and the lost person.

As is common in family therapy, we have found that the expression of anger is usually necessary before the patient forgives the deceased for some past wrongdoing. Many patients with unresolved grief remain attached to the deceased not out of love but through anger. The anger has blocked the full realization of the love they also hold toward the deceased. For this reason, grief-resolution therapy promotes the full expression of anger as a prelude to forgiveness and understanding.

In cases where there has been a symbiotic tie with an overly critical parent or spouse, it sometimes is useful (as Arkin and Battin, 1975, describe) to suggest that the deceased may have undergone a personality change for the better and is thereby more understanding and forgiving. However, this is usually not necessary if the therapist has elicited the full expression of both anger and love before requests for forgiveness are introduced.

During the guided imagery stage, the intensity of the emotional expression can be upsetting to the patient (and sometimes the therapist). Nevertheless, as Bowlby (1973, 1980) points out, anger and weeping appear to be necessary preludes to the recognition that the loss is final. For some patients, only a few tears with some terse statements are necessary; for others, extensive weeping and raging along with long dialogues are required. Weeping not only elicits caregiving from others but also promotes compassion for the self (Beck et al., 1979).

Having introduced some of these general processes that are facilitated during grief-resolution therapy, we are now prepared to discuss the specific treatment stages.

THE DECISION TO REGRIEVE

Most patients with unresolved grief are at least vaguely aware that they are hanging onto the past and that to continue to do this will bring further problems. Yet they resist letting go. To overcome this resistance, they must be encouraged to make a firm decision to regrieve and let go.

After detecting an unresolved grief reaction through history taking, the first task of the therapist is to establish sufficient rapport with the patient so that the patient feels he has a supportive guide who will help him grieve while finding new hopes. To do this, the therapist should empathize with the meaning of the loss to the patient and should acknowledge how difficult it will be for the bereaved to give up the deceased. A useful technique for sharing the meaning of the attachment is to prompt the patient to discuss positive exchanges with the deceased that occurred shortly before the loss, such as an affectionate embrace or the saying of kind words. The patient is then asked to close his eyes and attempt to reexperience the reciprocal feelings engendered by such exchanges. Reexperiencing the depth of the attachment in this way often revives the bereaved's lost sense of self and, although painful, engenders hope for the reemergence of parts of his or her identity. Suggestions of the necessity for grieving are then gradually introduced until the patient is finally prepared for a clear statement, such as: ''You have pinned all your hopes on him; now he is gone, and your hopes are there buried with him in the past. Do you think you can find the courage to let him go and find new hopes?''

Further cognitive structuring involves explaining the procedures used in the guided imagery and how the patient will gradually go through grief–hope transitions. For example: ''I will ask you to review what you experienced when you lost your loved one by seeing in your 'mind's eye' the events before and after his death. You will speak out loud in the present tense as though the events were happening right now. You will have your eyes closed, but you will be able to see the happenings in your mind. I will be there listening to your feelings and what happened to you. We will spend about 20 minutes each session to deal separately with each of the following scenes: your awareness of your relationship to the deceased shortly before the news of his death, then the arrival of the news and how you felt, then the happenings at the funeral home, then the funeral, and finally you will say 'goodbye' to him and walk away from the grave with the feeling that you can begin again. For each of these scenes, you will first relive what happened, then we'll rearrange the scene in your imagination so that you have removed obstacles to grieving, and after that you will revisit the scene and allow yourself to express feelings and deal with the conflicts which you previously have kept inside. Although your task will involve a lot of emotion—crying, perhaps anger—you also will experience a feeling of increasing freedom along with the awakening of parts of yourself that you have forgotten.''

The patient's decision to regrieve is often therapeutic in itself. How much time is devoted to the regrief work depends on the clarity of the patient's decision, his ego-strength, and the extent of his binds with the deceased. Usually, grief resolution therapy requires 6–10 half-hour or hourly sessions that are carried out as focal treatments within the context of other types of therapy. For outpatients, seeing the patient two times a week is usually necessary to maintain the intensity of the process and to allow time for discussion of other issues bearing on the regrief work. Past resentments and conflicts with the deceased are handled by psychoanalytically oriented psychotherapy. For severe depressive reactions associated with unresolved grief, which may require initial antidepressant medications in order to mobilize the patient, it is useful to hospitalize the patient, particularly if milieu therapy is available to support the patient's commitment to grieving. The regrief work can take place daily for inpatients.

GUIDED IMAGERY

The essence of the guided imagery method involves helping the patient progressively relive, revise, and revisit sequences of the loss as though they were taking place in the present. The essential steps are as follows: (1) *Reliving* sequences of the loss by viewing them in the "mind's eye" with eyelids closed as if the scene were happening now (for example, viewing the body at the funeral home); (2) *revising* the scene in order to remove barriers or binds that formerly inhibited full grieving (for example, the person is left alone at the funeral home rather than being with a crowd of people); and (3) *revisiting* the revised scene in the present tense as if it were really taking place in the here-and-now. It is important to encourage active visualization and to keep reminding the patient to use the present tense during each step.

The *reliving* stage gives opportunities for abreaction as well as provides information about obstacles which previously inhibited grieving. It has been found that the present-time imagery provides the quickest way to discover such obstacles, since the patient again feels he is actually confronting them instead of "talking about" them in the past tense.

In the *revising* stage, the patient is asked to remove the obstacles from the scene. Usually this involves creating solitary scenes with the deceased in which highly private material (for example, anger, secrets, binds) can be worked out in the absence of competing relatives and social constraints. Sometimes the therapist has to actively rearrange the scene (for example, opening the casket to let the person see that the deceased is really dead; removing a critical grandmother who is weeping over the body; allowing for dialogues which promote the exchange of feelings and forgiveness; having the patient view the casket being lowered into the grave as well as seeing the dirt fill up the grave after the patient has said his final ''goodbye'' and exchanged last words). As the patient revisits the scenes with the obstacles removed, the therapist may make further rearrangements as needed.

Occasionally, the patient did not attend the funeral or circumstances prevented opportunities for grieving with exchanges of ''last words'' and feelings. In such instances, the therapist and patient can collaborate in constructing some suitable imaginary scenes for the regrief processes. For example, a 42-year-old banker lost his beloved teenage son in an automobile accident, and the son's body was cremated shortly afterwards. The father estimated that his son probably died within four seconds after being hit by an oncoming train. This four-second period was expanded by pointing out that individuals while dying have a panoramic ''life review,'' and the father imagined that he was somehow in communication with his son during the life review. This was extremely helpful, allowing the father to become confirmed that he had been ''the best Dad'' that his son could have ever had. In the final second of the son's life, which was expanded for about 20 minutes of therapeutic time, last words moving toward the final goodbye took place, followed by much weeping and subsequent relief.

In the *revisiting* stage, the patient is encouraged to engage in ''dialogues with the deceased'' in order to acknowledge the finality of the loss, differentiate himself from the deceased, express tears and rage, deal with ambivalence and misdirected anger, tease apart interlocking grief reactions, emancipate himself from unspoken binds, reveal secrets and deal with unfinished business such as the expression of love and forgiveness, and get permission from the ''presence'' of the deceased to look for new relationships and options, especially those that seem to flow naturally from what the deceased would have wanted for the bereaved.

Toward the end of each of the revisited scenes in which dialogues with the presence have taken place, the therapist encourages the patient to exchange last words and asks whether the patient is ready to say goodbye to the deceased. In the earlier scenes, such as viewing the body at the funeral home or after the funeral, most patients are unable to utter a sincere goodbye, and the word seems to stick literally in their throats. The therapist should then recognize that the patient is not ready by prompting the patient to say "goodbye for now" while preparing the patient for the final goodbye when the deceased is lowered into the grave and covered with dirt (or the ashes being flung to the wind, in the case of cremation). The finality of this last scene usually has to be carried out in imagination, since most patients with unresolved grief have not in fact witnessed it. After this final scene, when the bereaved has "walked away" about 50 yards from the burial place, he is asked to "turn around and look back" in order to "feel if there are aspects of the deceased's personality that you choose to develop in yourself." Most often these are images of strengths, strands from the past that can serve as bridges to the future. These bridges are selective identifications that can be further amplified for identity reconstruction.

After the patient has finally said goodbye to the deceased, remarkable changes in relations to others are observed in milieu or family settings. When the patient is exposed to "linking objects," he reports a definitely different feeling (Volkan, 1975). For example, one patient reported that she could look at her husband's picture and wedding ring while no longer feeling "helpless and going to pieces." Encouraging the patient to revisit the cemetery can serve as an additional test; most common, after adequate grief resolution, patients report that the deceased is "no longer present with them in this life" and their reactions are more like memories tinged with sadness rather than expectant yearnings for reunion. Some therapists advise visiting the grave-yard with the patient (Volkan, 1975), but we have found that this is usually not necessary if the guided imagery has been thoroughly worked through.

In those patients who still cling to the deceased and do not experience a distancing effect on these tests, we have found that this is commonly due to inadequate expression of anger and ambivalence toward the deceased during the guided imagery which is a necessary prelude to the forgiveness leading to the final giving up. In such instances, we have gone back to selected scenes and had the patient rework them until the final goodbye is unfettered with unexpressed anger.

FUTURE-ORIENTED IDENTITY RECONSTRUCTION

The third basic stage of grief-resolution therapy involves helping the patient reconstruct his identity into the future. These future-oriented psycho-therapeutic techniques are discussed in detail in Chapter 12. The patient's conscious choices to be similar or different from the deceased in selective ways can serve as springboards into the future for the further crystallization and rehearsal of images about the self projected into the future. This provides a natural and effective extension of the guided imagery techniques of grief-resolution therapy.

The initial groundwork for the future-oriented psychotherapy can be laid when the patient has walked away, in his imagination, about 50 yards and looks back at the grave site in order to consider which strengths of the lost person he would choose to develop in himself. The therapist also can ask in which ways the patient chooses to be different from the deceased. The patient's choices to be similar or different are then recorded. The word choices are then later used as spurs to imaging the self in the future.

Another useful future-oriented technique is to create some time distancing between the present and the future. This can be done one day or so after the completion of the guided imagery phase of grief-resolution therapy. The patient is asked to imagine that he is visiting a place once cherished by himself and the deceased together. For example: "Imagine that it is now one year ahead in the future and you are visiting that special place in Michigan; be there alone: see the water, the rocks; feel the wind. Look back at this time now and tell me your feelings about letting him go. . . . What are your memories of him? How are you feeling now, in this place in the future?" If the patient can distance himself through imaginary time from the deceased, this can serve as a test of the adequacy of the grief-resolution work. Well-treated patients often say something like, "He is gone; he is only a memory; yet knowing him has helped me to become who I am." The therapist can then ask in what ways the patient has grown from the experience of grieving and whether he wishes to continue to grow along the same lines. His choices for identity reconstruction can be further reinforced with additional time-projections into the future in which he crystallizes his becoming self (see Chapter 12).

In similar fashion, the patient also can be projected to future times which are likely to prompt anniversary reactions of grief, such as the date of death of the deceased, Christmas, or birthdays. The patient is asked to imagine that these future times are taking place now. While empathizing with the patient's sense of isolation and loss during these times, the therapist can reinforce how the patient has grown by letting the deceased go and developing important new directions for himself. In addition, rehearsals of coping strategies for dealing with these anniversaries can be conducted.

Future-oriented identity reconstruction is particularly indicated for those patients who view themselves as victims. In this regard, the latent self-image of persons predisposed to pathological mourning is often that of a worthless person (Bowlby, 1980). This view of oneself as worthless and helpless appears to be held in check by a close relationship with another person who is deemed strong and dominant. With the loss of this other person, the patient's latent self-image as worthless and helpless becomes activated (Horowitz et al., 1980). That is, without this other person, the patient feels weak, helpless, and unlovable. Also, since the patient feels deserted by this other person, he often comes to feel not only worthless and helpless but also a victim.

The future-oriented psychotherapy can help the patient make a redecision about himself as a victim, as elaborated in Chapter 12. For those patients who are inveterate victim players, although grief resolution therapy can help resolve the grief, further psychotherapy of diverse types is usually necessary to help the patient overcome the victim role. Existential and cognitive strategies are particularly indicated in this situation as a prelude to further future-oriented work. For example, it is often useful to point out to the chronic victim player who is suffering from unresolved grief that not only has he lost the past but also he is losing the future if he continues to view himself as a victim. In addition, as discussed in the next section, family therapy is often necessary to interrupt undue reinforcement from others who may be highlighting the patient's sense of being victimized by a loss.

FAMILY THERAPY AS AN ADJUNCT

Family therapy may be useful before going through with the guided imagery in order to promote understanding and support of the difficult task of grieving and to make new attachments available. Also, the possibility of other family members having unresolved grief can be identified. Sometimes an entire family is conducting its affairs as though the deceased were still alive, and the dissolution of these binds and myths requires ongoing family therapy interspersed with individual regrief work. In many instances, one family member may refuse to give up the myth of ''the dead being alive somehow'' for fear that they will betray the illusions held by other family members. Here it is helpful to have the member who is most ready to go through grief-resolution therapy to be treated individually, and then later share with other members his ''dialogues'' which have freed him from the mythical binds. Other family members are then prompted to discuss how the deceased is still influencing the family's life plan and interactions. Resolving binding expectations, whether from the dead or between the living, is central to changing family systems.

ILLUSTRATIVE CASE VIGNETTES

The following case vignettes will be used to illustrate some of the key therapeutic exchanges employed in grief-resolution therapy.

Resolution of Ambivalence and Secrets

E.O. was a 27-year-old, married mother of two children who became acutely incapacitated with an uncanny fear of death when shortly after her husband's grandmother died, she revisited the same cemetery where her stepfather was buried three years previously. She had idealized her stepfather as being a "perfect man." During the regrief therapy, when she was reliving seeing her stepfather's body in the funeral home, she became aware of her anger toward him for having sexually fondled her as a girl, but she could not express this anger in the relived-remembered scene because her mother, from whom they had kept the secret, was there at the funeral home. The therapist asked her to revise the scene, removing the mother along with all other people, and encouraged her to express her anger and feelings. With the scene thus revised, she gave full vent to her anger and her guilt for having to carry this secret for so long. After that, she felt free to express her love for him, which she had refused to do during his terminal illness. She also acknowledged her complicity in the sexual activities, and then forgave him and subsequently felt he understood and forgave her for not caring for him during his terminal illness. With her guilt and anger dismantled, she felt immediately relieved, no longer "haunted" by the death phobia. In addition, she appropriately moved on to deal with some monetary "secrets" she had hidden from her husband, and these were dealt with in family therapy. On six-month follow-up and two-year follow-up, the patient was symptom-free and functioning "better than ever" at work and as a wife and mother.

Guilt and Interlocking Grief Reactions

A.K. was a 43-year-old, married mother of three children who presented for psychiatric hospitalization a bewildered, depressed, and suicidal state shortly after being rebuffed by a matronly fellow volunteer worker. History revealed that she had been severely depressed 10 years previously shortly after the death of her mother, and she required two psychiatric hospitalizations at that time and had repeated outpatient therapy for recurrent depressions since then. Therapy, including trials on adequate doses of different types of anti-depressant medications, had been to no avail, and her husband had become hopeless about the efficacy of psychiatric help. The patient stated that she had "talked about" the death of her mother with previous therapists, but this only made her feel worse, since she then began to feel acutely guilty and became "doubly perfectionistic." She had not cried at her mother's funeral and refused to cry about her mother, although she was profusely tearful when talking about her husband's aloofness and criticism of her. Her mother had been extremely hypercritical and controlling during her childhood. When the patient was age 18, her mother and father separated at the time that the father chose to leave the family and live with another woman whom he later married. Her father died 18 months prior to her mother's death 10 years ago. She had not adequately grieved his death since the mother and father's wife were constantly bickering about rights to the father's inheritance during the various funeral rites. The patient felt left out and angry at the greed and uncaring. Later, at her mother's death, the patient, who was an only child, was suddenly thrust into taking responsibility for quickly finding an alternative cemetery for the burial of her mother, since the father's wife vehemently prohibited the mother being buried next to her father, as had been planned. In the grief-resolution therapy, it was decided to deal first with the father's death, since this was not as complicated and the relationship was not so ambivalent as with her mother. The present-time guided imagery actually revealed many of the above facets which the patient was unable to recall when talking about her losses retrospectively. In the regrief work with regard to her father's death, the therapist had her progressively go through the various scenes of the funeral rites, but each time revised the scene so that her mother and her father's second wife were not there bickering; rather she was alone with the image of the deceased in order to allow for solitary exchanges, some of which turned out to be quite meaningful. For example: "I am angry at you for having left home when I was a teenager, since then mother kept beating on me mentally, making me feel guilty about everything, and I did not have your protection. . . . I wanted you for myself yet you left for another woman. . . . Now my mother and your wife are fighting over you, as though you are a piece of property, whereas in my heart I feel you have always belonged to me. . . . Part of me wanted you to die when you were so sick toward the end. . . . Do you understand all this? Can you forgive me? Can you understand why I was so confused after your death, still looking for you?" During the regrief work, the patient abreacted profusely with regard to her father's death and felt forgiven by him for her anger and her attraction to him, and in the imaginary scene of walking away from the graveyard after witnessing the lowering of her father's casket into the grave (which she did not experience in real life), she turned back and said, "I no longer have to search for you in every man I meet, nor in my husband." This was accompanied by considerable relief, her behavior on the ward became more spirited, and her hostile avoidance of her husband turned to a more open relationship. This opportunity was reinforced with family therapy.

One week later, the patient was finally ready to do grief-resolution work with regard to her mother's death. She had resisted this vigorously, but milieu and family therapy helped in giving her support to go through with it. The patient was amazed at how much the guided imagery brought back almost total recall of the circumstances and feelings related to this loss 10 years ago. For example, she could "see" the single rose which had been placed on her mother's coffin in the funeral home, and she again felt the resentment that "my mother does not deserve a rose." Some of the key dialogues took place after the funeral when the therapist suggested the revised scene of "being there alone with your mother, after all the other people have left, now with the casket open so you can see her face." For example: "Why did you have to drive my father away with your ugly nagging? No wonder he left the family; I forgive him for that. But then, when he died, you had to fight with his wife over his body, his property, yet you had no claim to him. When you couldn't nag him anymore after he left, you took it all out on me. I could never do anything right for you. How I tried to please you, yet I just ended up feeling I had not done enough ever. I hate you, mother, I hate you [followed by much sobbing]. No wonder my father's wife didn't want you buried next to him; you are a curse. Now I've had to find a place to bury you; you will not like it; it's too grubby. Even in death I cannot please you. But it's your fault; you made your own bed, your own grave. I am going to let you go, mother; along with all this guilt I will bury you. . . . Yet even now I feel I am disobeying you, leaving you alone; you needed to cling to me; in a way, I was your mother. Your mother, grandma, clung to you and made you feel guilty. Maybe that's the only way you knew. . . . Could you help it? [Much sobbing] MOTHER, I FORGIVE YOU! . . . *I forgive you—Now I can forgive myself* [followed by much relief]. I do not owe you anything. I am going to be different from you. I will not drive my husband away; I will be truly loving to my children. Gads, I have almost become like you. . . . Now that you are dead maybe you understand all this—I want to be free to be myself."

After witnessing the burial of her mother (which she previously had fled from) and after expressing her final goodbye with tears admixed with freedom to express love to her mother, the patient walked away from the grave and then, in her imagination, found a red rose (like the one she earlier felt did not belong on the coffin at the funeral), and went back to the grave to place the rose on it and said, "Thank you, mother, for loving me in the only way you knew how." She then walked away, feeling exhilarated and free.

After the above grief work, the patient's petulant behavior turned to open caregiving on the ward and toward her family. She was discharged from the hospital, and followed in couples therapy and future-oriented identity reconstruction. By six months after discharge, the patient was jocular and loving with her husband, had freed herself of excessive home obligations, and had obtained a responsible job. She also had taken a trip to visit her oldest daughter and felt pride when she could be caring without being "meddlesome" like her own mother. She had been tapered off all medications, including the imipramine that she had been taking for years. At follow-up one year after grief-resolution work, the patient repeatedly stated that "it was great to be alive." This brought tears of joy to her husband's eyes, since the patient had been chronically on the verge of suicide for the previous ten years. She left a poem with the therapist which contained the following phrase: "For what is guilt but feeling unable to be a way chosen or expected by another?" At three-year follow-up, the patient continues to do well.

CONTRAINDICATIONS AND COMPLICATIONS

The reactivation imagery of this technique is contraindicated for acutely manic or schizophrenic patients, although the guided imagery has helped severely depressed patients who have had recurrent hallucinatory images of a lost object. Also, reactivated imagery for patients who are recently grieving a loss is usually not employed, since the image of the loss is still fresh in their minds and usual modes of therapy (empathy, ventilation, and so forth) are often sufficient in such cases. Nevertheless, even with recent losses, the facilitation of the processes outlined in this chapter, such as mobilizing anger, weeping, forgiveness, and undoing binds, can be helpful in dealing with acute grief.

In our experience, there have been no lasting untoward complications of this treatment method. Short-term complications include resistance of the patient to go through the necessary emotional turmoil of grieving, emotional draining of the therapist in empathizing with the relived scenes, and insufficient building of alternative relationships so that the patient is left floundering after the regrief work. These complications usually can be managed by adequate pacing of the grief work, the use of a co-therapist to share the emotional impact and active restructuring of the patient's social network. The patient, the therapist, and the social network often have to be prepared for the patient to get worse, in terms of increased emotional turmoil, before getting better.

CLINICAL USEFULNESS

The guided imagery techniques outlined in this chapter have been used by the senior author in treating unresolved grief reactions in well over 100 patients.

The results have been good, sometimes dramatic after 6–12 sessions, particularly when the problem has been primarily unresolved grief uncomplicated by long-standing personality conflicts. Yet, even in the latter, the regrief work has brought to fore binds and clarifications that were constructive for subsequent therapeutic interventions. In most instances, the grief-resolution therapy has been integrated with other forms of therapy, including cognitive, milieu, and family therapy as well as the appropriate use of antidepressant medication for mobilizing severely depressed patients. Research is needed for finding what kind of therapy, or combination of therapies, is most useful for treating unresolved grief. Experience has indicated that the present-time guided imagery, or components of it, can quickly get at the core issues needing resolution. It serves to highlight the obstacles and binds which are often only dimly perceived when the patient talks about the loss in the past tense.

This method of grief-resolution therapy deals with similar dynamics outlined in Volkan's (1975) "re-grief therapy," but differs from it since we emphasize reexperiencing the grief in present-time imagery with the previous obstacles removed. Talking about the loss in the past tense is used only for initial history taking, since it has been found that the binds and affects emerge more vividly when the patient is actively encouraged to use the present tense and to reexperience the loss in the here-and-now. This, of course, requires that patients actively use their imaginations, even more so when the funeral scenes are revised. Whether an imaginary scene, rather than a remembered scene, can be therapeutic, and not discounted as being "make-believe" and unreal, has not been a concern of the patients we have thus far treated. Changing the patient's construction of reality, whether through reliving or reimagination, appears to be central to therapy (Kelly, 1955). Helping a patient change how he is construing his identity in relation to the loss is important for grief-resolution therapy.

Dealing with unresolved grief often highlights the patient's construction of his identity in relation to significant other people. During the regrief work, not only does the patient review the self vis-à-vis the lost person, but also there is commonly a review of relationships of other significant people who were either there or not there at the time of the loss and the funeral. This intermingling of times past with other people affected by the loss opens rich opportunities for further therapeutic work. Moreover, the loss of a close person brings to fore many of the key existential questions that face each person: death, freedom of choice, isolation, and meaning (Yalom, 1980). In this way, grief-resolution therapy, by telescoping times past, provides a window for looking at new future directions.

SUMMARY AND CONCLUSIONS

The major points of this chapter can be summarized as follows:

1   Grief-resolution therapy is indicated for the treatment of unresolved grief reactions that are incapacitating and have persisted for one year after the loss.

2   The dynamics underlying unresolved grief usually involve one or more of the following factors: persistent yearning for recovery of the lost object; over-identification with the deceased; the wish to cry or rage at the loss coupled with an inability to do so; misdirected anger and ambivalence toward the deceased; interlocking grief reactions; unspoken but powerful contracts with the deceased; unrevealed secrets and unfinished business; lack of a support group and alternative options; and secondary gain or reinforcement from others to remain grief stricken.

3   The processes involved in grief-resolution therapy involve removing the above binds and obstacles that previously have inhibited grieving while supporting the patient as he goes through cycles of attachment and detachment from the lost person.

4   The basic techniques of grief-resolution therapy consist of (a) cognitive structuring for the decision to grieve and give up the lost person, (b) present-time guided imagery centered on scenes of the loss, and (c) future-oriented psychotherapy for identity reconstruction.

5   The guided imagery phase of treatment involves reliving, revising, and revisiting scenes of the loss as though it were happening in the present. During the reliving stage, the patient becomes aware of the reality of the loss. In the revising stage, the patient is helped to rearrange the scenes of the loss so that he removes binds and obstacles that previously have inhibited grieving. He then revisits the scenes in his imagination, giving full vent to his feelings and actively dealing with binds to the deceased until he finally lets go.

6   After the patient lets go of the deceased, the stage is set for identity reconstruction through future-oriented psychotherapy. This helps the patient to regain his sense of control by realigning his futuring and temporal organization.

PART FIVE

Neurosis:
The Dread
of the Future

The neurotic individual dreads the future. In particular, he dreads his interactions with other people in the future since he fears that he might be rejected or controlled by them. To avert being rejected or controlled, he tries to appease others by meeting their expectations. But in trying to meet their expectations, he loses his own sense of self-direction. In this way, his future time perspective becomes owned by other people—by what he thinks they expect of him.

The term *neurosis* has had a checkered history in psychiatry. My use of the term, in keeping with DSM-III, emphasizes the central role of anxiety in neurotic disorders. Although there are many theories of anxiety, the view taken here is that anxiety reflects uncertainty about the future. In neurosis, this uncertainty about the future is particularly marked when the person anticipates his interactions with other people.

In terms of the hierarchy of time problems presented in Chapter 4 (Table 2), neurotic individuals are proposed to have problems with an imbalanced temporal perspective, particularly an over-focus on the past. It is proposed that the future is dreaded and uncertain since they fear that past uncertainties in relating to other people may recur in their present and future transactions with others. The dread of the future prompts them to avoid or misconstrue future transactions, and this draws them further into the past. In this way, a spiral ensues in which the dread of future induces a greater emphasis on the past, which, in turn, may augment the uncertainties of the future.

In terms of the hierarchy of time problems (Chapter 4, Table 2), it should be noted that time disorientation, the temporal disintegration of sequences, and rate and rhythm problems can disrupt temporal perspective. That is, these other time problems can produce imbalances of temporal perspective, such as misconstructions of the future from inappropriate transferences of the past, that may aggravate a person's neurotic anxieties and distortions. Thus these more severe time problems should be detected and treated before focusing on the person's neurotic expectations. In this regard, as is well known clinically, many psychiatric patients, whether schizophrenic, manic, or depressed, have degrees of neurotic distortions.

The neurotic dread of the future is easily distinguished from the psychotic loss of control of the future and the depressive block of the future. In an acute psychosis, the future is confused, the person lacks goal-directedness, and has difficulty with tracking sequences (Chapter 7), whereas the neurotic individual dreads specific situations in the future, remains goal directed, and has no difficulties with sequential thinking. The severely depressed patient feels hopeless about the future and is generally slowed down, whereas the neurotic person, although viewing aspects of his future with dread, has not yet given up, continues to strive actively, and has a normal rate of functioning which even may be accelerated slightly when anxiety is experienced.

More refined diagnostic discriminations have to be made when comparing neurosis with paranoid disorders and personality disorders. In nonpsychotic paranoid disorders and paranoid personalities, which do not have the marked tracking difficulties of an acute psychosis, the future is assumed to be known rather than uncertain and unknown as with neurotic disorders (Chapter 8).

There often is considerable overlap between neurotic disorders and personality disorders. Many personality disorders, which are held to be long-ingrained character patterns, have a good deal in common with neurotic disorders except that manifest anxiety is less prominent (Hine et al., 1972). It is rare to find a neurosis without a personality disorder or a personality disorder without some degree of neurosis. In this regard, as developed later in Chapter 11, the so-called paranoid personality can be likened to a paranoid neurosis: such a person dreads the future since he fears that other people might manipulate him.

A person with a neurotic depression also dreads the future: he fears that others will reject him. But unlike the severely depressed person who is hopeless about the future and slowed down, the neurotically depressed person has not yet given up and does not view the future as globally bleak. As developed later in Chapter 11, neurotic depressive disorders (now called dysthymic disorders) are perhaps better termed as *chronic low self-esteem*.

It is generally recognized that neurotic individuals can become psychotic, acutely paranoid, or severely depressed. They are then given two diagnoses. In this regard, neurotic individuals who become drained after long struggles with anxiety, guilt, sadness, or anger may become severely depressed and hopeless about the future. The neurotic person's long struggle with these emotions, as we will see, can be understood in terms of misconstrued expectations that induce an emotional vicious cycle (spiral).

Part V of this book will explore the neurotic dread of the future and its treatment. I will focus on the following central themes:

1 Emotional vicious cycles (spirals) occur when catastrophic expectations, stemming from the past, distort current and future interpersonal expectations.
2 Future-oriented psychotherapy, by helping a person to choose and rehearse expectations of himself, fosters self-direction and helps to overcome undue sensitivity to the expectations of others, thereby interrupting emotional spirals.

Chapter 11 deals with different types of emotional spirals that are seen in some common neurotic disorders. It is proposed that a key factor in these emotional spirals is that catastrophic expectations, such as fears of being rejected or controlled, prompt transactions with other people to become desynchronized, which, in turn, prompt further mismatched expectations. Since the person's future images are largely centered around what others expect of him, his plans of action are uncertain and his emotions are precariously tuned to how he thinks others are viewing him.

Chapter 12 deals with future-oriented psychotherapy as a treatment for emotional spirals. After identifying and interpreting the nature of a specific emotional spiral, the patient is helped to interrupt it by developing future images of himself toward which he organizes his plans of action. In this way, he becomes more self-directed toward his own expectations rather than focusing on the views of others. This helps make the interplay between his future images, plans of action, and emotions less uncertain and more internally harmonized.

CHAPTER ELEVEN

Emotional Spirals and Interpersonal Expectations

The role of anticipations in influencing feelings and action is far more dominant than is generally recognized. The meaning of a person's experiences is very much determined by his expectations of their immediate and ultimate consequences.

A. T. BECK (1976, pp. 40–41)

The neurotic individual often dreads the future. In anticipating future consequences, he tends to fear that something catastrophic will happen. He fears that he will become helpless vis-à-vis other people who might reject or control him.

This chapter will explore the role of catastrophic expectations in neurotic emotionality. As outlined in Chapters 4 and 5, I propose that neurotic emotional spirals often stem from an over-focus on the past that prompts the person to misconstrue his future with unrealistic and exaggerated fears stemming from the past. The person becomes vulnerable to emotional spirals since his dread and uncertainty about the future prompts him to avoid present and future transactions with others and draws him further into the grip of past expectations.

When people look ahead into the future, they usually have a host of expectations. Some of these expectations refer to the immediate future, others are short term, and still others pertain to the distant future. This amalgam of expectations is reflected in different types of emotion. That is, as outlined in Chapters 2 and 3, emotions reflect an overall appraisal of expected outcomes. If these outcomes are appraised to be favorable, then pleasant, optimistic emotions ensue. By contrast, if the expected outcomes are appraised to be unfavorable, negative pessimistic emotions are experienced. Extremely negative expectations, as detailed in Chapter 9, are reflected in the feeling of hopelessness.

The outcomes of importance to most people usually involve either valued accomplishments or relationships with significant other people. These may be called *achievement goals* and *affiliation goals,* respectively. Examples of achievement goals are getting good grades in school, becoming successful in one's career, and completing a creative task. Examples of affiliation goals include being able to share intimacy, power, and meaning with friends, colleagues, and family. These attachments to others are basic for human survival and growth (Bowlby, 1969, 1973, 1980). Affiliation and achievement are thus basic human goals. When Freud was asked what constituted the normal person, he described these normal human goals as the capacity "to love and to work."

Expectations about "loving and working" are involved in different types of emotion. These expectations may pertain to ourselves or to what we expect of other people. The simplest situation to analyze is the expectation of our own work in terms of success or failure of an achievement goal. However, the expectations get more complicated and ambiguous when they involve our loving and working with other people (Wachtel, 1973). In relating to other people, we commonly have to anticipate not only what the other person is expecting now but also what he might be expecting later. In the words of Bateson (1958, p. 176): "We have to consider, not only A's reactions to B's behavior, but we must go on to consider how these affect B's later behavior and the effect of this on A." In practice, these complicated expectations are rarely thought out step by step; rather, they are reflected in how we *feel* about another person and how we think they are feeling about us. In this sense, emotions can be thought of as a special language for interpersonal relationships. That is, our feelings guide our relationships with other people by providing summary signals of immediate, short-term, and long-term expectations. Thus I will emphasize the role of interpersonal expectations in emotion.

Our expectations about other people, and what we think they are expecting of us, are vulnerable to distortion. These misconstrued interpersonal expectations commonly underlie emotional vicious cycles. That is, there is a series of mismatched interpersonal expectations that prompts a negative emotional spiral, which, in turn, further desynchronizes the transactions between people. The purpose of this chapter is to outline some of the main ways in which these emotional spirals evolve.

EMOTIONS: NORMAL VERSUS ABNORMAL

When do emotions become abnormal? What is their normal function? These are key questions that are often avoided in major psychological theories.

Some theories of the mind have even attempted to exclude emotions from the domain of inquiry, largely because emotions are hard to manage as discrete entities that fit nicely into a precise logical theory of behavior. Nevertheless, following the leads of Darwin and Freud, some theoreticians of the mind have proposed the evolutionary importance of emotions in controlling thinking, perception, and behavior (Bowlby, 1969; Pribram and Melges, 1969; Plutchik, 1962). From a clinical standpoint, psychiatrists wrestle daily with questions about the function of emotions and whether they are normal or abnormal in a given patient.

Let me briefly review the proposals I have made about the function of emotions. As outlined in Chapters 2 and 3, the normal function of emotions is to attune the person to overall discrepancies between the present and the future so that he adjusts his plans of action to his future images. Different types of emotion reflect different appraisals of outcomes. Positive, optimistic emotions reflect favorable expectations. Negative, pessimistic emotions reflect unfavorable expectations. Different emotions also are associated with varying degrees of urgency about the interval between the present and an anticipated future event or goal. That is, emotions attune the person to urgency about time. As overall signals about expected outcomes, emotions help reorganize linkages between plans and future images (goals). Since emotions last longer than momentary thoughts or perceptions, they often set the stage or context for thinking and perception. The long-lasting, reverberatory nature of emotions is mediated by limbic-frontal circuits in the brain, whose circular structures are ideally suited for engendering amplifications of feedback and feedforward loops (Sommerhoff, 1974). The reverberatory nature of emotions makes them conducive to initiating deviation-amplifications (spirals) that form the basis of virtuous as well as vicious cycles. In other words, emotions can tip the balance toward either a positive or negative direction. That is, once an emotion is aroused, it reverberates for a while, like a ripple effect; and as it reverberates, it is apt to bring other changes into its swirl. In this way, emotions frequently bias the nature of thinking and perception so that the person's cognitions, including his subsequent expectations, become colored by whatever emotion has been aroused.

Although normal emotions outlast perceptions and thoughts, abnormal emotions are commonly defined as those which far outlast the circumstances that aroused them in the first place. For example, the reaction of fear is understandable when a person is faced with a tiger, and this will continue for a while afterward, but if the person remains fearful for weeks or months afterward, the fear is deemed unrealistic.

Emotions also are thought to be abnormal when it is difficult to find an external event that precipitated them. For example, the person is anxious "for no reason at all." Such an experience is called *free-floating anxiety* to suggest that it is disconnected with any apparent precipitating event. However, careful studies have revealed that the concept of free-floating anxiety is questionable, since the anxiety can usually be traced to an event that precipitated an expectation (usually in the form of a visual image) that continues to trouble the person (Beck, Laude, and Bohnert, 1974). Such precipitating events, as will be shown, may become unrealistically exaggerated.

The intensity of an emotion is another factor in determining whether it is normal or abnormal. If a person is overwhelmed by an emotion so that he is unable to think or act, the emotional experience is obviously nonadaptive. Lesser degrees of emotion, which ordinarily help the person to keep at a task until the problem is solved, appear to facilitate adaptation. In this regard, different degrees of anxiety have been most systematically studied (Lazarus, 1966; Izard, 1977). Low to moderate degrees of anxiety usually activate the person to perform better, whereas high degrees of anxiety are often incapacitating. From a clinical standpoint, a similar case could be made for different degrees of guilt, sadness, and anger. That is, a modicum of anticipatory guilt is necessary to keep aggressive and sexual impulses in check. Likewise, the experience of sadness in the face of a loss appears to be necessary in order to free the person from a past attachment and to prevent escalation to unresolved grief and severe depression (Arieti, 1978; see also Chapter 10). Also, the experience of "controlled" anger in the face of an infringement on one's rights may lead to adaptive assertiveness, whereas an uncontrolled angry outburst is usually fruitless.

In conclusion, emotions are usually considered abnormal when they unrealistically outlast the inciting event and when they are so intense that they overwhelm and interfere with the person's perceptions, thinking, and action. Once a person has become overwhelmed by an emotion, the recurrence of the emotion may become a feared outcome in itself rather than a signal about what the person expects of himself and others. This loss of the signal function of emotions, as with "fear of fear," may engender an emotional vicious cycle which intensifies and prolongs the emotional experience beyond that which is adaptive.

EMOTIONAL VICIOUS CYCLES

Emotional vicious cycles commonly underlie what is considered "neurotic" anxiety, guilt, depression, and anger. Neurotic individuals are vulnerable to overreacting to seemingly innocuous events with excessive and persistent emotion. There are a number of competing theories about why this is so. For example, psychoanalytic theory posits that neurotic emotions stem from conflict between unconscious wishes (usually sexual or aggressive in nature) and prohibitions against such impulses, whereas the behavioral tradition holds that neurotic emotion represents a conditioned response to stimuli previously associated with upsetting events. In this section, I will not attempt to resolve these controversies, but propose how neurotic emotions frequently represent vicious cycles of misconstrued interpersonal expectations. It will be seen that this model, even though oversimplified as presented here, incorporates key features of other theories of neurotic emotion.

The central thesis is as follows: *Emotional vicious cycles occur when catastrophic expectations, stemming from the past, distort current and future interpersonal expectations.* The catastrophic expectations usually are of being rejected or controlled by others. These expectations are catastrophic because the person fears he will become helpless and inadequate vis-à-vis other people. As he becomes preoccupied with the expectations of others, he loses self-direction, and then becomes even more under the influence of others' expectations, including the expectations of significant other people of his past. His emotions become tuned to meeting the expectations of others in order to prevent the catastrophic expectations from happening. His plans of action become geared to pleasing others, not himself, in order to avert the catastrophic expectations. But since it is virtually impossible to meet the divergent expectations of significant other people in his environment and of his past, there are frequent mismatches between his plans of action and the expectations of others. These mismatches arouse further catastrophic expectations of being rejected or controlled, and he becomes increasingly emotional as the catastrophic expectations further distort his current and future interpersonal expectations, making the prospects of relating to others seem dismal. In his interactions with others, he comes *to dread the future*. The emotional vicious cycles occur since the expectations feed into one another and breed further emotions, which, in turn, breed expectations of the self becoming emotionally crippled vis-à-vis other people. Eventually, he comes to expect that he will be overwhelmed by emotion—he expects that his interactions with others will be clouded by anxiety, guilt, depression, or anger. Attempts to defend against this expectation of undue emotionality disrupt his current relationships with other people, further augmenting his problems.

This thesis deals with factors that are within the person as well as those which happen between people. It is thus both an intrapsychic and interpersonal proposal. It takes into account that the vast majority of people who come for treatment of an emotional disorder do so because they are having conflicts with people in their current environment, but it also considers that these current conflicts frequently represent transferences of the past onto present and future relationships (Segraves, 1978).

Let us now examine the thesis in terms of different types of emotional spirals and interpersonal expectations. For heuristic purposes, the major interactions are presented in a condensed and oversimplified form in Table 6. That is, not all forms of neurotic emotion fit within the format of Table 6, and it should be obvious that each person has a highly unique constellation of expectations that requires considerable detective work to unravel. Nevertheless, as a general aid to such detective work, some common themes that often escalate anxiety, guilt, sadness, and anger into pathological vicious cycles can be gleaned from the table. Each emotional disorder will be discussed more fully in later separate sections. At this point, I will focus on the central thesis.

The immediate expectations that differentiate the various emotions reflect different appraisals of outcomes. That is, some event (external or internal) triggers questions about what is likely to happen in the immediate future and what the person can do to cope with the expected situation (Lazarus, 1966). With anxiety, the immediate expectation is danger of some kind (Freud, 1926; Beck, 1971, 1976). Anxiety reflects the dread of some future event (Krauss, 1967). With guilt, the immediate expectation is imperfection of the self, especially in the eyes of others. Shame is closely related to guilt; it reflects the immediate expectation of imperfection in terms of not meeting up to one's own standards. With sadness, the immediate expectation is loss—loss of an important person, of a body function, of an achievement, and so forth. With the loss of an important person, what is often most painful is that the other person will not be there in future situations for support, succor, and sharing. With anger, the immediate expectation is that of infringement on one's property, rights, beliefs, or self-esteem (Melges and Harris, 1970). Thus far, the occurrence of these various emotions is understandable as normal emotional responses to different types of expected outcomes. The proposed relationships between the various emotions and the different appraisals of outcome are supported by a number of studies on emotion, as reviewed by Beck (1976), Arnold (1960), and Pribram and Melges (1969). At this initial stage, since the emotional responses serve as signals about immediate expectations, they are normal processes that are not pathological.

The pathological vicious cycles begin to arise when the person's immediate expectations become overly influenced by how he expects significant others will react to his initial emotional state. These expectations of other's intentions are often distorted by catastrophic expectations that the self will become helpless and inadequate in relation to others, like a small child relating to a rejecting or critical parent. The catastrophic expectations frequently represent transferences of the past onto the present and future. They are aided and abetted by the person's unwitting acceptance of past "script" messages. The

Table 6 Emotional Spirals and Interpersonal Expectations

Emotion	Immediate Expectation	Expectation of Others' Intentions	Catastrophic Expectation	Past Script	Present S–O Message[a]	Preventive Schemes	Escalated Clinical Syndrome
Anxiety	Danger	Uncertainty	S–helpless O–abandonment	Don't be yourself	Take over	Avoidance Escape	Anxiety neurosis Phobic neurosis
Guilt (shame)	Imperfection	Disapproval	S–incompetent O–humiliation	Be perfect	I'm in control	Perfectionism Rituals	Obsessive-compulsive neurosis
Sadness	Loss	Rejection	S–unlovable O–total rejection	Don't exist	Kick me	Self-reproach Obedience	Depressive neurosis
Anger	Infringement	Manipulation	S–entrapped O–domination	Don't trust	Bug off	Suspicions Revenge	Paranoid personality

[a]S refers to self; O refers to others.

225

latter are usually parental commands, given nonverbally or verbally, that told the person how he should be (or not be) as a child in order to meet the parents' expectations. (The script messages also can come from surrogate parents and dominant siblings.) If the person becomes controlled by these past script messages, he may send messages to people in his current environment that places them in a parental role similar to when the person was a child. If others comply with his message, this confirms his catastrophic expectations. If they do not comply, then the current interpersonal situation seems unfamiliar and uncertain, prompting further anxiety. The person may attempt to help himself with various preventive schemes (defenses) in order to avoid or dampen the emotional vicious cycle. Yet these defenses are often self-defeating since they impair the person's capacity for intimate relationships with other people in the here-and-now. Eventually, this swirl of expectations, warped by the past, escalates to a full-blown clinical syndrome called a neurosis. The interaction of these factors can be visualized as a snowball effect involving the variables listed at the top of Table 6.

Thus in these formulations, it can be seen how normal emotions can escalate to emotional vicious cycles when they become distorted by mis-construed interpersonal expectations, particularly by catastrophic expecta-tions stemming from the past. The invasion of the past into the future is perhaps the most common neurotic time warp.

In the course of these emotional spirals, the catastrophic expectations are rarely well formulated and, most common, the person is only partially aware of their occurrence. Frequently they take the form of visual images. That is, the person gets a glimpse of a dire consequence and suddenly becomes more emotional (Beck, Laude, and Bohnert, 1974). For example, one anxious patient who was fearful of flying got glimpses of himself screaming for his mother as the plane took off, and these glimpses just upset him more. At other times, the catastrophic expectations take the form of self-statements, such as, "I can't go on" or "They will ridicule me."

It should be pointed out that, once a negative emotional spiral starts, it tends to foreshorten future time perspective (see Chapter 2). This tends to close off considerations of other future alternatives. It also throws the patient back into the past where he may be gripped by catastrophic expectations shaped by past script messages.

In summary, the neurotic person is overconcerned with the expectations of other people, and these concerns reflect catastrophic expectations stemming from the past. This overconcern with a distorted view of the future often prompts him to neglect positive aspects of the future, as well as the present, that could help counterbalance his negative expectations.

ANXIETY SPIRALS

Let us now look at how anxiety can get caught in a spiral of misconstrued expectations so that it eventuates in an anxiety disorder. It is well known that anxiety is at the core of most neurotic problems, and that a given patient often has combinations of phobic, obsessive-compulsive, and depressive (dysthymic) features along with recurrent anxiety (Detre and Jarecki, 1971). For this reason, I will devote more discussion to anxiety than to the other emotional spirals that can be considered, at least in part, as derivatives of anxiety spirals.

Common themes that feed into one another in the escalation of an anxiety spiral are listed in Table 6. Initially, some event triggers the immediate expectation of danger. This event can be an external circumstance that threatens one's security, or it can be an internal impulse that the person believes is alien to his self-image (Kelly, 1955). His personal domain is threatened (Beck, 1976). Such experiences of anxiety have been felt, at one time or another, by everyone. The normal person uses the signal of anxiety as a spur to cope with the danger. He may do this by generating future alternatives (futuring) and developing plans of action to solve the problem (temporal organization). He often shares his anxiety with others and attempts to enlist their help in meeting the danger. By contrast, the neurotic individual is vulnerable to being thrown back into the past when he starts to generate expectations about the danger. The initial anxiety stirs catastrophic expectations that the self will be helpless, like a child who becomes panicked when abandoned by his parents. The neurotic person doubts whether he can help himself deal with the anxiety, and he is uncertain whether other people will turn away from him if he reveals his anxiety. Yet he feels highly dependent on the expectations of what others want of him, since his past script messages have drilled him to try to please others, not himself. That is, his past script message can be codified as ''don't be yourself,'' or some version of this, such as ''don't feel what you feel,'' ''be like me, not you,'' and so forth (Goulding and Goulding, 1978, 1979). Thus the neurotically anxious person feels uncertain about his capacity to depend on himself, yet he also feels uncertain about whether other people will abandon him if he reveals that he is anxious. The mounting uncertainty augments his anxiety. Moreover, he begins to fear the recurrence of anxiety and its escalation to panic.

It should be pointed out that the arousal of catastrophic expectations, such as being helpless and abandoned in the face of anxiety, may stem from what is called ''state-dependent learning.'' That is, the initial experience of anxiety reinvokes previous experiences associated with the state of anxiety, such as being helpless or threatened with abandonment as a child. The reverberatory nature of emotions makes them good candidates for generating such state-dependent spirals.

Even though the anxious person may want to conceal his anxiety from others, his anxiety is usually revealed to others by nonverbal signs such as jitteriness, sighing, sweating, and so forth. These signs are often read by other people as a message to "take over" for the afflicted person. If they do attempt to take over, this confirms the person's catastrophic expectation that he is becoming helpless. On the other hand, if they do not take over, he may feel that he will be abandoned. Either way, he foresees himself as helpless. In attempts to avoid the recurrence of anxiety and the interpersonal factors that seem to escalate it, he begins to avoid situations that bode risk, particularly the uncertainties of relating to other people. Here is seen a full-bown anxiety disorder, where the person feels highly vulnerable to becoming anxious, particularly in unpredictable interpersonal situations.

The emotional spiral of expectations involved in a phobic disorder is similar to that of an anxiety neurosis. The main difference is that the phobic patient has developed a set of preventive schemes (defenses) which ensures his attachment to significant others and prevents the escalation of anxiety so long as he can escape from certain situations. The phobic person fears certain places, such as being in water, or certain objects, such as bottles. More precisely, he fears the possible future implications of these places or objects (Serban, 1974). For example, it is not water per se that he fears but rather the possibility that he will drown. Or it is not the bottle per se that is feared but rather the possibility that the bottle could break, explode, and somehow harm him. These are elaborations of normal fears (Beck, 1976). For the phobic, mere possibilities are reacted to as though they were probabilities. In severe phobias, the endless elaboration of these fearsome possibilities often appears to be a way for them to maintain a dependent relationship with a significant other person, thereby preventing the catastrophic expectation of being abandoned. In other words, phobics do not feel helpless so long as they can get others to take over.

GUILT SPIRALS

Whereas anxiety and fears of becoming anxious are central to anxiety neurosis and phobias, anxiety about becoming guilty or ashamed are common emotions in obsessive-compulsive disorders. With guilt, the immediate expectation is that the person believes he has not fulfilled his duties to others or society; he expects others will judge him to be imperfect, unworthy, or wrong. With shame, the person's immediate expectation is that he will find himself wanting or imperfect according to his own internal standards. So far, these are normal experiences. However, in the neurotic, guilt and shame begin to snowball when the person begins to worry excessively about other people disapproving of his imperfections. This is spurred by catastrophic expectations that the self will become incompetent and that others will humiliate or ridicule one's self for being inadequate. These catastrophic expectations often come from the acceptance of past script messages to ''be perfect,'' so flawless that there is no need to be close to other people in order to depend on their help. Moreover, the experience of emotions and feelings is often thought to be alien to this ''be perfect'' script. In this regard, spontaneity and risk taking are anathema to the obsessive-compulsive (Salzman, 1979). The message that such patients usually send to other people is ''I'm in control,'' but also they are aware of an isolated, mechanical existence because of lack of intimate contact with other people. To prevent the escalation of their sense of guilt or shame for not being perfect at all endeavors, they commonly become perfectionistic with regard to a narrow range of orderly tasks. This is commonly manifested in attempts to gain rigid control over clock time (Pettitt, 1969; Campos, 1966). That is, they become extremely punctual, engage in doubting and indecision before attempting any task whose outcome might be unpredictable, and perform rituals, such as counting or hand washing, as superstitious ways of preventing dreaded consequences. Moreover, they become fearful of unfilled future time spans, since such unstructured time might bring uncontrollable events. In these ways, defensive attempts to prevent the escalation of guilt or shame may culminate in a full-blown obsessive-compulsive neurosis. These interactions between guilt, expectations of being found imperfect, and perfectionistic behavior are portrayed in Table 6.

It should be noted that persons with an obsessive-compulsive disorder often have the ''narrow future'' that predisposes them to a severe depression when aspects of this constricted future seem doomed to failure or seem lost (see Chapter 9).

DEPRESSION SPIRALS

With regard to depressive neurosis (now called dysthymic disorder), I have already dealt with the spiral of hopelessness involved in depressive illness (Chapter 9). At this point, I will therefore only highlight the common themes of Table 6 to illustrate the emotional vicious cycle involved in depressive neurosis, which might better be termed ''chronic low self-esteem.'' These individuals frequently interpret a loss as a rejection from others, and their feelings of rejection prompt catastrophic expectations that the self is unlovable and that other people will totally reject the self. These catastrophic expectations hark back to the past. The person with chronic low self-esteem has usually accepted the past script message of "'don't exist'" or some version of this such as "if you weren't around, I could have had a successful career" (Goulding and Goulding, 1979). The acceptance of such messages makes the child within the person feel unworthy and unlovable. In obedience to these past messages, the person may provoke rejecting behaviors from others in his current environment just to prove that this negative view of the self and his expectations of being rejected are correct. As Berne (1961, 1972) points out, the transactional message to others frequently takes the form of "'kick me.'" If others comply with this message, the person's catastrophic expectations are confirmed. If they do not comply, the situation seems unfamiliar and anxiety provoking. The person may then engage in self-reproach and self-criticism as a way of rejecting himself (Beck, 1976). The self-reproach also might serve to prevent total rejection from others, with the expectation that if the person is blaming himself, then others might be less harsh. Another preventive scheme seen commonly in this disorder is extreme obedience to other people's wishes and expectations. It is almost as though the person fears rejection so much that he is afraid he will offend others even when he is reasonably assertive. In this way, the sense of self-efficacy becomes further undermined.

ANGER SPIRALS

Whereas anxiety, guilt, and depression are emotions commonly associated with the term neurosis, recurrent bouts of anger have traditionally been conceptualized as clinical syndromes other than a neurosis. Paranoid personalities, paranoid states, and other nonpsychotic forms of paranoia, such as occurs in the borderline syndrome, are the labels given to people who are vulnerable to emotional spirals of anger. Paranoid disorders often are preoccupied with threats of being controlled, which makes them unduly suspicious (Chapter 8). Also, it should be recognized that anger often covers anxiety, but unlike excessive anxiety, the spiral of anger is likely to mobilize the person toward action (Melges and Harris, 1970). Whatever label one gives these disorders, angry spirals are frequent in clinical patients. Moreover, spouse, friends, and extended family are commonly caught in their swirl.

The dynamics of an angry emotional spiral is similar to the development of a paranoid ideation as outlined in Chapter 8. The important differences are that there is less fear of loss of self-control and more concern with thwarting manipulation from others at the instant when it is perceived. As listed in Table

6, the immediate appraisal of outcomes reflected in anger is that of an infringement on one's personal domain (Melges and Harris, 1970; Beck, 1971, 1976). Anger is a normal response to such an interference or offense. However, the emotional spiral of anger ensues when the person misconstrues others as being intentionally manipulative. This often relates to catastrophic expectations that the self will be entrapped while others will dominate the self. These catastrophic expectations stem from past script messages of "don't trust" or from actual experiences wherein the person was played for a "sucker." The angry individual essentially tells others to "bug off," but in so doing may provoke retaliation and control from them, thereby confirming his expectations that they are out to manipulate him. To prevent being controlled by them, he becomes suspicious and wary. Moreover, if he believes that he has been infringed upon, he may announce his intentions of revenge, which prompts his adversaries to become cautious and manipulative in self-defense. In this way, the anger snowballs into a tangle of distorted interpersonal expectations (Table 6).

AMBIVALENT ATTACHMENTS AND DESYNCHRONIZED TRANSACTIONS

From the discussion thus far, it can be seen that a major predisposing factor to an emotional vicious cycle is overconcern with what other people expect of the self. In attempting to please others, the neurotic person often loses his self-direction. He becomes molded by what others expect of him rather than pursuing his own future goals and images. When he does meet others' expectations, he often feels that he has somehow sacrificed his own identity and autonomy. This may prompt him to begin to push others away just at the time when others feel everything is going fine. These mismatched expectations frequently lead to desynchronized transactions between people. When transactions are desynchronized, they are "out of phase" with one another. The result is a lack of reciprocal intimacy between people. A host of interpersonal "games" and "rackets" evolve that distance people from each other just at the times when they appear to be getting closer. In this section, I will explore some common themes underlying these desynchronized transactions.

The most general problem is that getting close to someone carries the threat of being controlled by the other person. Attachment to another person means that some degree of personal autonomy has to be given up. This is an almost universal experience and, as such, is normal. In relating to other people, individuals have to work out a balance between attachment and autonomy, between what Satir (1967) calls relatedness and individuality. This polarity is the basis for what might be considered as normal ambivalence in interpersonal relationships.

However, this ambivalence becomes accentuated in neurotic individuals, where getting close to another person often arouses catastrophic expectations of being abandoned, humiliated, rejected, or dominated. That is, getting close to another person reawakens the risks of being a child who is attached to but also controlled by his parents. Commonly, the more attached the neurotic person gets to someone in his current environment, the more threatened he becomes by the possibility that the other person will reject or control him, as his parents did in the past. He is usually not aware of this past source of his threats. Moreover, he usually exaggerates or distorts some fault in his current relationship in order to justify pushing the other person away. He either avoids, rejects, alienates, or attempts to control the other person as ways to prevent the past catastrophe from recurring (Ezriel, 1952). In attempting to detach or distance himself from closeness to the other person, he usually is aware only of his discomfort at being with this other person and is not aware that he is attempting to prevent a past catastrophe from recurring. Interpretations aimed at making the person aware of his hidden agenda commonly take the following general form: You are avoiding a close relationship for fear of being controlled by this other person, but underneath you may fear closeness because it gives others the power to hurt you, like a parent who can control or reject his child.

The person on the receiving end of these distorted expectations is frequently mystified. He may be able to discern a recurrent pattern but does not understand it: just as they are getting closer, everything suddenly backfires. Of course, the other person usually also has ambivalent feelings about attachment implying control from the other. This may prompt him to respond in kind to the other's attempts at distancing just when they are getting closer.

The overall pattern of such transactions, as seen in marital discord and troubled families, is a series of interactions moving toward reciprocal synchrony until, at some point, the participants are suddenly out of phase with one another, where almost every statement or act is interpreted as having an ulterior motive aimed at controlling the other person. At this stage, each participant usually is transferring his or her past onto the present relationship and freezing the nature of any future interactions with catastrophic expectations. Once they are sufficiently distanced from each other, there is usually a reemergence of desires for attachment. In analyzing families, this ambivalent cycle between attachment and distancing has been called "distance regulation" by Kantor and Lehr (1975).

Ambivalence frequently gets expressed in terms of time issues. Being late, procrastination, and "dragging one's feet" are common examples of ways that a person can undermine the expectations of another person without directly opposing him. On the other hand, rushing the other person and expecting things "done yesterday" are common ways of assuming an authoritarian mode of relating. Mismatched expectations and miscommunications about time issues are frequent opening ploys in many interpersonal "games" described by Berne (1961, 1972), such as "uproar," "hassle," and "now you made me do it." That is, these games are often started by a crossed transaction about time, with one person rushing and the other dilly-dallying. The ultimate payoff for such games is to distance the participants in order to avoid the threat of control that comes with intimacy.

Unless people find ways of handling ambivalence in a marriage or family (or work group, for that matter), relationships are apt to become desynchronized at one time or another. It is those who try to force utopian goals of total bliss on a relationship that set themselves up for disappointment. Negative emotions, attendant to any close relationship, become submerged under the utopian myth, and begin to build up and contaminate the positive feelings. In time, there is only ambivalence. Transactions are desynchronized because the participants not only cannot agree but also cannot agree to disagree (Satir, 1967).

A good example of the submergence of ambivalence under a utopian myth occurs in women with psychiatric difficulties shortly after childbirth. The birth of a new baby is expected by all involved to be a joyous occasion, yet new mothers are about five times more vulnerable to psychiatric illness during the postpartum period (Melges, 1968). These women often feel that they must give a flawless performance as a new mother in order to meet the utopian expectations of their husbands and families, particularly their own mothers. When they find themselves resenting or rejecting the infant, this fills them with guilt, yet because of the utopian myth surrounding childbirth, they feel unable to share their ambivalence with others. They begin to feel that they are "bad mothers," and they desperately turn to others for advice. The advice is often conflicting. For example, the patient's mother and mother-in-law may cross swords about when and what to feed the baby. If the new mother attempts to meet these conflicting expectations, she soon becomes confused about her own identity as a mother. As she begins to vacillate, other people, such as her husband, begin to question her capabilities as a mother. This further undermines her self-esteem. Meanwhile, while the caretakers are doubting and fighting with each other, the baby is not getting fed on time. His screams of hunger augment the tangled ambivalences surrounding the scene. This series of desynchronized transactions during the postpartum period is unfortunately quite common.

When an individual loses his own identity, as is common in postpartum psychiatric problems (Melges, 1968), it is often because the person is attempting to define himself or herself in terms of others' expectations. That is, self-identity becomes compromised when an individual looks primarily to others for direction rather than being inner-directed toward his own chosen goals (Riesman, 1968). Without self-direction, the person is easily swayed by others. If the other people in his social network are ambivalent and unable to work through both their positive and negative feelings, the person who lacks identity is apt to become even more confused, since he cannot get a clear reading from others as to what they expect him to be. In short, a person who defines himself in terms of how others view him is likely to be poorly defined when others are markedly ambivalent.

Finally, it should be mentioned that ambivalence about getting too close to another person frequently underlies what is called "triangulation" in family interactions (Bowen, 1976). That is, as two people become threatened when they get closer, they involve a third person in order to diffuse the closeness. The third person is triangulated as either the go-between, rescuer, scapegoat, or accomplice to the conflicts arising between the original pair. For example, a daughter may be triangulated between mother and father as a way to keep them from getting too close.

The occurrence of triangulation at times when people are getting too close accounts for rather baffling role switches. Common role switches between three people who are enmeshed with one another have been described by Karpman (1968) as the "drama triangle" that is composed of the following roles: victim, persecutor, and rescuer. These roles are useful for describing who is doing what to whom at a given time, and for how the role positions may shift. For example, a victim player advertises that he is being persecuted by a persecutor, enticing a rescuer to rescue the victim; the rescuer often rescues by persecuting the persecutor, who becomes victim and who then may be persecuted (or rescued) by the former victim. In these drama triangles, it is uncanny how an accomplished victim player can manipulate others and win from an underdog position. That is, the victim player often gets a rescuer and persecutor to fight with one another while the victim player ostensibly remains helpless and victimized. This payoff of being able to control others through assuming the role of a victim is another factor that may perpetuate and reinforce neurotic behavior. Other ways of describing such payoffs are "secondary gain" or transactional "rackets," in which the person is using emotional expression in order to control others. A chronic victim player represents an extremely entrenched form of neurosis, yet the person is often unaware of the power he obtains from the victim role. That is, he indeed views himself as a victim, and this may have become intrinsic to his identity. Underneath he usually does not want to give up his emotional vulnerability, since to do so would mean relinquishing part of his identity and his ability to control others. In short, ambivalent attachments and his concept of himself as a victim have become a familiar way of life. Strangely, when rescuers get close to him and attempt to dislodge him from the victim role, he often transforms them to being persecutors, since his basic modus operandi is being threatened. Well-intentioned therapists, attempting to rescue such an inveterate victim, are often mystified at how they are suddenly viewed as persecutors just as they were getting closer to such a patient.

The combinations and permutations of these ambivalent attachments are legion and would require a treatise on family therapy to be covered adequately. Suffice it to say that, as a general rule, ambivalence about becoming attached to another person is commonly fraught with misconstrued expectations, stemming from the past, which prompt people to interact with one another as though they were dealing with ghosts of their pasts rather than the people moving with them in the present and future.

THEORETICAL COMMENT

This proposal about neurotic emotionality and interpersonal behavior has selectively focused on the role of misconstrued expectations. In order to emphasize the role of the future in neurotic emotions, the proposal deliberately neglects some important variables in neuroses, such as constitutional drives (for example, sex and aggression), inhibition of drives states, approach–avoidance conflicts, and reaction formation to opposite forms of overt behavior as ways of hiding inner drives and conflicts from oneself and others. A sophisticated integration of these multiple variables, couched in terms of a downward spiral of interacting personal and interpersonal factors leading to greater and greater misery, is given by Hine et al. (1972).

Why does neurotic misery persist? In terms of instrumental learning theory, behavior which proves to be nonrewarding and provokes punishment should eventually discontinue and become extinguished. Yet, in neuroses, misery-producing behavior and thinking continue despite the misery. This is called the "neurotic paradox" (Mowrer, 1960). One explanation for the neurotic paradox is that short-term rewards (for example, the immediate relief of anxiety) overrides long-term outcomes (Dollard and Miller, 1950). For example, with an anxiety disorder, the person often gets immediate relief of anxiety by avoiding anxiety-producing situations, but by so doing restricts the range of his behavior such that, in the long run, it becomes recurrently maladaptive. Another explanation is that the neurotic person often provokes feedback from other people that confirms his catastrophic expectations.

Although this may produce misery, it can be strangely reinforcing, since the feedback confirms the person's expectations. It can be seen that these explanations of the neurotic paradox are consistent with the proposal about the role of immediate, short-term, and long-term expectations in neurotic emotionality.

THERAPEUTIC IMPLICATIONS

If these proposals about the role of distorted personal and interpersonal expectations in emotional vicious circles are correct, it would follow that therapies designed to interrupt the interaction between the expectations would be helpful. It is interesting that various types of treatment for emotional disorders focus on one or two of these interactions. For example, the use of tranquilizing or panic-blocking medications helps to dampen the physiological concomitants of anxiety and related emotions and lessens the patient's expectation that the later recurrence of the emotion will overwhelm him (Zitrin et al., 1980). That is, he has less "fear of fear." In similar fashion, behavioral techniques for relaxation in the face of provocative stimuli give the patient a way to cope with expected bodily perturbations that formerly have overwhelmed him. Also, direct exposure to the fearsome event under the guidance of the therapist helps overcome the expectation of helplessness (Marks, 1978). Cognitive therapies commonly focus on modifying the patient's catastrophic expectations by challenging beliefs about the self interacting with others (Ellis, 1962; Beck, 1976). In particular, cognitive therapies attempt to modify the patient's self-statements and visual images that are aggravating the catastrophic expectations (Meichenbaum, 1977). The focus of psychoanalytic therapy is primarily on past experiences, particularly one's relationships with parents, which are being inappropriately transferred to the present. The patient also learns to recognize the ways he habitually defends against anxiety and other emotions. The "script analysis" of transactional analysis has a similar focus on the past, but there is also an interpersonal approach to modifying how the past script is played out in current interactions with other people. Along this line, family therapy and other social network types of therapy attempt to help patients streamline communications, work through ambivalences, and alter the nature of the patient's interpersonal support system so that, rather than being an aggravating factor, it serves as a buffer against anxiety (Pattison, Llamas, and Hurd, 1979).

Most of the above therapies focus on past and present interactions. It is assumed that improvement of past and present assumptions about the self relating to other people will have an indirect effect on future expectations. By contrast, future-oriented psychotherapy attempts to deal directly with a person's future expectations (Melges, 1972).

Future-oriented psychotherapy is designed to interrupt emotional spirals by helping the person develop sets of future images toward which he can organize and rehearse his plans of action. By enhancing self-direction, it helps overcome the neurotic tendency to be controlled by the expectations of other people. The person's emotions become tuned to his own futuring and plans of action rather than being overly concerned with the expectations of others. This approach is described in Chapter 12.

SUMMARY AND CONCLUSIONS

The central thesis explored in this chapter is as follows: Emotional vicious cycles occur when catastrophic expectations, stemming from the past, distort current and future interpersonal expectations. Points relevant to this thesis are summarized below:

1   The normal function of emotions is to serve as signals about expected outcomes, particularly with regard to interpersonal expectations.
2   Emotions become abnormal when they unrealistically outlast the inciting event and when they overwhelm, rather than guide, thinking, perception, and action.
3   Abnormal emotions usually represent vicious cycles that involve escalated interactions between the following factors: immediate expectations, expectations of others' intentions, catastrophic expectations, past script messages, present messages from self to others, and self-help preventive schemes.
4   In emotional vicious cycles, there also is the perpetuating fear of later becoming overly emotional. That is, fear of becoming anxious, guilty, depressed, or angry compounds the problem.
5   A neurotic individual's vulnerability to catastrophic expectations is often rooted in his tendency to meet the expectations of others rather than being self-directed toward his own goals. If a person loses his self-direction, his sense of identity becomes compromised.
6   Getting close to another person carries the risk of being controlled by the other person. This is a common source of ambivalence in interpersonal relationships. The ambivalence is heightened if the person equates getting close with catastrophic consequences, such as being a child who might be abandoned, humiliated, rejected, or dominated by a parental figure.

7   The inability to handle ambivalence is often the basis for unexpected rifts between people. Just as they are getting closer, the transactions suddenly become desynchronized. Distance is created between the participants as a way to decrease the hidden threats associated with getting closer.

8   The modification of distorted interpersonal expectations is important for the treatment of emotional vicious cycles.

Thus emotional spirals commonly involve an interaction between personal and interpersonal expectations as follows:

1   The transference of catastrophic expectations of being rejected or controlled by parental figures onto present and future interpersonal relationships

2   Fears that others might reject or control the self

3   Defenses to prevent others from rejecting or controlling the self

4   Ambivalence about being with others

5   Desynchronized transactions with others, giving rise to further interpersonal uncertainties and further emotion

In these ways, the person may become further drawn into the grip of catastrophic expectations of the past, and a spiral ensues from the inappropriate feedforward of these fearful anticipations. He comes to dread the future since his future images are misconstrued, his plans of action are uncertain, and anxiety mars his interpersonal relationships.

CHAPTER TWELVE

Future-Oriented Psychotherapy

When the individual is dominated by segmental drives, by compulsions,
or by the winds of circumstance, he has lost the integrity that comes
only from maintaining major directions of strivings.

GORDON ALLPORT (1955, pp. 50–51)

The essential purpose of future-oriented psychotherapy is to help people synthesize and organize their personal strivings (Melges, 1972). Although future events are inevitably uncertain and unpredictable, a person can decide now what kind of person he chooses to become so that he maintains his identity regardless of what happens in the future.

Future-oriented psychotherapy is designed to interrupt and prevent emotional vicious cycles. As described in Chapter 11, these emotional spirals occur when catastrophic expectations, stemming from the past, distort current interpersonal expectations. As the person becomes preoccupied with the expectations of other people, he loses his self-direction. He may then become increasingly controlled by others' expectations and further drawn into the past. In a sense, his personal future becomes owned by others, not himself. His emotions become tuned to meeting the expectations of others, rather than serving as signals that guide the reorganization of his plans of action toward his own goals and expectations. Future-oriented psychotherapy counteracts these emotional vicious cycles by helping patients become self-directed toward their own future choices rather than being unduly swayed by the past or the expectations of other people.

Various types of psychotherapy differ according to the attention given to the past, present, or future (see Chapter 6). These different temporal foci include helping the patient to (1) free up inappropriate adhesions to his past, (2) modify his present responses and interactions, and (3) develop effective

239

plans of action to meet realistic future goals. Although an integrated treatment approach would involve all three temporal stages, the future-oriented approach has been relatively neglected.

The central aims of future-oriented psychotherapy are to help patients (1) choose and clarify realistic personal goals and (2) develop and rehearse plans of action that will achieve their chosen goals. Its main methods consist of using visual imagery to create a realistic future self-image and employing time projection for integrating plans of action with the future self-image. These processes are based on the principles of futuring and temporal organization, as described in Chapter 3. That is, as images of the future are brought into the psychological present, plans of action are generated to meet the evolving images.

Although future-oriented psychotherapy incorporates information from the past and present, its main focus is on reconstructuring future expectations and strivings in order to interrupt vicious cycles. This *future-oriented reconstruction* is reflected in its abbreviation as FOR therapy. FOR therapy helps patients crystallize their identities, as well as what to do next and how to go about it. Emphasis is placed on what the person is striving *for*.

Before describing the treatment procedure and its application to patients with problems with identity diffusion, low self-esteem, and various types of emotional vicious cycles, some of the major points of this book will be reviewed in order to outline the rationale of future-oriented psychotherapy.

THE RATIONALE OF FUTURE-ORIENTED PSYCHOTHERAPY

The processes and techniques of FOR therapy are designed to crystallize a person's core identity so that he will have a set of constructs about the self that will serve as useful guides into the future. It is postulated that the crystallization of an identity directed toward the future will make him less vulnerable to undesirable influences from the past.

As outlined in Chapter 11, emotional vicious cycles occur when catastrophic expectations, stemming from the past, distort current and future interpersonal expectations. A lack of future orientation may make individuals more vulnerable to these catastrophic expectations from the past. On the other hand, the development of self-direction toward the future is likely to interrupt emotional vicious cycles and help transform them into virtuous cycles of self-fulfillment.

Considerable experimental work has demonstrated that behavior is controlled by its consequences. Since humans have an extended time sense, a person's behavior is particularly under the control of anticipated consequences (Bandura, 1974, 1977; Melges and Harris, 1970). Such anticipations guide his current behavior and beliefs (Kelly, 1955; Bannister and Mair, 1968). It would therefore appear that changing a person's view of his own future would modify his behavior and beliefs about himself and others.

An extended and positive future orientation is associated with coping, high ego-strength, the capacity to delay gratification, high self-esteem, pleasant emotions, and the belief that skill, rather than fate, determines one's destiny. By contrast, a foreshortened and negative future orientation is associated with a failure to cope, low ego-strength, impulsivity, low self-esteem, unpleasant emotions, and the belief that chance and luck, rather than skill, determine what happens to a person. The negative future outlook and associated factors may culminate in hopelessness (for review, see Chapters 2, 3, 9, and 11).

The restoration of hope is fundamental to all forms of psychotherapy (Frank, 1974). This is accomplished primarily through helping the patient achieve greater self-control while he modifies unrealistic expectations of himself and other people (Strupp, 1970). These directions appear to be facilitated by certain qualities in a therapist, such as genuineness, compassion, accurate empathy, and warmth, which do not engulf or possess the patient (Meltzoff and Kornreich, 1970; Lazarus, 1978). Besides these important therapist qualities, it would appear that specific techniques designed to help patients become more self-directed toward the future would raise hope, enhance self-control, and modify unrealistic expectations.

In light of the above considerations, a central therapeutic question is, How can a patient be helped to develop an identity that is more self-directed toward his own future goals? Aside from recognizing self-defeating past patterns and deciding to change them, there are two interrelated factors that appear central to this endeavor: (1) structuring the ego-ideal and (2) enhancing self-reinforcement.

Structuring the ego-ideal is important for developing a core identity that is not just a reflection of past identifications and the expectations of other people. It involves prompting the patient to clarify the kind of person he chooses to become. Erikson (1959, p. 149) states that "the imagery of the ego ideal could be said to represent a set of to-be-strived for but forever-not-quite-attainable ideal goals for the self." According to Erikson (1959, p. 89), a clear image of the ego-ideal gives rise to the sense of identity through confidence in "one's ability to maintain inner sameness and continuity" and also enhances self-esteem through the "conviction that one is learning effective steps toward a tangible future, that one is developing a defined personality within a social reality which one understands." In support of this, research has shown that the discontinuity of past, present, and future is associated with the fragmentation of identity (depersonalization), and also that changes in future outlook and self-esteem wax and wane together (see Chapters 7 and 9). It would therefore appear that helping patients to attain "inner sameness" with a feeling of continuity toward a hopeful future would be therapeutic for establishing identity and raising self-esteem.

In order to help a patient restructure his ego-ideal with a feeling of continuity toward the future, future-oriented psychotherapy prompts the patient to make choices as to the kind of person he wants to become, and vivifies these choices through visual images that are time-projected into the future. The therapeutic usefulness of guided imagery has been pointed out by Leuner (1969), Shorr (1972), Susskind (1970), Kosbab (1974), and Singer (1974). The use of visual images may have the advantage of bypassing erroneous beliefs about the self maintained through verbal self-statements (Beck, 1976; Ellis, 1962). In this regard, the use of visual images might be conceived as facilitating change predominantly by right cerebral hemispheric functions rather than by the linguistic modes of the left hemisphere (see Chapter 2). Another therapeutic advantage to the restructuring of visual images is that they may mitigate the impact of catastrophic expectations from the past, which are often visual flashbacks (Beck, Laude, and Bohnert, 1974; Horowitz, 1976). That is, well-structured, positive visual images about the self may help overcome traumatic past images, thereby interrupting emotional vicious cycles.

Thus helping the patient develop clear images of the kind of person he wants to become is a fundamental method of FOR therapy. It is called self-futuring. Specific techniques for the creation, synthesis, and imprinting of this restructured ego-ideal will be described later. Once this future self-image has been formulated and appropriately revised as realizable internal values for the self, the stage is set for the temporal organization of plans of action that will meet the patient's chosen goals. That is, with well-defined criteria for the future self-image, the person's plans of action are more likely to become self-reinforcing since he is in a better position to appraise whether or not his intentions and actions are approaching his chosen goals. As a person becomes more self-reinforcing, he becomes less dependent on the expectations or views of others for his sense of worth (Bandura, 1969, 1977).

A person becomes more self-reinforcing when his plans of action become increasingly congruent with his goals. When the outcomes of his plans meet his goals, positive and optimistic emotions occur (Pribram and Melges, 1969). The induction of positive emotions, in turn, prompts the person to generate further goals and plans and to explore potential links between new potentialities and opportunities. In short, the temporal integration of goals and plans may induce virtuous cycles of self-reinforcement.

This process is deliberately enhanced in FOR therapy by helping patients to organize their plans of action temporally toward their chosen goals. As explained later, techniques for doing this largely involve helping patients link anticipated events with their chosen future images. This is done by time-projected rehearsals that streamline present plans of action toward the chosen goals. These connections through time are fostered by a setting of expectancy that there will be a match between the goals and the outcomes of the plans. Research has shown that the temporal juxtaposition of events within a setting of expectancy fosters conditioning in humans (Bandura, 1974, 1977; Mischel, 1973). In FOR therapy, the intent is to help patients make new time connections between the present and the future in order to overcome self-defeating past patterns.

Another reason for temporally organizing plans of action toward the patient's future self-image is to endow the visual images with a sense of time. That is, the visual images are given both duration and succession. When the visual images are woven into the fabric of time, they appear to have a greater sense of reality as compared to fleeting fantasies about the future. In this way, the patient familiarizes himself with new ways of reaching out into the future.

In summary, future-oriented psychotherapy is based primarily on the principles of futuring and temporal organization (see Chapter 3). Self-futuring is the process of bringing the future into the psychological present in order to choose and clarify realistic personal goals. Temporal organization involves the sequencing of plans of action in order to meet the chosen goals. In future-oriented psychotherapy, self-futuring is synthesized with temporal organization in order to provide the patient with new coping strategies.

ESSENTIAL STAGES OF FUTURE-ORIENTED PSYCHOTHERAPY

There are five essential stages of future-oriented psychotherapy: (1) assessment and selection of patients; (2) interpretation of vicious cycles; (3) redecisions to overcome past patterns; (4) self-futuring; and (5) temporal organization. The uniqueness of FOR resides in the last two stages, but as outlined below the earlier stages are essential for priming the patient for the later interplay between self-futuring and temporal organization.

An overview of the important steps involved in FOR therapy is outlined in Figure 2. The nature of these steps will become clear in the discussion below.

Figure 2 can serve as a checklist for guiding the conduct of FOR therapy, once the steps are understood.

Figure 2   Flow Sheet of Procedures for Future-Oriented Psychotherapy

1 *Assessment and Selection of Patients*
Rule out psychosis and organic brain syndromes.
Consider patients with low self-esteem, emotional (neurotic) spirals, and identity disorders.
Obtain baseline tests, especially (see Appendix A):
    Eriksonian semantic differential of the self (ESD)
    Short future outlook inventory
Check for capacity to visualize.
Check for hypnotizability, and explore use of hypnosis as adjunct with patient.
Do interview with family or social network, and explore combination of individual and family treatment.

2 *Interpretations of Vicious Cycles*
Formulate interaction between current expectations, catastrophic expectations, and past script messages that may be feeding into an emotional vicious cycle.
Discuss and check out formulation with patient.
Revise as necessary.

3 *Redecisions*
Prompt patient to redecide whether he wishes to continue to obey his past script messages.
The redecisions include taking a stance against:
    Destructive past script messages
    Catastrophic expectations
    Collecting payoffs (for example, bad feelings or feeling superior or inferior)

4 *Self-futuring*
Decide on uncontaminated day about three months ahead.
Time-project patient to that day:
    Activate visual imagery as though taking place in present.
    Go through entire day as patient generates images (choices) about himself:
        Morning: Focus on images that flow from redecisions.
        Afternoon: Dimensionalize some choices according to bipolar scales of ESD and redecisions.
        Evening: Allow patient to generate unique images pertinent to his chosen ego-ideal.
    Record future choices (ESD and otherwise).
In subsequent sessions, crystallize images:
    Check for realizability.
    Challenge social expectations.
    Reconcile conflicts.
    Encourage homework.

5 *Temporal Organization*
Feedback: Help patient to appraise whether he is meeting his chosen goals and whether he is becoming more self-reinforcing.
Linking images with the past:
    Energize future choices with activation of "free child" experiences.
    Use metaphors.
Cueing images with the present:
    Self-stroking reminders.
    Color reminders.
    Clock time reminders.

Rehearsals toward the future:
   Short-term:
      Anticipatory alternativism: positive coping imagery
      Future autobiography: retrospective view of future week
   Long-term:
      Temporal role–playing (for example, dialogue between present and future self)
      Psychodrama of future (for example, time-telescoped stage setting or "life review" at time of
      death)

ASSESSMENT AND SELECTION OF PATIENTS

Patients are assessed according to the interviewing and assessment strategies outlined in Chapter 5 and the mental-status examination (Melges, 1975). Also, they are given a battery of brief tests, such as the Eriksonian semantic differential of the self (ESD), the future outlook inventory, the modified internal–external control scale, the semantic differential of emotions, and the temporal integration inventory. These tests are listed in Appendix A. The patient is instructed to fill them out according to his experiences of the preceding few days. The tests are used not only for assessment but also for evaluation of progress during therapy, as explained later.

Patients who are suitable for FOR therapy are those whose primary problem is an imbalanced or fragmented temporal perspective, particularly with regard to future time perspective. That is, as outlined in Table 2, patients with time disorientation, temporal disintegration, and rate problems are, for the most part, excluded, whereas those with problems of temporal perspective and desynchronized transactions with others are considered for FOR therapy.

The reason for excluding actively psychotic patients is that the time projection techniques of FOR are difficult to conduct with a person who is temporally disintegrated. That is, a person has to be able to distinguish past, present, and future before he can usefully project himself into the future. Furthermore, time projection may confuse a person who cannot keep track of sequences. It should be noted, however, that after a patient has recovered from a psychosis, some aspects of FOR therapy may be useful, particularly for establishing identity.

In terms of standard psychiatric diagnoses according to the DSM-III (1980), patients who are diagnosed as having one of the following conditions can be considered for FOR therapy: identity disorder, depersonalization disorder, anxiety disorder (including generalized anxiety, panic, phobic, and obsessive-compulsive disorders, formerly termed "neuroses"), dysthymic disorder (formerly depressive neurosis), and adjustment disorder. Also, some personality disorders (dependent, antisocial, and borderline) as well as a few cases of multiple personality have been treated successfully with FOR therapy.

In general, FOR therapy is indicated for nonpsychotic patients whose predominant problems are lack of identity, low self-esteem, and recurrent emotional spirals of the neurotic type. Other indications for FOR therapy include a foreshortened or incoherent future time perspective, an over-concern with the expectations of other people, and a past so rife with repeated traumata that it appears that working with the present and future will be more expedient than delving into the past.

With a patient who has unresolved grief, grief-resolution should be conducted before proceeding to FOR therapy (see Chapter 10). The patient usually has to let go of such preoccupations with the past before he can fully engage in the future.

It is wise to interview the family and social network during the assessment stage (see Chapter 5). This helps the therapist become aware of specific social conflicts that the patient has to deal with during the course of FOR therapy. Also, it helps pave the way for the family and social network to be supportive of the patient's self-futuring. As explained later, when there are prominent desynchronized transactions with others, individual future-oriented psychotherapy can be usefully combined with family therapy.

Patients who benefit the most from FOR therapy are those who can readily produce visual images. Although 95% of people are capable of doing this to some extent (Horowitz, 1970), I have found that about 20% of my patients have difficulty with visual imagery and predominantly process information in the auditory mode. For these latter patients, traditional verbal and cognitive forms of therapy are more appropriate. Testing for the capacity for visual imagery can be done clinically; for example, check the clarity with which a patient can visualize looking at himself in the mirror that morning or whether he can recapture a scene in his "mind's eye" from an earlier part of the interview. Another test is to have him visualize himself eating an apple; while doing this, if he gets concomitant impressions of taste, texture, and smell, he is probably a good visualizer.

Since hypnosis can be a useful adjunct to FOR therapy, the patient's wish to use hypnosis and his degree of hypnotizability should be assessed by the usual means (Hilgard, 1965; Spiegel and Spiegel, 1978). Hypnotic time distortions can be used to imprint visual images and facilitate time projection (see Chapter 6). The use of hypnosis in FOR therapy will be explained later.

Finally, it should be noted that those patients who do extremely well with FOR therapy are similar to those found suitable for short-term dynamic psychotherapy (Marmor, 1979; Davanloo, 1978). In general, such patients are psychologically minded, responsible, reasonably trusting, aware of their feelings, and, most important, motivated to change. Such patients can make significant changes within 12–30 sessions. It should be emphasized, however, that FOR therapy is certainly not restricted to such "ideal" patients, and that difficult, long-standing problems have responded well to FOR therapy, even after traditional modes of therapy have failed.

INTERPRETATION OF VICIOUS CYCLES

After the assessment and selection stage, the next stage of FOR is the interpretation of vicious cycles. Much of the information relevant to the nature of a particular patient's vicious cycles usually has been already gleaned from the assessment interviews. The main purpose of formulating and expressing these vicious cycles to the patient is to work out a rationale that will serve as a common background shared by both therapist and patient for proceeding to subsequent stages of FOR therapy. Providing a rationale is conducive to effective psychotherapy (Frank, 1974). Since it is necessary for the patient to understand the rationale, the therapist should obtain feedback from the patient about the interpretations of the vicious cycles. Ideally, the formulation should be a collaborative enterprise.

The key to pointing out a vicious cycle is to show the patient how one change augments other changes, leading to a snowball effect that I term a *downward spiral*. The patient is told that the first task of both therapist and patient is to discover what factors feed into these downward spirals and when the downward spirals are most likely to occur. This task will require joint detective work. After this, the next task will be to find ways of forestalling the downward spirals and inducing upward spirals. In short, the overall rationale of the therapy will be to transform vicious cycles into virtuous cycles.

A straightforward way to introduce the idea of a downward spiral is the example of "fear of fear." That is, a person who becomes anxious often becomes fearful of becoming anxious again, and his fear about becoming anxious may snowball into panic. Most patients grasp this process immediately.

Next, the therapist can introduce the idea that expectations can feed into one another, leading to a snowball effect. That is, in interacting with another person, an individual has immediate expectations of himself, short-term expectations of what the other person will do or say, and also long-term expectations of the nature of their relationship. These expectations may be in conflict or they may augment one another. This idea is best introduced by simply commenting about a connection that the patient has revealed during the interview. For example: "You become anxious when you are unsure of how other people will react to you," or "You expect perfection in yourself since you don't want other people to think that they can control you." If the patient grasps these ideas, it is then opportune for the therapist to make a brief statement about how expectations govern behavior and emotion.

Ideally, after a few gentle probes and explanations, the patient himself will begin to formulate his particular spiral of expectations. In such instances, the therapist serves mainly as a coach, giving feedback when necessary but allowing the patient to make the important connections himself. If the patient can define the problem largely by himself, he is in a better position to initiate problem solving on his own rather than expecting the therapist to do it for him.

Compromises usually have to be made with the above ideal. That is, the patient has to be gently guided into relevant areas (see Chapter 5). In doing this, it is useful for the therapist to keep in mind the key expectations and variables that commonly feed into an emotional vicious cycle as outlined in Table 6. In guiding the patient to make such connections, it is wise to progress from current expectations and behaviors toward the catastrophic expectations related to the past script messages.

For example, with a patient with chronic low self-esteem (that is, a depressive neurosis), the progression of interpretations might go as follows: "From what you say, you are feeling low about yourself because you expect other people will reject you. . . . Does it sometimes seem that you beat on yourself as a way to prevent others from beating on you further? . . . Perhaps sometimes you are setting yourself up to get put down by others as a way to confirm your expectation that they will reject you. . . . Have you noticed that your fears of being rejected become greater when you get closer to someone? [Finally:] When you get close to someone, do you expect that something catastrophic will happen? . . . Like when you got close to your mother, and then felt rejected by her? . . . When your mother left you as a child, it was like giving you the message of 'don't exist.' . . . When the little kid in you obeys that message, you expect to be rejected. . . ."

Such interpretations, of course, have to be tailored to the individual. The reasons for working gradually toward the catastrophic expectations and past script messages include the following considerations: First, the patient is often unaware of the influence of his past on his current expectations. If he becomes aware of these influences too abruptly, he either becomes frightened by his lack of control over his thinking or he becomes resistant to the idea that these factors may be controlling him. Second, once he experiences the impact of the catastrophic expectations and past script messages, he commonly is at an impasse; he is at a loss as to how to get out of their grip. He may begin to wallow in the past in an effort to redo it somehow; he wants to turn back time, which is not only impossible but also interferes with current coping (Mann, 1973). Third, when the patient realizes his impasse, he is primed for discovering alternative ways of feeling, thinking, and behaving. In other words, he is ready for the reconstruction stages of FOR therapy.

Before proceeding further, the therapist should summarize the particular interaction of expectations that feed into the patient's downward spiral. The patient should be encouraged to disagree, revise, and modify the formulation. It is most important that both therapist and patient have a common understanding of the nature of the emotional vicious cycle. In particular, both should be aware of factors or situations that often trigger the downward spiral so that each is alert to preventing its escalation.

After the summary, a brief rationale for the reconstruction stages of FOR is explained. This can be done in a straightforward manner without getting into details. For example: "So we've agreed that you are caught in a web of expectations. The question is how to get out of them, if you choose to do so. Of course, your being alert to when these expectations begin to feed into one another may help forestall a downward spiral. But there are some other methods which may be of further help. These methods are aimed at changing the nature of your expectations according to your own choices. There are essentially three steps. First, we will see if you can make some "redecisions" about some of the past messages you seemed to have bought about yourself. Second, you will construct a future self-image, something that you will see so clearly in your mind's eye that it will be like a guide or inner gyroscope. Third, you will do some 'time traveling' in order to rehearse plans of action that will meet the goals you have chosen for yourself. Again, the basic idea is to help you change your expectations about yourself so that you can stop the downward spirals and start some upward spirals."

At this point, the patient is told that the reconstruction process usually takes from 12–30 sessions, his questions are answered, and he is then asked whether he would like to proceed. Patients' reactions are diverse. Some are enthusiastic, others are skeptical and want to think it over, some are afraid of giving up old familiar ways (even if they have been painful), and still others are reluctant to decide anything about themselves in the future for fear that this would rob them of the leeway of controlling others through their symptoms. These factors have to be handled sensitively while emphasizing that future-oriented psychotherapy will not transform the person in any way other than to facilitate the realization of one's own personal choices.

REDECISIONS

In each of us as adults, there are remnants of our past that have not changed with the passage of time. In transactional analysis, these remnants of the past are referred to as the "child" ego-state (Berne, 1961, 1972). The child within us is highly impressionable, sensitive, and vulnerable to being influenced by past script messages from parental expectations. In addition, the child within us is a source of fun and energy and, if we have thrived long enough to become adults, was probably smart enough to learn how to survive. The Gouldings (1978, 1979) emphasize that an important way that the child learns to survive is to go along with the parental expectations. That is, the child *decides* to obey the parental script in order to survive. What was once decided can be *redecided*. This is the basis for "redecision" therapy, which attempts to free the child within us from parental expectations no longer appropriate to our present and future (Goulding and Goulding, 1979).

Since redecision therapy has been well described in the Gouldings' books, only some major points will be outlined here. Within the context of FOR therapy, redecision therapy is useful for prying patients away from the past and for helping them take a firm stand against catastrophic expectations.

In formulating an emotional vicious cycle with a patient, the nature of the patient's catastrophic expectations have already been assessed. These catastrophic expectations usually are tied into the past script messages. That is, according to the oversimplified outline of Table 6, the relationships between the patient's past script messages and his catastrophic expectations are as follows: Accepting the script message "don't be yourself" gives rise to the catastrophic expectation that the self will be helpless if abandoned by others, since the person believes he cannot rely on his own resources. Accepting the script message of "be perfect" gives rise to the catastrophic expectation that if the self is somehow incompetent, others will humiliate the person. Accepting the script of "don't exist" gives rise to the catastrophic expectation that the self is unlovable and deserving of total rejection by others. Accepting the message of "don't trust" makes the self fear that if he is entrapped, he will be dominated and controlled by others.

Aside from the above script messages, the Gouldings also list some other common variants, such as don't feel; don't belong; don't succeed; don't grow up; don't get close; and so forth. The task is to get the patient's child within him to reverse his early decision to obey these script messages. He is prompted to make a redecision.

In order to activate the child ego-state, the patient is asked to take a recurrent emotion, such as depression, and take it back into the past to a scene when he was a child feeling depressed with parental figures. He is prompted to be and feel like the child he once was, and to reenact the scene as though it were taking place in the present. The patient's child within him is encouraged to confront the script messages and to make a redecision about them. For example, if he received the message of "don't exist," rather than accepting and obeying this script by chronically entertaining ideas of suicide, he makes a redecision. The redecision can be dramatized through role-playing techniques. For example, the image of the patient's mother may say to him, "Get lost!" but the child within him retorts: "I won't obey that; I will exist; I will take care of myself, regardless of what you want." As is known to many transactional therapists who have used the Gouldings' methods, the dramatization of these redecisions can be emotionally moving. The redecisions also can have long-lasting therapeutic benefit, especially with patients who are psychologically minded and motivated to change.

In my experience, the most effective redecisions are those where the child within the person takes a firm stance against the following: (1) the destructive script messages, (2) the catastrophic expectations that are expected when the script messages are disobeyed, and (3) collecting the "payoffs" that stem from obedience to the script messages, such as familiar bad feelings about oneself or feeling one-up or one-down in relation to others. In this regard, it is important to point out that one of the quickest ways to discover a destructive script message is to consider a patient's recurrent bad feelings with others as a kind of "payoff" for following a script (Goulding and Goulding,1978, 1979). That is, the bad feelings are signals that the patient is obeying his parental dictates; they are a twisted kind of payoff since they help him maintain his position in relation to his parents; even though he feels bad, he feels protected by his parents; his emotions are related to the past, not to the present or future. To decide not to collect the payoff for feeling bad (for example, getting attention or strokes) is an important aspect of redecision work.

For many patients, however, these verbal redecisions are just beginnings which must be given further structure and reinforcement through time-projected visual imagery in order for the patient to overcome self-defeating patterns. In FOR therapy, the person is helped to structure his future self-image in line with his redecisions. The chosen future self-image is designed to serve not only as a buttress against catastrophic expectations stemming from the past but also as an internal guide for exploring new opportunities for personal growth. Moreover, the visual imagery helps elaborate the redecisions made by the child ego-state. In this regard, Berne (1972) emphasizes that the parental script messages are usually auditory (verbal), whereas the child's mode of thinking is largely visual.

A useful way to bridge redecisions with future images is to prompt the patient to differentiate himself from major identification figures. For example, a young man who complained of feeling "dead and unreal" felt engulfed by his mother whom he viewed as "dead, eerie, and not belonging to this world"; the patient was asked whether he wanted to remain similar to his mother or to make some redecisions as to how he would choose to be different from his mother; he chose to differentiate from his mother by becoming "alive, free, and belonging." These initial choices were then projected into the future as he visualized himself being and behaving as "alive, free, and belonging." Thus out of his redecisions to be different from his mother came the initial nidus for his identity reconstruction, which was elaborated further by the last two stages of FOR therapy: self-futuring and temporal organization.

SELF-FUTURING

The patient's redecisions provide the general framework for the next stage of FOR therapy, called self-futuring. This involves helping the patient bring anticipated scenes of his personal future into the psychological present so that he can make choices about his becoming self. These choices are transformed into internal goals or values by vivifying them through visual imagery. The aim of self-futuring is to help the patient construct a nurturant and realistic ego-ideal so that he can maintain his identity regardless of the expectations of others in the past, present, or future. Through creating a unique synthesis of personal choices, the patient is prompted to establish a core identity that will thwart downward spirals and hopefully instill upward spirals.

It is remarkable how people with recurrent emotional problems have difficulties imagining themselves in the future. When they are prompted to view themselves in the future, the pictures they get are often hazy or negative. The negative projections into the future frequently represent the extrapolation of a self-defeating life script. Even when pressed to conjure up a positive image of themselves in the future, many of them quickly return to negative images, while others get only a vague and an ill-defined image of a global-feeling state, such as happiness. It would seem to follow that if a person is unable to imagine positive images of himself in the future, his personal future is likely to be a replica of his negative past. Similarly, if a person has difficulty in delineating specific images that define the self in the future, his feeling of identity in the future is likely to be vague and diffused.

The techniques of self-futuring are designed to counteract the above difficulties by helping patients construct specific future images of themselves according to fundamental dimensions of the self-concept. These fundamental dimensions are captured in brief form in what is called the Eriksonian semantic differential of the self (ESD—see Appendix A). The bipolar scales of this test were derived from Erikson's (1959) epigenetic life stages and were subsequently refined for research and clinical purposes (Melges et al., 1971). During the earlier assessment stage, the patient has already depicted himself

in terms of "My Own View of Myself Now" on the bipolar scales of the ESD.
He has done this by checking one of the spaces interposed between each of the
following bipolar scales:[1]

TRUSTING	__:	__:	__:	__:	__:	__:	__:	DISTRUSTING
SELF- CONSCIOUS	__:	__:	__:	__:	__:	__:	__:	SELF- ASSURED
ASSERTIVE	__:	__:	__:	__:	__:	__:	__:	DEFENSIVE
INADEQUATE	__:	__:	__:	__:	__:	__:	__:	COMPETENT
REAL	__:	__:	__:	__:	__:	__:	__:	UNREAL
DISTANT	__:	__:	__:	__:	__:	__:	__:	WARM
CARING FOR OTHERS	__:	__:	__:	__:	__:	__:	__:	SELF- ABSORBED
PHONY	__:	__:	__:	__:	__:	__:	__:	SINCERE
STRONG	__:	__:	__:	__:	__:	__:	__:	WEAK
PASSIVE	__:	__:	__:	__:	__:	__:	__:	ACTIVE
GOOD	__:	__:	__:	__:	__:	__:	__:	BAD
FEMININE	__:	__:	__:	__:	__:	__:	__:	MASCULINE

[1]In the bipolar scales of the ESD, it can be seen that the socially desirable, or positive, pole of each scale is
alternated from left to right so as to avoid response sets. Also, with the last scale of feminine versus
masculine, it is assumed that for a woman the feminine pole is positive, whereas for a man the masculine
pole is positive. The total ESD score is derived from giving each space between a bipolar scale a value of
one to seven, with seven representing the positive pole, and then summing the values of all the bipolar
scales; see Appendix A. The total ESD score can serve as a rough idea of overall change during FOR
therapy. On the other hand, the most important use of the ESD scales in FOR therapy is not necessarily to
induce socially desirable changes but rather to help patients choose and crystallize their own personal
choices regardless of whether they are socially desirable. In addition, the patient's idiosyncratic choices,
such as those that spring forth from his redecisions, should be put into the form of the seven-spaced
semantic differential test. For example, the choice to be "free" can be dimensionalized as free versus
constricted, with seven spaces in between so that the patient can indicate the degree to which he presently
feels free as well as the degree to which he wishes to feel free in the future.

To begin the process of self-futuring, the patient is again shown his baseline depiction of himself on the ESD that he made during the assessment stage, and words reflecting his redecisions are reviewed. This is done to remind him of these important dimensions of the self. Also, it serves as a format for a brief discussion of how his redecisions, if carried out, might alter his self-depiction. He is then told that he will soon be time-projected into the future and, after this, he will use the scales of the ESD as well as those derived from his redecisions as initial prompters for describing how he would like to realistically choose to view himself in the future.

Before the time projection into the future, the therapist must be careful to guide the patient to choose a realizable ego-ideal, not standards of perfection that would vex the patient with repeated frustrations (Horney, 1950). In explaining this, the therapist may show the patient William James's (1892) simple but profound equation:

$$\text{Self-esteem} = \frac{\text{success}}{\text{pretensions}}$$

This provides a cognitive framework for making the choices of the ego-ideal realistic: to decide for oneself which goals are valued and reachable and to give up pretensions about striving for anything else.

The patient is then asked to select a day about three months in the future to which he will be time-projected. Three months is far enough away for most patients to expect some change by then, yet it is not too far off that they become discouraged about the length of time necessary for changing. Also, research indicates that most therapeutic changes occur within about three months (Meltzoff and Kornreich, 1970). It is usually best for the patient to choose a holiday about three months ahead, especially if the patient expects to be interacting with significant other people on the holiday. This facilitates the imagination of specific scenarios in the future. For some patients, holidays are not appropriate because they are contaminated with troublesome associations, such as anniversary reactions. Whatever future day the patient selects, it is important that it be a day in which the patient anticipates meaningful interactions with other people. This enhances self-reflection from images of other people, which is a process important for conceiving the self (Rosenberg, 1979).

The patient is then time-projected to the future day he has selected. This is done with guided imagery. The patient is told to close his eyes, and he is given some brief relaxation exercises, such as deep breathing and progressive muscle relaxation. (If the patient has chosen to use hypnosis to facilitate the time projection, and if he is hypnotizable, hypnosis may be used at this point, as explained later.) When the patient is sufficiently relaxed, he is then gradually age-progressed toward the day three months ahead. In doing this, the therapist obtains feedback from the patient as to whether he is experiencing scenes of his personal future as though they were happening in the present. For example: "You are now time traveling into your future. Now it is tomorrow; you see yourself there in a situation that seems almost as real as the present; you move, talk, and see people interact with you. . . . When you see yourself vividly interacting with other people, raise your right forefinger. . . . Fine. . . . Now let yourself travel further ahead into the future, to one week ahead from now. Again picture yourself interacting with people as though everything were happening in the here-and-now. Again, raise your right forefinger when you have captured the feeling of being there in the present. . . . Fine. . . . Now let yourself move on to one month ahead. . . ." The patient is then taken ahead to two months and finally to the day he has selected three months in the future. This gradual age progression primes the patient for vivid imagery during his selected future day. Most important, it provides a "warm-up" for experiencing this *future day as though it were happening in the present*. This "making present" of the future endows self-futuring with a feeling of reality. The "presentification" of the future (or past) is necessary for adequate time projection therapy.

On the future day three months ahead, it is usually best to guide the patient to start the day with some solitary scenes that enhance self-reflection. For example: "You wake up; you feel well-rested. You get up and look in the mirror. . . . You remember the redecisions you made three months ago; you say them silently to yourself as you're looking at yourself in the mirror. . . . You see the expression on your face—your eyes, your mouth, the way you hold your head. . . . Now, when you're ready, when you've captured the image of seeing yourself in the mirror, state aloud to your image in the mirror your redecisions. . . . [At this point, the patient usually murmurs a redecision, such as "I will exist; I will take care of myself" or "I don't have to be perfect; I will feel good about myself being just who I am."] Can you say that to yourself more convincingly. . . . Say it with enough emotion so that it shows on your face as you look in the mirror. . . ."

At this point, the patient either states his redecisions with gusto or gets frightened, saying that he cannot do it. In the latter instance, the self-futuring has to be temporarily postponed, and more work has to be done on the redecisions. If the patient does convincingly state his redecisions to himself in the mirror, these redecisions provide the framework for the creation of visual images about the self as the future day unfolds. For example: "Now you are going to live this day according to your redecisions. . . . See yourself eating breakfast with someone close to you. . . . Be the person you choose to become. . . . The way you talk, the way you move, your posture, the way

you feel inside—all are in line with the way you choose to become. . . .
Observe how people respond to you when you are what you choose to
be. . . . Go through the whole morning's activities seeing yourself being
comfortable with the ways you have chosen to become. . . .''

The patient does all this with his eyes closed. He is encouraged to use vivid
visual imagery and to imagine concrete situations where he feels himself
engaged with others in active, emotionally meaningful exchanges. By instilling movement and emotion into his visual scenes, a feeling of duration—of
time unfolding—is created. This also lends a feeling of reality to the scenes.
The therapist allows the patient a period of about 10 minutes to create on his
own, without talking aloud, the scenes of the morning's activities. When the
patient signals that he feels he has completed the morning scenes, the therapist
tells the patient that he will now go through the afternoon with a few more
guidelines for forming his chosen images about himself.

As the patient imagines scenes of the afternoon on this future day, he is
instructed to create images of himself that seem to fit comfortably with his
becoming self according to the dimensions of the Eriksonian semantic differential (ESD) and words reflecting his redecisions. For example, the therapist
states one of the bipolar ESD scales, such as "trusting versus distrusting,"
and the patient is to create an image of his future self that is somewhere
between or to one side of these poles. The patient is encouraged to see himself
acting in the present with significant others according to his choice to be
trusting, distrusting, or somewhere in between. He should not think too much
about his choices; he should just let the images spontaneously emerge,
making sure that he feels comfortable with them. When the patient has
sufficiently captured an image that fits his choice, he is asked to signal his
readiness to move on to another dimension. His signal can be verbal or
nonverbal, as with raising his forefinger. The therapist then states another
bipolar dimension, such as "self-assured versus self-conscious," and the
process is reiterated until all the ESD and redecision scales are completed.

Next, the patient is asked to go through the evening of this future day,
creating other images of his future self that are particularly unique to his
personality. Some of his unique images may represent what he has always
been; if so, he should firmly establish them by seeing himself interacting with
others in that particular way. Finally, as the day ends, he is to look back and
review the images and scenes that gave him the most satisfaction on this future
day.

The patient is then asked to open his eyes. Immediately thereafter, he is
given a blank form of the ESD and redecision scales with "How I Want to
View Myself Three Months from Now" written at the top. He is asked to fill
out this form according to the images and feelings he just experienced during

the time projection into the future. He should do this rapidly so that his choices reflect the images.

After the patient fills out the future scales, he is then interviewed about his experiences during the time projection into the future. The therapist takes notes on important images and scenes. He also notes troublesome or conflictful areas. For example, in some instances, the patient may not have been able to form an image along a particular ESD or redecision dimension. (This is usually already known to the therapist since during the time projection, the patient did not signal he had captured a fitting image.) Brief inquiries are made about these difficulties but they are not discussed at length at this point. The therapist should emphasize the positive and rewarding images at this stage. This raises hope for change and helps the patient to believe that he can choose alternative ways of construing himself.

There are some practical issues that should be mentioned at this point. It is wise to set aside about 1½–2 hours for this guided imagery into the future. If the therapist is confined to the customary 55 minute session, then the time projection may have to be done in two sessions. During the first session, it may be possible to cover only part of the ESD, and the patient should fill out his choices for as far as he has gone. For the second session, the same future day or a date near to it can be used for the completion of the ESD dimensions, the redecision scales, and the genesis of other pertinent images. Another problem is that some patients get caught up in the meaning of the words on the scales. If this happens, the words have to be defined or simplified, and the whole procedure may have to be repeated since the primary aim of the time projection is to create visual images, not verbal quibbling. Of course, the intellectualization of the choices may represent a defense against making the choices. This has to be handled with traditional psychotherapy before repeating the time projection into the future.

The completed future ESD and redecision scales provide a format for further cognitive and image therapy. In subsequent sessions, the therapist reviews the patient's choices and associated imagery. Choices that appear to reflect social, therapist, or parental expectations should be challenged. For example, the patient may have chosen to become moderately trusting as follows:

TRUSTING   __: X: __: __: __: __: __: DISTRUSTING

But the visual imagery associated with this choice may be vague, or the patient's nonverbal communication may reveal discomfort with this choice. The therapist asks, "Are you sure that 'moderately trusting' is your own choice? . . . Or is it what you think society expects of you? . . . Or what your mother expected of you? . . . What I expect of you? . . . Regardless of what other people expect of you, is it your choice to become 'moderately trusting'? . . . Is this something you feel you can realize with those people you want to be close to? . . . Do you want to revise your choice? . . . Now close your eyes and gradually drift into that future day again; create a visual image of yourself that fits your choice. . . .'' In this way, the patient is helped to rework his choices as realistic goals of his ego-ideal.

In addition, possible inconsistencies, such as the choice to be ''warm'' but also ''self-absorbed,'' should be reconciled. Sometimes such apparent conflicts represent poles of existence evoked by imagery specific to certain situations. For example, a woman chose to be ''warm'' when with her husband but ''self-absorbed'' during her creative work as a writer. Such poles of existence, if they are understandable, should be respected and reinforced. A guiding rule for resolving inconsistencies is that the patient should make his own choices with respect to his relationship to himself or with significant other people (for example, spouse, boss, and so forth); he may choose to be different with strangers.

Once a particular choice has been worked out, the patient must practice evoking images congruent with the choice. Ideally, this should be done each day. The words representing the choices (for example, ''slightly assertive'') should serve only as prompters for the creation of visual images in which the self is seen in the mind's eye interacting with significant others. After all the ESD and redecision choices have been appropriately revised, the patient can be given a copy of his choices to carry in his wallet in order to remind him to practice visualizing as often as possible. This can be done unobtrusively during the course of daily activities. Many patients do it while being driven or waiting in lines; others have usefully combined practicing the visual imagery while exercising, such as swimming or running. Of course, words other than those of the scales can and should be used if they prompt mental images more pertinent to the patient's own sense of becoming. Also, it is often useful for the patient to find a mnemonic that captures some of his key choices. For example, one person used his name, BILL representing boyish, industrious, loving, and laughing. The words of the mnemonic are used as convenient reminders for practicing the visual imagery.

With a bright and hardworking patient, the major therapeutic work of self-futuring for the initial reconstruction of the ego-ideal can be completed within about four to five sessions. Thereafter, the patient continues to practice his visual imagery on his own. When the patient can readily evoke visual images congruent with his choices, he usually experiences a sense of centrality. One patient expressed it as follows: ''It's like having a solid center, like I know here I'm going.'' When the patient's ego-ideal appears to be crystallizing along these lines, he is then ready for the next stage of FOR therapy: temporal organization.

TEMPORAL ORGANIZATION

Whereas self-futuring involves bringing the future into the psychological present in order to choose between desired images and goals, temporal organization entails the planning of sequences in order to meet the images and goals which have been selected. Thus as discussed in Chapter 3, whereas futuring employs the simultaneous visualization of options, temporal organization refers to the linear arrangement of sequences of the past, present, and future toward the preferred future options. In FOR therapy, temporal organization helps give the patient's chosen images the reality of time in terms of duration, succession, and temporal perspective.

There are essentially four techniques that are used to enhance temporal organization: (1) feedback, (2) linking images with the past, (3) cueing images with the present, and (4) rehearsals toward the future. In actual practice, these techniques are usually interwoven, but they will be discussed separately below.

Feedback

The formation of clear personal goals during self-futuring aids the process of feedback. With clear goals, the patient is in a better position to determine whether, and to what degree, he is meeting his goals during his daily living. The therapist facilitates the process of feedback by prompting the patient to review recent life events in terms of his chosen goals. That is, from session to session (which are usually weekly) as the patient reports activities and interactions with others during the intervals, the therapist helps the patient focus on his goals and register to what degree he is meeting them.

The therapist facilitates feedback mainly by asking questions. For example: ''During the past week, which of your chosen images about the future self did you actualize to some degree? . . . Give me an example of how you were 'caring' toward your mother? . . . How did doing that make you feel? . . . At times the therapist has to actively point out that the patient is not registering feedback. For example: ''You seem to be discounting yourself; you're not giving yourself credit for being what you choose to become. . . . Replay the scene in your mind, and allow yourself to feel this time. . . . How does it feel to get closer to this image you have chosen for yourself? . . .'' In these ways, the therapist assists the patient to become attuned to detecting and registering feedback in terms of his own appraisals of outcomes and associated emotions. Through giving himself feedback, the patient becomes more self-reinforcing.

Practically every experience that the patient has is grist for the mill for feedback in terms of his chosen goals. The task of the therapist is to help the patient evaluate the experience in light of his goals. If a patient describes an event in which he acted contrary to one or more of his goals, the therapist can ask: "What thoughts and images were running through your mind at that time? . . . Did you bring your chosen image into mind at the time? . . . If that circumstance were happening right now, how could you remind yourself to bring your future image to mind? . . ." Even dream experiences can be handled in this way. For example: "Which chosen aspect of your future self is revealed in the dream? . . . What's in the dream that is contrary to your future self? . . . Do you anticipate difficulties in meeting these goals? . . . Suppose that you could reenter the dream and direct your actions according to your future self; how would the dream turn out? . . ."

At times the therapist has to point out that the patient is overlooking or distorting sources of feedback. For example: "Out of the whole week, you had this one upsetting experience in which you believe you 'blew it'—what about the rest of the time during the week? . . . You seem to be using your future image of yourself like a standard of perfection; even though you moved closer to your chosen goals, you felt frustrated because you were not perfect. Your future image is like a friendly guide, not a tyranny of 'shoulds.' Can you give yourself credit for those things you did which *to some degree* were in the direction of your future self? . . . You seem to be thinking in terms of absolute 'either-or' ways of evaluating your actions; that is, *either* you are totally trusting all of the time *or* you view yourself as a failure. This is not only unrealistic but also may start a downward spiral, like 'I'm a failure; nothing will work out; there's no use to try; see I'm a failure.'. . ." In this regard, many of the techniques of cognitive therapy can be used to help patients realistically appraise feedback and monitor their expectations of themselves (Beck et al., 1979).

The therapist also should be realistic. He should not expect that the patient's future image, even if well crystallized, will by itself bring about behavioral change. The future image is only a beginning. It is like an embryo that is faced with changing a lifetime of habitual ways that the patient has previously construed expectations of himself and others. Backsliding into the grip of these expectations stemming from the past is to be expected and anticipated. When backsliding occurs, it should be interpreted in terms of the patient's life script and catastrophic expectations. This helps deter the escalation of a downward spiral. These interpretations also help the patient to understand himself. The understanding promotes a feeling of forgiveness for the self. When a patient can forgive himself, rather than just further downgrading himself, he is more ready to start afresh again. In addition, helping the patient to identify and interrupt a vicious cycle that reappears during the course of therapy provides a form of practice for the patient's coping with these tendencies after therapy has ended.

The patient's report of his progress (or lack of it) provides the therapist with information as to which images may need strengthening by integrating them through the past, present, and future. Techniques for enhancing the images by giving them a sense of continuity through time include linking the images with the past, cueing them with the present, and rehearsals toward the future. These special strategies for helping patients to organize their images temporally are outlined below.

Linking Images with the Past

The past provides a wealth of memories which can be replayed as visual images. These past images may be positive or negative. Patients are prone to focus predominantly on negative images of the past, and traditional modes of therapy accentuate this negative focus by attempting to get patients to work through childhood traumata. While such an approach may be helpful in overcoming catastrophic expectations that stem from the past, it also may distort the reality of the past by neglecting important positive experiences during childhood. In particular, in contrast to the view that the child is entirely helpless and must obey parental dictates, the child within us is also a source of strength, energy, fun, and freedom (Goulding and Goulding, 1978, 1979). In transactional analysis, this fun-loving, spontaneous, and playful aspect of the child within us is called the "free child." The free child is relatively autonomous and is capable of making its own decisions. It is an important aspect of a person's identity which is often submerged in patients with emotional problems.

In FOR therapy, an attempt is made to reawaken the patient's free child and to link these positive experiences of the past with the patient's future self-image. The intent of this procedure is to imbue the future self-image with a feeling of continuity from the past. This helps reestablish the person's identity by making him aware that what he is striving for, he once was. In particular, as a free child, he did not always feel restricted and put down, but felt autonomous, free to make his own choices. He can rekindle this feeling of autonomy as he fashions his future self-image. Also, he can reconstruct his views of his past by choosing to highlight those experiences that are congruent with his future self-image.

The technique for linking free-child experiences with the future self-image is as follows: The patient is asked whether he ever experienced something similar to one (or more) of his future choices when he was a playful child. He is then time-projected into the past in order to recapture the relevant free-child experiences and to relive them in his mind's eye as though they were happening in the present. After this, while keeping the feelings of being a free child alive, he is again time-projected into the future so that the visualization of his future choices is bolstered by his free-child experiences. Finally, after debriefing the patient about his experiences during the time projections, cognitive therapy is conducted, emphasizing that what the person once was as a child can energize what he chooses to become.

Past scenes that are most useful for activating free-child experiences are those with the child playing by himself or with peers. In general, it is wise to avoid scenes in which parental figures are present, since this often inhibits the feeling of autonomy. Typical examples of useful free-child experiences include roller skating, swimming, swinging in a swing, playing in a sandbox, playing hide-and-seek, and so forth. The more self-created activity and fun, the better.

The linkage between the free-child experiences and the future self-image can be facilitated by metaphors. For example, one patient, who chose to become more "self-assured" in the future, had a feeling of liberation when she recaptured feelings of "sure-footedness and grace" while ice skating as a child. She also recaptured a feeling of "spunkiness" when she relived playing with her favorite doll. When she was time-projected into the future to a day three months ahead, she was asked to visualize herself as being self-assured with significant others with the same feelings of sure-footedness and spunkiness. In this future scene, she imagined herself wearing invisible ice skates and that her doll was nearby. After the session, she went out to buy a replica of her doll and placed it in a central chair in her living room to remind her of her basic spunkiness.

It should be noted that with patients who have great difficulty in imagining themselves in the future to be any different from their present negative self-image, this technique of activating free-child experiences can be used earlier in FOR therapy as a way of building a platform for more positive self-futuring. That is, the free-child experiences can be used as a springboard for the creation of the future choices. This helps overcome a negative mental set by demonstrating to the patient that what he once was, he can become again.

Cueing Images with the Present

With this technique, cues in the present environment are used to remind the person of his chosen future images. The present cues also can serve as reminders of free-child experiences associated with the future images. In these ways, cueing images with the present enhances the temporal organization of past, present, and future.

The key to this technique is to use ubiquitous external stimuli as cues for triggering the recall of certain future images. These cues can be colors, clock times, or forms of self-stroking. The latter include habitual ways of touching one's own body, such as stroking one's hair, beard, or cheek. When these idiosyncratic mannerisms occur, it usually means that the person is showing that he cares for himself. After discussing this possibility with the patient, he is then asked to choose a future image that he would like to be evoked by his particular form of self-stroking. For example, one patient chose to associate "being sincere" with the gesture of brushing his hair off his brow. This was practiced during the therapy sessions, and he did daily homework in order to activate the image of being sincere whenever he stroked himself in this way.

Colors are ubiquitous present stimuli that can be quite useful in this regard. The patient is taught to associate one of his favorite colors with an important future image of himself. For example, one patient chose the image of "being free" with his favorite color of blue. He practiced visualizing himself as being free and spontaneous whenever he saw the color blue—blue skies, blue walls, blue shirts, blue pens, and so forth. Also, as a boy, the blue expanse of the ocean with him running freely in the splashing waves was particularly appealing to him. This image of himself as a free child was repeatedly paired with his seeing blue in his present surroundings. From four to five of the patient's favorite colors can be paired with different future images in this way.

Clock periods are useful present stimuli for activating different future images during particular times of the day. For example, a lawyer wanted to be "hardheaded" during his working day, but "warm" and "trusting" during the evenings and weekends when he was with his family. In line with this, he practiced seeing himself as being hardheaded whenever his clock or watch gave readings of between 8 A.M. and 5 P.M., but at other times he visualized himself as being warm and trusting. This technique also can be used to help manage recurrently stressful or troublesome periods of the day, such as when children return from home in the afternoon or a person's tendency to indulge in excessive food or drink in the evening.

Rehearsals toward the Future

The temporal organization of future images of the self is greatly enhanced by rehearsals toward the future. These rehearsals can apply to the short-term or long-term future. It is usually best to start with short-term rehearsals, since the patient can easily imagine specific situations in the near future that he will have to cope with. In other words, the short-term future has a greater "reality" than the long-term future. However, with some patients who feel locked-in by their present and near-future circumstances, it is sometimes useful to begin with long-term rehearsals, especially when the distant future seems less binding. Also, the person's view of himself over the long run is the most growth-producing perspective for the development of plans of action consistent with the continuous goals of the future self-image.

For both short-term and long-term rehearsals, role-playing techniques are commonly used. Sometimes the patient plays all the roles in creating dialogues between his present self, his future self, his past self, his mother, his father, and so forth. The "double-chair" setup, popularized by Perls (1973), is useful for this purpose. Here the person talks to an empty chair in which sits an imagined person, which may be his future self, a parent, and so forth. He then switches chairs and talks back to his present self, creating a dialogue. The therapist acts like a coach on the sidelines, facilitating the exchange. Most patients require some coaxing to begin double-chair work, but once started it can be quite meaningful since it helps concretize different views and their resolution. At other times, the therapist may play the role of the patient's past self, mother, husband, and so forth. This is usually necessary when patients are unimaginative or otherwise inhibited, as is common with depressed patients.

Short-term rehearsals toward the future pertain to anticipated events one day to one week ahead. There are essentially two forms: anticipatory alternativism and future autobiography.

Anticipatory alternativism refers to rehearsing alternative plans of action that are different from one's previous ways of coping with a situation yet consistent with one's future self-image. For example, a woman was apprehensive about her mother coming to visit her from out of town the next day. Previously, she felt she had always "lost her center" when her mother visited, putting on a "phony" show of being an immaculate housekeeper and dutiful mother in order to impress her mother. This contradicted her choice to become "sincere." After the patient revisualized her imagery of being sincere three months in the future, she was asked to close her eyes and act according to this imagery in her mind's eye during her mother's upcoming visit. In her imagination, she told her mother that she wanted to be a "friend" rather than a "good little girl who keeps an immaculate house." She rehearsed scenes like this for about 10 minutes, including images of how she would maintain her sincerity in face of her mother's disapproval of her less-than-perfect housekeeping. The next day, to her surprise, her mother replied, "I always wondered why you fussed so about my coming; I resented fussing over my mother in the same way, and I don't want you to resent me."

During anticipatory alternativism, it is important that the anticipated scenes are as specific as possible and that the patient sees himself moving, acting, and talking in the scene as though it were taking place in the present. A motion film analogy often helps. For example: "Feel yourself moving, as though you stepped into a movie of what you anticipate to be happening. Make things happen by your actions." In addition, once the patient has developed some momentum in line with his future self, the therapist can interject some typical challenges that he knows from the patient's history. For example: "Now your mother is frowning at you, saying that you should show her more respect. How do you keep that sincerity going?" The therapist also can role-play the part of the troublesome person. Sometimes such challenges are too much for the patients so that they become upset and lose sight of their future choices. When this happens, the anticipated scene has to be replayed and again rehearsed until the patient is satisfied with the imagery. These anticipatory rehearsals are similar to the constructive alternativism of George Kelly (1955) and the use of positive coping imagery for inoculating a person to withstand stress (Meichenbaum, 1977).

Future autobiography is another short-term rehearsal technique that helps patients structure their plans of action according to their chosen goals (Melges, 1972). In effect, the patient gives an autobiography of his future. The patient is asked to project himself ahead in time, usually one week ahead to the next appointment with the therapist. Both patient and therapist pretend it is actually that time ahead. The therapist then takes a detailed "history" of what supposedly "happened," and the patient describes how he coped with imagined situations in this future time span, now viewed as "past." In this way, the patient discovers options and rehearses plans of action that help him reach the goals he has chosen for himself.

In executing the future autobiography, it is important that the patient pretends it is one week ahead (or more) and looks back. This enhances a greater differentiation of what is likely to happen and also reduces the uncertainty of future events by making them seem as already accomplished facts. By contrast, if the patient talks about coming events of the week ahead by using the future tense, there are a host of *ifs, ands,* and *buts.* Thus the therapist has more to work on if he insists that the patient use the past tense to describe the one week ahead. If the patient describes a stultifying event, the therapist asks: "What did you do then, what options did you find? . . . And when you did that, how did you feel inside? . . . Which chosen-goal for yourself did you feel closer to? . . ." The therapist can also introduce events that have been recurrently stressful for the patient into this retrospectively viewed future week. For example, he can say: "When your mother criticized your type of housekeeping, what did you say? . . ."

The future autobiography technique often reveals elements of the patient's unwitting life script. These script elements may show up in the patient's report of ordinary, mundane events. For example, the therapist asked a patient what she did (in the future) after she left the therapist's office, and the patient replied, "Oh, I felt pretty good for a couple of hours. . . . Then I went home and found my husband engrossed in the newspaper. . . . I felt rejected. . . . To get his attention, I picked a fight with him and started to nag at him. . . ." Since this was a repetition of how she used to get her father's attention by creating some sort of uproar, and since her behavior (in the future, viewed retrospectively) contradicted her choice to become "straight," the therapist had her listen to the tape recording of this segment of her future autobiography so that she could see how she was projecting old ways into her future. Then the future autobiography was repeated until the patient's report matched her choice to become more direct in her ways of communicating and getting attention. The important point is that unless a patient's projected plans of action change in the direction of his chosen images, it is unlikely that his actual behavior will change.

Although anticipatory alternativism and future autobiography are usually short-term forms of rehearsal, they also can be used for long-term rehearsals. More common, however, long-term rehearsals include what is called temporal role-playing and psychodrama of the future. These latter procedures can be applied to spans of future time three months ahead, one year, or five years into the future. In FOR therapy, long-term rehearsals are commonly directed toward spans of future time of about three months to one year ahead, since such spans of time are not too far into the future as to seem unreal to the patient.

Temporal role-playing means that the patient assumes the role of his future self, present self, and past self, and creates dialogues between these various selves. In addition, dialogues between the future self and past identification figures (mother, father, and so forth), as well as current significant others (spouse, friend, boss, and so forth), can be created.

One of the most useful forms of temporal role-playing is the creation of dialogues between the future self and the present self. This method is particularly productive when it creates empathy for the self in the future as well as nurturance of the future self for the present self. The technique involves role-playing. This can be done with the patient's eyelids closed with his taking the part of his future self, then his present self, back and forth, in his mind's eye. But the procedure is also effective if the patient can engage in "double-chair" work, as previously described (Chapter 6). That is, after rekindling the imagery and associated feelings of the future self by a brief time projection three months ahead with revisualization of the patient's choices, the future self sits in one chair and talks to the present self who is imagined to be in the other empty chair. At appropriate times, the therapist asks the patient to switch chairs, so that the patient becomes his present self again talking back to his future self. While switching back and forth between his present and future selves, the patient creates a dialogue that hopefully fosters plans of actions, emotions, and other temporal connections between the present self and the future self.

Below is a condensed version of the kinds of exchanges that can be fostered by this method:

Future Self (*to Present Self*):	"Hello, how are you?"
Present Self:	"Not as well off as you are."
Future Self:	"Am I too much for you?"
Present Self:	"Well, sometimes I think I'll never become like you. . . . But I created you—you're my own doing; I can change you if I want, even drop you. . . . How's that make you feel?"
Future Self:	"Scared. You're pretty powerful. . . . Yet I also feel compassion for you. You lost your beloved daughter, and you think life will be just a downhill course after that. . . ."
Present Self:	"Compassion? (*Begins to cry.*) How can you feel compassion for someone like me? I'm so pitiful. I don't deserve it. . . ."
Future Self:	"I want to take care of you, to nurture you, like you took care of your daughter. . . . I feel your daugher would have wanted me to do this. What do you feel?"
Present Self: (*Crying.*)	"She would have wanted me to go on. . . . I hope you understand how difficult it is for me. . . . You know, I do feel more secure with you there, nearby. . . ."

The above patient experienced feelings of relief, as well as recommitment, after the above exchange and stated, "I realized I had someone to care for; I could nurture myself!" The creation of a nurturant ego-ideal is an optimal outcome.

This creation of a nurturant future self that takes care of and guides the present self is usually facilitated by guided imagery in which the patient, with eyelids closed, looks back in time from his future self toward his present self. The person is time-projected into the future about three months ahead, and the images of the future self are fully activated as though the person is now his future self. This can be enhanced with hypnosis. Also, imagery of the past can be used to kindle the spontaneity and nurturance of the future self. Once the future self is recaptured, in order to enhance mutual empathy between the future self and the present self, it is appropriate for the therapist to suggest that the future self feels ''warmly'' and ''wants to take care of'' the present self, to serve as a ''guide'' and ''friend'' to the present self. Moreover, it can be suggested, if it is the patient's choice, that this nurturant future self will bring out the free child in the present self and help the patient to become free from catastrophic expectations of being controlled or rejected by parental figures. Then after switching the patient back into his present self, he is asked whether he can engender feelings of warmth toward his future self. The patient goes back and forth, creating an emotional tie between his present and future selves in this way. Some patients, especially those with a romantic bent, have responded to this procedure by ''falling in love'' with their future self. This has often produced dramatic improvement. For example, a severely phobic woman who had been housebound for seven years overcame her fears the very day she fell in love with her future self.

Another long-term rehearsal technique is called *psychodrama of the future*. Here the person, from the standpoint of his future self, creates a drama in his mind's eye. The drama involves significant people of his past, present, and future. This telescoping of time is often useful toward the end of FOR therapy, since it helps a patient to resolve unfinished business with archaic figures and to crystallize new directions emerging from the future self.

Psychodrama of the future is applied to a time three months to one year in the future, but it can refer to three to five years in the future, and even longer future time spans. It is best for the patient to select the future time span according to when he estimates his future self will have become an intrinsic part of him. The technique involves guided imagery. After the patient is relaxed, he closes his eyelids and is time-projected into the future. His own choices are reviewed, and he is to see himself in his mind's eye as already being what he has chosen to become. Then he is to imagine that he is on a Shakespearian round stage surrounded by significant people from his past, present, and future in the audience. He then creates a moving scene in his mind's eye as he invites certain people from the audience to join him on stage. He is the stage director who determines the cast of characters and the situations to be created. He sees himself being his future self as he interacts with others who have joined him on stage. He speaks to them; they speak to him; looks and embraces are exchanged; and a great deal of emotional expression and feedback takes place. The therapist guides the patient to get feedback from others about the person he has become. He is encouraged to deal with past figures with whom he has not resolved important issues. He speaks to them from the standpoint of his future self, expresses feelings never said before, forgives when necessary, and establishes a new sense of identity by generating new responses to archaic problems.

These psychodramas of the future are often dreamlike in the way that time becomes telescoped. For example, a patient chose to introduce his beloved grandfather, who died when he was a boy, to his wife, and then asked his grandfather for advice as to how to work out problems with his marriage. Another patient saw herself helping her daughter (who in reality was about to get married) give birth to her first child. Another patient, after the therapist suggested that she set the tempo of the scenario to music of her liking, reported that she envisioned "close-up faces with wonderful expressions, like a 'happening' in a Fellini film."

Toward the end of the psychodrama of the future, the patient is asked to say goodbye to each person he has invited on stage and to finish off the situation to his liking. This may involve saying "last words" to certain individuals or asking some people to be seated in the periphery of the audience while asking others to be nearer. It is best to end the scenario with the patient standing alone and giving a soliloquy, stating to the audience who he has become and the kind of person he has self-actualized.

A variant of psychodrama of the future is to have a patient extrapolate to the time of his death. This is useful for highlighting priorities while viewing one's affiliations and achievements over the long run. However, it should be used cautiously, usually after the person has a firm sense of identity. The patient is told that while he is dying, he has entered a serene state and has a multitude of visions about his accomplishments and relationships, similar to the "life review" that has been reported to occur in some people as they are dying (Stevenson and Greyson, 1979). He is to experience this life review from the standpoint of having truly become his future self by the time of his death. The technique makes use of a paradox intrinsic to the writings of many existentialists (Yalom, 1980): Through the emotional realization of death, people commit themselves more fully to living.

Thus in FOR therapy, temporal organization serves to help patients integrate their chosen images over time. This is accomplished by (1) feedback, (2) linking images with the past, (3) cueing images with the present, and (4) rehearsals toward the future. The latter include (a) short-term rehearsals, such as anticipatory alternativism and future autobiography, and (b) long-term rehearsals, such as temporal role-playing and psychodrama of the future.

PRACTICAL ISSUES IN FUTURE-ORIENTED PSYCHOTHERAPY

Variation in Technique

Although FOR therapy usually proceeds according to the essential stages outlined above (that is, assessment and selection of patients, interpretation of vicious cycles, redecisions, self-futuring, and temporal organization), the order of these stages is sometimes altered depending on what the patient needs at a particular time.

For example, if suicidal tendencies are discovered during the assessment stage, it is sometimes useful to deal with this in terms of a psychodrama of "the aftermath of suicide," particularly when there are suggestions that the patient is attempting to manipulate others through threatening suicide. The patient is projected to the time after he is found dead. Who finds him? What are their reactions? How long do their reactions last? How painful is their grief? Does the suicide change their lives forever? What does he see when he is looking down at his own funeral? What do people say about him? What are their thoughts? Did he achieve the desired effect on other people by committing suicide? In viewing the aftermath of suicide, many patients find that the intended consequences of suicide are short lived or discounted by the people they wish to hurt. On the other hand, if the patient reports serene fantasies of death and relief after ending hopelessness and pain, then strict precautions to prevent suicide should be mobilized, including, in some cases, hospitalization.

As previously mentioned, another variation in the order of techniques is to use the activation of free-child experiences early in treatment in order to build a platform for the genesis of the future self-image. This is particulary indicated for difficult patients who are locked in to beliefs such as "my whole life has been total misery," "I never have been happy and I never will be happy," and so forth. The activation of the free-child experiences demonstrates to them that before their current negative mental set, they did have fun in the past and this makes it possible in the future again.

A brief form of FOR therapy consists of (1) activation of images of the free child, (2) time projection into the future for the development of the future self-images kindled by the free-child experiences, and (3) guided imagery and rehearsals to build mutual empathy between the future self and present self, emphasizing the nurturant and guiding functions of the future self. In cooperative patients, this can be accomplished in one session. This brief form of therapy is often a useful introduction to the more extensive procedures.

As suggested in Chapter 10, the guided imagery techniques for grief-resolution therapy can be productively followed by future-oriented identity reconstruction. In this regard, a useful way to generate future choices for the self after grief therapy is to have the patient look back, in his imagination, after he has walked about 50 yards from the grave site and to ask himself whether there are strengths or traits of the deceased that he chooses to develop in himself. In addition, he can decide how he would choose to be different from the deceased. These choices can serve as the images for self-futuring in FOR therapy. This combination of grief-resolution therapy with FOR therapy is a natural and an effective linkage.

FOR therapy can be combined with many other treatment approaches, or it can be used as an adjunct for the future-oriented completion of past- and present-oriented therapies (Melges, 1972). It can be used in conjunction with group therapy, milieu therapy, and psychoactive medicines. Although it is usually an outpatient procedure, it has been used successfully with hospitalized patients, particularly those with identity diffusion or depression. Antianxiety medicines can be used in conjunction with FOR therapy for those patients who need to interrupt the "fear of fear" cycle as they are forming new directions. Antidepressant medicines also can be used for mobilizing the energy of depressed patients so that they become more engaged in structuring their futures. In addition, as discussed later, with suitable patients, FOR therapy can be productively combined with hypnosis as well as family therapy.

Frequency of Sessions

With outpatients, FOR therapy is usually conducted weekly with each session lasting 55 minutes. However, during the self-futuring stage, it is often useful to have some sessions of 1½–2 hours long and to increase the frequency to at least twice per week. This is done to start the process of imagery on the right track and to help the patient gain momentum. Also, the importance of daily homework can be reinforced by more frequent meetings during this stage.

With hospitalized patients, FOR therapy is usually conducted daily for half-hour sessions that are rounded out by milieu therapy and nursing staff collaborators. The integration of the treatment plan with the nursing staff cannot be overemphasized. In this regard, FOR therapy is readily teachable, and clear communications are enhanced since therapist, resident, nurse, technician, medical student, and, most important, the patient can all speak "the same language" when planning and executing FOR therapy.

Time-Limitation

Future-oriented psychotherapy is a short-term form of psychotherapy, which is usually limited to 12–30 sessions. For most patients who are well motivated and appropriately selected according to the guidelines outlined previously, about 12 sessions is usually sufficient for the self-futuring and temporal organization stages fundamental to FOR therapy. Depending on the patient and his problems, variable periods of time are necessary for building to these latter two stages in terms of interpretation of vicious cycles and prompting the patient to make redecisions.

A strict time limitation, agreed upon in advance by both patient and therapist, is useful for mobilizing intensive work during the allotted time and for dealing with issues of separation–individuation right from the start of therapy (Mann, 1973; Chapter 6). It also helps prevent excessive dependency on the therapist by giving the patient the expectation of having to make it on his own after a preset date. Although I previously used a time limitation of 12 sessions with almost every patient, in recent years a more flexible time limitation of 12–30 sessions is now communicated to the patient at the start of therapy. There are two major reasons for this more flexible time limit: FOR therapy is now being applied to more difficult types of patients, and also, it is being integrated with family therapy, which requires more sessions, as described later.

As with other forms of cognitive psychotherapy, termination of treatment with FOR therapy is not as complex as with the ending of the therapeutic relationship after a prolonged psychoanalysis (Beck et al., 1979). Nevertheless, the therapist should be aware of similar dynamics around termination, such as the recrudescence of symptoms, regression, and resistance, as a means of maintaining the relationship with the therapist. These factors should be handled with the usual interpretations. They also can serve as springboards for future rehearsals beyond the time of termination. For example, if the patient is anticipating a sense of loss and helplessness after therapy ends, he can be time-projected three to four weeks ahead in order to rehearse plans of action that will maintain his future image on his own. If he is projected to the hour and day of week that he has customarily met with the therapist, this highlights issues of making it on his own without the therapist.

By the time of termination, it should be obvious that most patients feel they have some way to go before they have reached their desired future image. They are told that this is to be expected, since the goals of the ego-ideal are never quite attainable but are with them as spurs toward growth. They are told that FOR therapy was aimed at giving them a start—that is, a way of working on problems by themselves. For them to continue to grow, they will have to build on what they have learned during FOR therapy by making the visual imagery and rehearsals an almost daily habit.

In order to reinforce daily practice and to evaluate progress, it is wise to schedule about 3–4 "booster" sessions at monthly intervals after the last regular session. During these sessions, the most important message to convey to the patient is that he now has ways of helping himself.

It should be noted that the time limitation may have to be rescheduled in order to deal with significant crises in the patient's life, such as death of a family member, sickness, and major life decisions involving one's career or marriage. Unlike some forms of psychotherapy that advocate no major life decisions be made until treatment is completed, FOR therapy encourages problem solving and decision making in terms of envisioning both short-term and long-term consequences.

EVALUATION

Throughout the course of FOR therapy, which usually lasts from 12–30 sessions, both therapist and patient review evidence with regard to how well the patient's thoughts, images, emotions, and behaviors are approximating his choices for his future self-image. This feedback is obtained clinically as well as through readministering the Eriksonian semantic differential of the self (ESD) and redecision scales in terms of the patient's "Own View of Myself Now." The scales provides systematic feedback in terms of movement toward the future choices as well as movement away from the baseline depiction at the start of therapy.

Toward the end of therapy, the patient's progress is evaluated according to the following criteria:

Systematic Assessment (see Appendix A for nature of tests):

1 Differences between present and future self-image in terms of the ESD scales.
2 Changes in hope in terms of the short future outlook inventory. The Hopelessness Scale by Beck et al. (1974) also can be used for this purpose.
3 Changes in the degree of internal control in terms of the modified internal–external control inventory.
4 Changes in the semantic differential test of emotions.
5 Changes in the degree of temporal integration, particularly in goal-directedness.

Clinical Assessment:

6 Changes in central symptoms, presenting problem, and recurrent past problems.
7 Ability of patient to maintain future images despite challenges.

8 Changes in the nature of the patient's self-statements, particularly his expectations about himself.

9 Changes in the nature of the patient's social interactions, especially with his family.

These outcome measures are usually discussed with the patient in order to enhance the process of feedback. The use of brief forms of measuring outcome in this way during clinical practice not only serves to monitor progress but also may pinpoint areas in need of further work (Melges, 1972). The therapist (or his secretary or other trained assistant) can administer the tests. Of course, if systematic research is being conducted, it is best to have testers who are not involved in the therapy in order to elicit unbiased reports, and the tests should be used purely for measurement rather than feedback to the patient. In this regard, in a study at Stanford that compared FOR therapy with client-centered therapy for the treatment of depression and incipient heavy drinking, FOR produced significant pre–post changes after 12 treatment sessions in 28 of a total of 30 variables, whereas client-centered therapy produced 15 significant changes in the control group over the same time period. Eighty-nine percent of the patients showed positive changes, and most of these were sustained at one year follow-up.

THE USE OF HYPNOSIS IN FUTURE-ORIENTED PSYCHOTHERAPY

As previously outlined (Chapter 6), hypnosis can be used to alter duration (rate), sequence, and temporal perspective for therapeutic purposes. In FOR therapy, with patients who are hypnotizable, the patient is given the option as to whether he wants to use hypnosis as a means of accelerating therapy. He is told that there is nothing magical about hypnosis, but it can be useful for inducing a "ribbon of concentration" that may help "imprint" his chosen images and "firm up his plans of action." Since the techniques and precautions for inducing hypnotic time distortions have already been described (see Chapter 6), they will not be repeated here, but I will point out how they can be incorporated into FOR therapy.

The process of self-futuring can be enhanced by the hypnotic "slowing down of inner time." As inner tempo is slowed down, the person experiences an altered state of consciousness that seems unfettered by extraneous thoughts, and the patient appears more receptive to present input. The heightened focus on the present facilitates time projection into the future whereby the future is experienced as though it were taking place in the present. That is the person feels he is "there" in the future, which has a reality akin to the present. In addition, the slowing down of inner time makes the person's images appear to last longer in the mind, since the images are separated in time from other thoughts and images and also are invested with more psychological duration than normally. Thus both the heightened focus on the present and the prolongation of inner duration appear to enhance the "imprinting" of the patient's chosen future images.

The temporal organization strategies of FOR therapy also can be facilitated by hypnosis. Age regression into the past can be used for activating free-child experiences in order to link the patient's future images with positive past experiences. Posthypnotic suggestions can be given for linking the future images with ubiquitous present stimuli, such as colors or clock times. In addition, rehearsals toward the future can be given the sense of time unfolding through age progression into the future. The combination of age regression into the past followed by age progression into the future can provide the patient with a feeling of continuity of his reconstructed self-image. Establishing this sense of continuity is particularly indicated for patients with identity problems and depersonalization.

When hypnosis is used in FOR therapy, the patient is taught to hypnotize himself so that he can use this tool for rehearsing his imagery and related plans of action in his daily homework. During the therapy sessions, he is told that he will always maintain his sense of control and freedom of choice. In this way, hypnosis and self-hypnosis are used as a vehicle toward self-mastery.

COMBINATION OF FOR WITH FAMILY THERAPY

Although FOR therapy was originally developed as an individual form of therapy, it is now being increasingly combined with family or marital therapy. This is usually done on an alternating basis, with the therapist (or co-therapist) treating individual members separately and then conjointly. The individual treatment focuses on helping a patient to become more self-supporting so that he can later support the other family members, who, in turn, have worked on their own future directions. When family members obtain autonomy, what Bowen (1976) calls "taking the 'I' position," this helps free them from enmeshed expectations of one another so that their relationships can become more freely synchronized. With this approach, the entire family is not always seen conjointly, as is advocated by some family therapists, but the alternating individual and conjoint sessions seem to work well. Here I will give a few guidelines for this combined approach, while realizing that space does not permit discussion of the full complexities of family therapy.

The major reason for combining FOR therapy with family therapy is that there are often binding expectations that interfere with each member's self-futuring. These binding expectations have been given different terms by various schools of family therapy (for example, enmeshment, mystification, undifferentiated ego mass, rigid homeostasis, and so forth), but they all point to the same phenomenon: interpersonal control via expectations. The expectations are usually mediated by indirect or direct threats of harm, separation, reduction of privileges, or withdrawal of love. Helping patients resolve these binding expectations is fundamental to family therapy.

Another reason for involving the family is that one's immediate social network is perhaps the most powerful source of reinforcement for initiating, as well as maintaining, new directions. The growth-producing functions of a family have been highlighted by Speer (1970, p. 274): "Families need to be constructively responsive to change, able to change with change, and capable of learning to learn to give up obsolescent constraints." In FOR therapy, these growth functions of a family are enhanced.

The essential stages of FOR therapy can be synchronized with the family approach. That is, the treatment of individual members, as well as the family unit, can focus progressively on the interpretation of vicious cycles, redecisions, futuring, and temporal organization. The application of these stages to family therapy is briefly outlined below.

Interpretation of Vicious Cycles

Vicious cycles can occur within an individual or between individuals. As previously outlined (Chapter 8), a common individual vicious cycle occurs when hopelessness leads to inactivity, which leads to lack of reward, and the latter, in turn, leads to further hopelessness. Vicious cycles that occur between people are often subtle and difficult to pinpoint unless one observes the timing of the interactions. Having the family members there together facilitates the observation of the timing of interactions. For example, as one family member tries to get closer to another person, this latter person may then attempt to distance himself by expressing negative feelings, and he, in turn, is rescued by a third member, thereby reinforcing the distancing process and the negative emotions. In this way, an individual's own emotional vicious cycle, such as hopelessness, may be subtly reinforced by well-intentioned family members attempting to rescue the situation.

A general framework for understanding some common factors involved in interpersonal vicious cycles has already been presented in Chapter 11. To recapitulate briefly, as people get closer to one another, there is often a concomitant increase in ambivalence since attachment may mean being vulnerable to being controlled or rejected by the other person. In order to diffuse this threat, people invent ways of distancing each other. This is commonly done by fault finding (the role of the persecutor) or advertising one's own sense of misery (the role of the victim). When the persecutor–victim interaction escalates, a third party is usually brought into the fray in the role of a rescuer. The rescuer then sides with the victim against the persecutor, who may then feel victimized and seek out another rescuer in order to form another coalition against his persecutors. This process may escalate into a complex series of vicious cycles that spread beyond the family to friends, clergymen, and police.

In family therapy, once sufficient rapport has been established, the interpretation of these vicious cycles can be fairly direct. A good way to start is to ask the family, as a whole, what the "payoff" might be for all the negative feelings cycling through its members. They usually answer this question in terms of other people not meeting up to what is expected of them. This opens the way for a discussion of how they are caught in a web of expectations, including the expectation that closeness to one another may mean being vulnerable to control or rejection from other persons. Role switches between victim, persecutor, and rescuer can be pointed out, and these terms can be explicitly used, especially if the therapist can inject irony and humor as the family members examine their interactions. Usually families who come for therapy are so mystified and confused as to what is going on between them that they are hungry for some way to understand their problems. The interpretation of their vicious cycles is often quite revealing to them and makes them aware of the times that their spirals are likely to escalate.

Redecisions

In future-oriented family therapy, redecisions commonly involve decisions to stop playing a role that was scripted by one's family of origin. For example, a father, who as a boy was reinforced for rescuing his mother from his brutal father, firmly decided that he would no longer play the role of rescuer when his wife and daughter fought with one another. This helped stop a vicious cycle and eventually brought the wife and daughter closer together. Sometimes a family script will go back several generations. For example, a mother wanted to "lock up" her 13-year-old daughter who had run away from home on a number of occasions. History revealed that the mother, grandmother, and great-grandmother had actually run away from home around age 13. The daughter's redecision not to follow this trans-generational script had to be matched by the mother's redecision to tolerate her daughter's burgeoning sexuality, something the mother's mother had found to be abhorrent when the mother herself was a teenager.

An individual's redecision may have to be openly communicated to other family members in order to mitigate catastrophic expectations. For example, a young woman with identity diffusion had been given a strong message of "don't grow up" by her father. In individual FOR therapy, she made the redecision to no longer obey this injunction, but she feared that this would mean that her father would withdraw his love from her. In family therapy, she announced to her father that she would no longer be "Daddy's little girl." At first the father denied that he wanted her to stay a little girl, but later he admitted that he wanted to "bottle her, have her stay the way she's always been." His redecision was to grieve the loss of his "little girl," but he reassured her that he would always love her as a father, thereby mitigating her catastrophic expectations.

In marital discord, perhaps the most common form of interlocking scripts is a wife with a "don't exist" message and a husband with a "don't feel" message. Here, when the husband does not show overt feelings for his wife, she takes this to mean that she should not exist in his eyes. And when she becomes emotional, he just further closes off his feelings. Getting each of them to make redecisions about the early script injunctions is a start toward unraveling the pathological interaction.

Futuring

In family therapy, it is crucial to find out from each participant the differences between the current and desired interactions within the family. This provides a framework for beginning to resolve the differences in expectations. Some of these differences may never be resolved. In that case, as Satir (1967) emphasizes, people have to agree to disagree. That is, rather than being caught in a quagmire of unexpressed expectations, by stating the differences in their expectations, the individuals differentiate from each other on some issues and come together on others. In this way, there is a better chance of finding an optimal balance between autonomy and affiliation within the family.

An individual's self-futuring, initiated during one-to-one therapy, can be shared with other family members, if the person so chooses. Likewise, other family members can describe their own time-projected images of the personal future. This provides a format for feedback about the realizability of the images. In addition, if a person's self-futuring meets with conflicting expectations from family members, these differences have to be worked through. On the other hand, there may be a surprising degree of reinforcement for each other's evolving images. Sharing images of the future often produces commitments toward mutual growth.

Sometimes it is possible to engage a family in conjoint futuring. That is, the therapist prompts the entire family to project themselves three months into the future in order to visualize how each would like their interactions to be different at that time. The therapist asks them to try an "experiment." They are to close their eyes, relax, and drift into the future about three months ahead. In their mind's eye, they are to see themselves interacting in desired ways that are realistically possible for them. In order to give the imagery some specificity, some common dimensions of family functions as outlined by Fleck (1980), such as leadership, maintenance of boundaries, emotional support and expression, and communication, can be mentioned by the therapist. For example, as the family is visualizing the future, the therapist can ask: "Who do you see in the leadership roles? How do you see the leaders leading, and the followers following? How is the power shared?" After each dimension, the family can then open their eyes, and discussion can take place about their different images.

Procedures such as the above often produce lively discussion. The therapist should acknowledge and respect differences, but he should emphasize points of agreement. The latter can serve as conjoint goals toward which the family can temporally organize their plans of action. If they can learn to synchronize on some issues, they can learn to grow together.

Temporal Organization

Once conjoint goals are crystallized, strategies for temporal organization within a family can follow along similar lines to those outlined for individual FOR therapy. These include feedback, linking images with the past, cueing images with the present, and rehearsals toward the future.

In family therapy, it is important for the therapist to make sure that each family member receives full feedback from other members about whether his plans of action are approximating his chosen goals. The most common interferences with feedback are as follows: not listening, discounting compliments from others, jumping ahead of the other person with one's own thoughts and internal speech, and "mind reading." The latter means the assuming of what the other intends to communicate or is feeling, usually on the basis of posture or facial expressions, without fully hearing him out (Bandler, Grinder, and Satir, 1976). These miscommunications have to be pointed out repeatedly in order to instill proper feedback.

Videotape playback of segments of family interactions is a powerful way to provide the entire family with feedback. Brief playbacks of audio recordings also are useful. The therapist can interrupt an interaction midstream, play it back, and ask the family members whether they are interacting in line with their chosen goals.

Linking images with the past also can be accomplished within a family or marital setting. The activation of free-child experiences may be rekindled by review of the courtship period of husband and wife. Some couples are so embroiled in their current conflicts that they literally have forgotten what they once had. In the terms of transactional analysis, they have "excluded their child," and are interacting mainly on the levels of critical parent or cold-calculating adult. If the therapist can get family members to start "playing" with one another, even with experiments like imagining themselves to be kids in a sandbox together, major headway is often made.

Cueing images with the present in family therapy usually involves contractual trade-offs. That is, one person agrees to remind the other when he is getting out of hand, and vice versa. Or each person agrees to compliment the other when the other's behavior becomes consistent with his chosen goals.

In future-oriented family therapy, rehearsals toward the future are particularly useful for generating plans of action that are likely to meet both individual and family goals. The entire family can engage in rehearsals in the form of anticipatory alternativism and psychodramas of the future. With anticipatory alternativism, the whole family decides in advance about alternative ways of coping with an impending stressful event. For example, in anticipating the second anniversary of the death of a son, a family carefully structured their time during that day so that they would be mutually supportive to each other. Psychodramas of the future are useful for dealing with anticipated life-cycle changes in the family, such as the children leaving the home. For example, a daughter "sculpted" how she wanted her mother, father, and sister positioned at the time of her wedding; and then the mother and father enacted how their relationship would change once their favorite daughter had left home. Family sculpting is a good way to portray visually anticipated changes in relationship (Papp, Silverstein, and Carter, 1973). In addition, the effect on the family of a given person becoming his future self can be appraised by having the person act as though he has become his future self at some time in the future, such as Christmas. The whole family pretends that it is now Christmas, and they react to, as well as challenge, the person's future self-image. Of course, there can be many modifications and variations of these psychodramas of the future. For example, each family member can enact his future self-image in consecutive fashion, or all family members can assume the role of their future selves at the same time. These exercises provide a fertile ground for dovetailing plans of action with the chosen future images.

THE FUTURE OF FUTURE-ORIENTED PSYCHOTHERAPY

The explicit emphasis on structuring the personal future is unique to FOR therapy. Also, the techniques of visual imagery and future time projection make it different from the usual verbal modes of psychotherapy that concentrate on the past or present. Nevertheless, FOR therapy does incorporate components of other forms of therapy. These include the modification of beliefs as in cognitive-emotional therapy (Beck, 1976; Beck et al., 1979; Ellis, 1962), short-term dynamic psychotherapy for the understanding of how the past invades the future (Marmor, 1979; Davanloo, 1978), principles of behavioral modification for engendering self-reinforcement and self-efficacy (Bandura, 1969, 1977), and transactional analysis for synchronizing interpersonal relationships and for making redecisions (Goulding and Goulding, 1978, 1979). In addition, hypnotic techniques and family therapy can be combined with FOR therapy. Thus FOR therapy can be considered as a synthesis of various future-oriented psychotherapeutic strategies.

From a theoretical standpoint, FOR therapy is rooted primarily in Kelly's (1955) psychology of personal constructs and Miller, Galanter, and Pribram's (1960) theory of plans and the structure of behavior. The development of FOR therapy took place while formulating a neuropsychological theory of emotion (Pribram and Melges, 1969). Thus in light of these theoretical underpinnings, FOR therapy may be considered to be a cognitive-emotional form of therapy. It is a practical extension and integration of these theoretical foundations.

FOR therapy also has been influenced by transactional analysis (Berne, 1972; Goulding and Goulding, 1978, 1979). In terms of transactional analysis, some of the emotional vicious cycles described in Chapter 11 are initiated because the person is overly concerned with the "critical parent" of others' expectations, and then from his "adapted child" ego-state either complies or rebels against these demanding expectations in order to maintain an early decision about his position in life vis-à-vis others. Future-oriented psychotherapy addresses this critical parent and adapted child interaction by helping the patient to develop an internal "nurturant parent" who guides and rewards the free, or natural, child.

The diversity of approaches synthesized in FOR therapy enhances its application to a wide variety of clinical problems but also, from a research standpoint, may confound comparisons with other forms of therapy. Nevertheless, besides its clinical usefulness, the future of FOR will be determined by impartial investigators who will ask precise questions about how it can be effectively used for specific problems. To date, FOR therapy has been successful in treating identity diffusion, low self-esteem (neurotic depression), anxiety disorders, and well-motivated patients who have sociopathic or borderline features. From a clinical standpoint as well as in terms of systematic evaluative measures (see Appendix A), over 80% of such patients show substantial improvement after 12–30 sessions of FOR therapy. This compares favorably with other forms of short-term dynamic psychotherapy or cognitive therapies (Davanloo, 1978; Rush and Beck, 1978). About 15% of patients have required further psychotherapy, such as group, family, or psychoanalytic psychotherapy.

Research in psychotherapy is fraught with the difficulty in teasing out the influence of the therapist's style of relating versus his techniques or theoretical orientation (Strupp, 1978; Lazarus, 1978). The personal qualities of the therapist, such as compassion, accurate empathy, and positive regard for the patient, appear to be very important. Yet one has to ask if it is these qualities that enable a therapist to be flexible in applying different techniques at times when the patient needs them the most. In other words, does a therapist's sensitivity to the patient allow for a more flexible and timely execution of various techniques? In this regard, an appropriate research question would be to ask if past-oriented, present-oriented, or future-oriented techniques are more effective at particular times for different kinds of problems that arise within the same patient or family over time (Melges, 1972). Psychiatry's attempts to define the indications for different types of psychotherapy in terms of broad clinical syndromes have been too imprecise (Strupp, 1970). What is needed are guidelines for executing specific techniques for specific problems at specific times during the course of treatment. Knowing what to do when is basic to skillful psychotherapy; this includes knowing when to focus on the past, present, or future.

SUMMARY AND CONCLUSIONS

Future-oriented psychotherapy (FOR) helps people structure their personal futures by (1) choosing and clarifying personal goals and (2) developing and rehearsing plans of action that will meet their chosen goals. Through the use of visual imagery and time projection, FOR therapy helps individuals reconstruct a realistic ego-ideal and to become more self-reinforcing rather than being overly influenced by the expectations of others. FOR therapy is based on the rationale that a positive and extended future orientation is associated with coping and may prevent the escalation of vicious cycles initiated by catastrophic expectations stemming from the past. The techniques of FOR are designed to enhance an interplay between futuring and temporal organization. That is, as images of the future are brought into the psychological present, plans of action are generated to meet the evolving images.

The essential stages of FOR therapy are as follows:

1   *Assessment and selection of patients.*   FOR therapy is indicated for nonpsychotic patients with identity diffusion, low self-esteem, anxiety

disorders, and certain types of personality disorders. Optimally, patients should be good visualizers.

2 *Interpretation of vicious cycles.*   These show the patient how catastrophic expectations are distorting his views of the personal future and leading to downward spirals.

3 *Redecisions.*   The person is prompted to take a stand against his past script messages that contribute to his catastrophic expectations.

4 *Self-futuring.*   Through visual imagery and time projection into the future, the person chooses and crystallizes personal goals and values that are important to him.

5 *Temporal organization.*   This involves the organization of plans of action in line with the person's chosen future images. The techniques entail feedback, linking images with the past, cueing images with the present, and rehearsals toward the future.

The important steps of FOR therapy are outlined in Figure 2. This figure can serve as a checklist for guiding the conduct of FOR therapy.

Hypnotic time distortions can be used in FOR therapy in order to imprint the future images or to give them a feeling of continuity through age regression and progression.

Individual FOR therapy can be combined with family therapy in order to resolve binding expectations. The essential stages of future-oriented family therapy are the same as those in individual therapy, but the techniques are modified to fit the family approach.

The emphasis on restructuring the personal future is unique to FOR therapy. Yet FOR therapy also can be considered as a synthesis of future-oriented strategies inherent in other forms of psychotherapy. By assisting the patient to learn how to bring about changes in himself, future-oriented therapy provides the patient with techniques that he, as a self-directed individual, can continue to use.

Conclusions

This conclusion collates the central themes of this book. Since more specific summaries are given at the end of each chapter, they will not be repeated here.

In the normal person, anticipatory control over thinking and behavior is largely achieved through an interplay of futuring, temporal organization, and emotion. Futuring is the process of bringing future images of possibilities into the psychological present in order to appraise options and select goals. Once the goals are selected, this sets the stage for temporal organization to take place so that sequences of plans of action become organized and revised in order to meet the goals. Emotions attune the person to discrepancies between future images (including goals) and plans of action, thereby providing the context for the reciprocal interaction between futuring and temporal organization. Mismatches between future images and plans of action are reflected in negative emotions, prompting the person to reorganize his plans of action or revise his future images and goals. By contrast, matches between future images and plans of action, as when the plans of action are effective in meeting goals, are reflected in positive emotions, prompting the person to continue on his present course and to elaborate his present plans of action and goals. Thus within an emotional context, as images of the future are brought into the psychological present, plans of action are generated to meet the evolving images. I propose that this is how people attempt to gain control over their personal futures.

This normal interplay between future images, plans of action, and emotion depends on the proper timing and temporal coordination of mental events as related to ongoing changes in the environment. That is, the basic components of psychological time—sequence, rate, and temporal perspective—have to be intact for anticipatory control to be effective. On the other hand, disturbances in psychological time can disrupt this normal interplay between future images, plans of action, and emotions. Disturbances in psychological time can give rise to inappropriate mismatches or matches between the person's future images, plans of action, and emotions, leading to a lack of anticipatory control and making him vulnerable to vicious cycles (spirals). The time problems can induce spirals by obscuring goals, diminishing feedback, amplifying feedforward, or producing the mistiming of feedback and feed-forward. Thus when a time problem hinders the person's ability to make timely corrections in order to reach goals, this results in lack of anticipatory control and vicious cycles may ensue.

Vicious cycles are like snowball effects in which the person becomes progressively alienated from his goals. These downward spirals are quite common in psychopathology. The psychopathological spirals of the major psychiatric syndromes appear to involve different problems with time and the personal future. Correction of the problems with time and the personal future is likely to restore anticipatory control, thereby interrupting psycho-pathological spirals. The treatment of problems with sequence, rate, and temporal perspective can take place at the biological, psychological, or social levels of intervention.

Different psychopathological spirals can be conceptualized in terms of a hierarchy of problems with time and the personal future. This hierarchy, which is presented in Table 2, Chapter 4, goes from the most severe and pervasive problems to those of lesser severity as follows:

1 Time disorientation reflects pervasive problems with sequence, rate, and temporal perspective. It is common in organic brain diseases.

2 The temporal disintegration of sequences refers to intermittent lapses of sequential thinking. It is common in the group of schizophrenias. The sequential difficulties appear to give rise to oscillations in mental rate as well as the episodic telescoping of larger time sequences, such as past, present, and future.

3 Rate and rhythm problems are common in the affective disorders, such as mania and depression. In mania, rate is fast; in depression, rate is slow. These rate problems may be mediated by deranged biological rhythms.

4 Problems with temporal perspective, such as an over-focus on the past, present, or future, are common in neurotic and personality disorders. These imbalances of temporal perspective can result from or give rise to misconstruction of the personal future.

5 Desynchronized transactions refer to interactions between people that are mistimed, out of phase, or at cross purposes. They can stem from any of the above time problems but also can occur per se, usually as a reflection of ambivalent relationships with other people.

In terms of this hierarchy, psychopathological spirals are proposed to occur (1) between different types of time problems, as when sequential difficulties induce changes in rate and temporal perspective, and (2) between a time problem and a misconstruction of the personal future. For an example of the latter, in depression, slowness of mental rate may induce hopelessness about the future, which, in turn, may aggravate the slowness. Thus the treatment of psychopathological spirals should be directed at correction of the time problem as well as helping the patient to reconstruct his personal future.

By way of conclusion, I will recast this hierarchy of problems with time and the personal future in terms of the cybernetic concepts about anticipatory control, as outlined in Chapter 3. That is, for the major psychiatric disorders, I will attempt to show the nature of the psychopathological spirals in terms of an incoordination or disturbed relationship between future images, plans of action, and emotions. This disharmony is proposed to stem from problems with sequence, rate, and temporal perspective. The reframed hierarchy of spirals is presented in Table 7. The hierarchy is ordered from top to bottom to indicate that the most severe spirals often involve spirals of lesser severity.

In line with the central themes of this book, I propose that for each major psychiatric disorder listed in Table 7, a particular type of time problem disrupts the timely interplay of future images, plans of action, and emotions, thereby inducing different psychopathological spirals. The nature of these spirals can be understood in terms of progressive and excessive mismatches or matches as a person projects into the future. That is, the person's feedforward into the future entails excessive mismatches or matches between future images, plans of action, and emotions, or there may be confluence and incoordination of these anticipatory factors because of a time problem. Moreover, the excessive or incoordinated feedforward mismatches and matches may become insufficiently counterbalanced by feedback from present outcomes because of a time problem that disturbs the temporal integration of feedforward and feedback processes (see Chapters 3 and 4). For each psychiatric disorder, the nature of these spirals is summarized below in terms of the format of Table 7.

1   In organic brain disease, because of the pervasive problems with sequence, rate, and temporal perspective, the person's future images are confused, his plans of action are disorganized, and his emotions usually are labile although they may be impoverished. This confluence and confusion of future images, plans of action, and emotions give rise to a spiral of pervasive loss of control over the future.

2   In schizophrenic disorders, because of the intermittent problem with keeping track of sequences, the person's future images are fragmented and incoherent, the sequences of his plans of action are incoordinated and poorly organized toward goals, and his emotions are incongruous since they reflect the disharmony and lack of coordination between the future images and the plans of action. The spiral consists of intermittent episodes of mental incoor-

Table 7 Spirals of Impaired Anticipatory Control in Psychiatric Disorders

Psychiatric Disorder	Future Images	Plans of Action	Emotions	Spirals
Organic brain diseases	Confused	Disorganized	Labile	Pervasive loss of control
Schizophrenic disorders	Fragmented	Incoordinated	Incongruous	Intermittent incoordination of future images, plans, and emotions
Affective disorders: Mania	Over-expanded	Accelerated	Euphoria	Feedforward matches exceed feedback mismatches
Depression	Constricted	Slowed	Depression	Feedforward mismatches exceed feedback matches
Neurotic disorders	Misconstrued	Uncertain	Anxiety	Feedforward of fearful anticipations
Adjustment disorders	Mismatched interpersonal expectations	Desynchronized with others	Ambivalence	Mismatched interpersonal feedforward and feedback

dination in which there is a jumbling of future images, plans of action, and emotions that unpredictably merge and augment one another during experiences of time telescoping.

3   In the affective disorders, because of opposite problems with mental rate, there is either excessive feedforward or restricted feedforward. In mania, there are a host of future images that are overly expanded into the future, the sequential plans of action are accelerated, and the anticipated matches between the future images and plans of action are reflected as euphoria, which, in turn, prompts further extensions into the future. By contrast, in severe depression, there is a dearth of future images that are constricted in scope, the plans of action are slowed, and the discrepancies between the future images and the plans of action are reflected in emotions of depression and hopelessness, which, in turn, further constrict the personal future. The spiral consists of excessive feedforward mismatches, such as anticipated dysjunctions between plans and goals, that override whatever feedback matches which occur as present outcomes.

4   In neurotic disorders, the future images often are misconstrued by catastrophic expectations from the past, the person's plans of action for dealing with these contaminated future images become uncertain, and the combination of misconstrued expectations and uncertain plans of action is reflected primarily in the emotion of anxiety. The anxiety, in turn, may further impair the person's confidence about coping with the personal future. The spiral mainly consists of excessive feedforward of fearful anticipations that feed into one another.

5   In adjustment disorders, such as marital or family discord, a person's future images often are mismatched with other people in his social network, conjoint plans of action with other people become desynchronized, and the emotion often is ambivalence about the expectations and intentions of other people as related to the self. The ambivalence, in turn, may prompt further mismatched interpersonal expectations and desynchronized transactions with other people. The spiral consists of progressive, mismatched interpersonal feedforward as well as feedback.

I believe that this temporal approach to psychiatric disorders, as cast in cybernetic terms, offers a useful and practical paradigm for understanding psychopathological spirals. It also provides a framework for the initial treatment of these spirals by highlighting the importance of correcting problems with time and the personal future in order to restore anticipatory control.

Epilogue

What follows is a personal glimpse of my own recent struggles with time and the future. I originally wrote this on an early morning in February of 1980 in an attempt to gain perspective on my recent past as related to my inner future. I was unsure whether this personal reflection belonged in this book, but friends have encouraged me to put it in as an epilogue. It may help to extend some of the academic and clinical themes of this book by highlighting the existential meanings of time and the inner future, at least in one man's life.

While I was writing this book, my own future was under almost constant threat. The spectre of death made time ever so precious.

Since I had been conducting studies on time and the mind for 18 years, and since I had come to realize the importance of time and the personal future in clinical work with my patients, I had a great desire to complete this book before I died.

The year that I started the first draft was the very year that the long-term complications of my juvenile diabetes began to take their greatest toll. First there was the threat of blindness. Black spiderlike forms, stemming from hemorrhages in my retinae, occluded my vision. My eyes were treated with lazer beams. The green jolts of light into my eyes seemed like a final countdown.

Then the nerves in my legs became impaired. As a former athlete who still loved to run, swim, golf, and play tennis, the weakness undercut whatever pride I had left in my physical prowess. I grieved the loss of perfect health. I felt I did not deserve this fate, since I had tried to control my diabetes as well as anyone I knew. Others, perhaps with less brittle forms of diabetes, had escaped these complications. Why me?

Next came the biggest threat of all: kidney failure. I searched the medical literature and consulted national experts. I found out that I had about 10 months to live. Dialysis might give me another six months to a year, but for a diabetic it was often complicated by blindness and paralysis. A kidney transplant would give me a better bet, but the overall odds were about fifty-fifty for surviving one year.

In the midst of all this, I noticed that my 12-year-old son, Kurt, was losing weight and drinking copious liquids. I tested his urine for sugar. My worst fears had come true. He had come down with diabetes. Sensitive and intelligent, he was aware of my situation and what this might mean for him. In agony, we embraced and cried.

I resolved to make the most out of the time I had left. I would help Kurt with his diabetes. I would show him how to cope with an uncertain future. I would continue to contribute—to teach, to treat, to complete this book. I would go for a kidney transplant. I would kindle hope and laughter to quell the poison of gloom surrounding my family.

It is difficult to describe the bewilderment that a whole family goes through when a member is getting a kidney transplant. For a diabetic the odds are much better with a living, related donor. Our hopes were raised when my brother turned out to be a perfect match, but then he was ruled out as a donor because of being prediabetic. My sister was a fair match, but she was understandably reluctant since she had become the only breadwinner of her family. This left my parents, who were in their mid-seventies. Because of age, they were excluded by one medical center. This left a cadaver transplant. With a cadaver transplant the chances for survival for a diabetic were at that time somewhere between 25–50%. We all did not like the odds.

After some deliberation, my nephrologist, Dr. Robert Gutman, decided to evaluate carefully my parents as potential donors. This was done at Duke Medical Center in the summer of 1979. Time was getting short, since my kidney failure was getting worse. My parents' incredible willingness to give me a kidney at their age filled me with awe. I was thankful, yet I felt guilty for even asking them to donate. I scoured the literature and pressed their doctors to rule out every possible risk to them.

Finally, my 75-year-old mother was selected to be the donor. The image of her loving, benevolent face had always been a source of courage for me. Now, 43 years after I was born and 27 years after I left my childhood home in Michigan to live in Princeton, and then in New York City, Stanford, and Duke, her love persisted: she would give me a kidney. My mother's love felt like the most timeless element ever known.

In the final weeks before the transplant I pounded out the remaining chapters for the first draft of this book. With the tremendous support of my good friend Dr. Keith Brodie, I arranged for the book to be polished and, I hoped, published should something happen to me during the transplant or afterwards. I knew the book could give a different perspective on mental illness. But the contribution seemed more than that. The recent events in my life had convinced me at a deeper level than ever before of the importance of time and the personal future in a person's emotional life.

During this time my wife, Connie, became ''born again'' as a Christian. Her belief in the ultimate salvation of mankind and in an afterlife was a source of great comfort to her. Although I did not share some of her beliefs, I became even more aware of the godliness of nature's order. I marveled at how, in the fall, the leaves turn red. Or how a drop of blood dries and then forms a scab to protect the body. To me these are the great miracles.

On September 5, 1979, I underwent surgery for the transplant. My mother, with the grace of God, tolerated the surgery well. Seven days later I felt well enough to walk one flight up to visit her in her hospital room.

On the tenth day of postsurgery, I began to have fevers as high as 106°F degrees. I was rejecting the kidney. All sorts of medicines were poured into my veins.

During this time my mother told a friend, ''You tell him that he'd better not reject my kidney since that kidney has known him even before he was born.''

Today is February 17, 1980, five months after the transplant. My mother is fine. Her kidney is serving me well. I have a lot more polishing to do on this book. Yesterday Connie and I watched Kurt star in a basketball game. Today my son Rick talked to me about his girlfriend troubles. Tomorrow we all plan to play golf together. Nothing is so precious as these little times together.

When we fully realize that we are not eternal in this life, each instant has eternal significance. On the other hand, if we believe that somehow we will live beyond death, then what we do now in this life may reverberate forever. In either case the concept of eternity makes time precious.

I remember going to Point Lobos National Reserve, California, just south of Carmel, shortly before my transplant. It is my favorite spot in the world. I went there to grieve. It is the place where I want my ashes flung to the sea.

I sat on a huge rock and watched the waves splash below. In a quiet inlet where the waves were calmed by an undertow, the waters glistened and a family of seals played with each other. The young ones, floating on their backs, clapped their flippers and squealed into the howling wind. If they drifted too near the rocks, the old ones would nuzzle them back to safety.

Right there I felt my ashes being flung to the wind. Tears filled my eyes. The waves kept crashing on the rocks. The seaweed swayed below.

I was there for an hour, but it seemed like a lifetime. Images of my boys, my wife, my parents, my triumphs and defeats reeled through my mind.

The sun lay a golden blanket over an island of rocks where hundreds of seals and walruses were cawing and mating with each other. As I watched the sun sink beneath the horizon, the seals and walruses bleated louder and louder. Their mournful cries heartened me. Life with all its cycles would go on.

Postscript June 7, 1982: And life has gone on. My mother is fine, and my health is good. Looking back, except for the physical hardships, I wish that somehow I had had an experience like that of the transplant much earlier in life. It has helped me to live more fully in the present toward the future regardless of what might happen in the future.

Glossary

altered state of consciousness   A change in the stream of awareness that feels different from the normal waking state.

anticipation   The attempt to foretell the nature and timing of an expected event; that is, the intuition of not only what might happen but also when it might happen; the grasping beforehand of what and when an event might happen in the future with only minimal present cues signaling an expected event. Compare *expectation*.

anticipatory control   The attempt to master a situation before it happens; the generation of plans of action that will meet anticipated images of future situations so that one is prepared to respond appropriately to the events once they do occur.

biological rhythm   An innate capacity for cycles of certain biological functions to become synchronized with certain periodic changes in the environment.

biopsychosocial   Pertains to the interaction of biological, psychological, and social factors impinging upon a person.

change   An observable difference between the past, present, and future.

circadian   Refers to a type of biological rhythm that roughly follows a 24-hour periodicity; for example, the activity–rest cycle that occurs in phase with changes of light to dark during a 24-hour day.

coincidence   The occurrence of two or more events that appear to take place at the same time. An "uncanny coincidence" refers to the feeling that events have coincided in time beyond that which would be expected to occur by chance or as a result of a series of previous sequences.

construct   A way of framing reality. A *personal construct* is a bipolar way of anticipating events; that is, before an event occurs, a person's idiosyncratic beliefs determine, in large measure, whether the event is construed to be good or bad, strong or weak, and so forth (Kelly, 1955).

construe   To put a construction or interpretation upon events.

control   The correction of deviations from a goal; that is, control is achieved when the outcomes of plans of action serve to reduce discrepancies from a goal.

cybernetic   Refers to processes involved in "steering" a system toward control, such as the counteraction of deviations from a goal that has been detected through feedback.

deja vu   The current experience that events happening now have occurred before in the exact same way; French for "already seen."

delusion   A false belief that is difficult to falsify; a personal conviction that is unshared by one's social network and is resistant to modification by logical argument or subsequent experience.

depersonalization   The feeling of strangeness about one's self.

desynchronized transaction   An exchange between two or more people that is out of phase or mistimed. Desynchronized transactions occur frequently when there are mismatched expectations about the intentions of other people.

discontinuity   The fragmentation and incoherence of the timeline of past, present, and future.

duration   The interval (time-gap) separating two successive events. The experience of duration usually applies to the interval between the present and a future event of concern.

ego-ideal   Optimal characteristics and goals constructed for the self.

expectation   Looking forward to a future event as about to come due, usually when present cues arouse memories of past sequences that are likely to recur in similar situations.

feedback   The detection of deviations from a goal; that is, the perception and registration of how and to what degree an organization has currently deviated from its goals.

feedforward   The expectation or anticipation of deviations from a goal. In contrast to feedback, which refers to present outcomes, feedforward refers to future outcomes.

future   That which has not yet occurred. In contrast to the past and present, the future is like an open context, a container to be filled.

future time perspective   The time span of awareness extended into the future.

future-oriented psychotherapy   A form of psychotherapy that focuses on the construction and rehearsal of a person's choices for his identity extending into the future.

futuring   The process of bringing images of the future into present awareness. Futuring involves the simultaneous visualization of options and possibilities.

geophysical time   Time as an independent metric system of equal units of duration; roughly equivalent to world or clock time. The Newtonian concept of time holds that time equals distance divided by velocity.

goal   A desired end-state, like a target; in humans, part of a future image of a situation.

goal correction   The organized process of counteracting deviations from a goal. Compare *control*.

goal-directedness   The orientation of an organization toward making adjustments to reach a goal. Similar to *goal correction*.

guided imagery   A semistructured way of guiding a person's imagination (mainly visual images) for the purpose of psychotherapy.

grief-resolution therapy   A form of psychotherapy that uses guided imagery to help free a person from a past attachment.

hope   The expectation or anticipation of desirable outcomes; similar to optimism but entails more active yearning for a positive future outcome.

hopelessness   The loss of hope; the belief that the future is bleak and devoid of desirable outcomes; pessimism, with loss of sense of efficacy about self's ability to change future outcomes.

identification   The process of taking an image of another person as a model for one's own self-image and behavior.

identity   Core views and beliefs about the self that are sustained through time; that is, self-sameness and continuity through time.

image   The perception of spatially arranged events. A ''future image'' is the construction of holistic patterns, usually involving the synthesis of various expectations and anticipations.

inner future   A person's inward outlook on his personal future.

inner–outer confusion   Mistaking events inside the self to be coming from outside the self, for example, hallucinations.

intensive design   A form of research design that makes use of changes that occur within a person as he is studied longitudinally over time.

memory   The re-presentation of past events. Immediate memory refers to events that occurred just seconds ago, short-term memory to events from minutes to hours ago, and long-term memory to events days, years, or decades ago.

paranoid   Generally, a person's unwarranted conviction that other people are intending to do him harm; literally, ''beside one's mind.''

paranoid connectivity   The feeling that there is an interconnected global conspiracy or plot directed against the self.

past   That which has already occurred, that is, the after-now. Compared to the present and future, the past is usually experienced as fixed and unchanging.

personal future   An individual's unique outlook on the future of his own life.

plan   A prearranged sequence of intended actions designed to meet a goal.

precognition   The supposed capacity to foretell future events beyond that which can be logically inferred or statistically forecasted.

present   That which is perceived to be happening now. In contrast to the fixed past (after-now) and the open future (before-now), the present is continuously perceived to be changing, and the changes usually occur simultaneously in all five senses. The duration of the present is difficult to define, but usually lasts only about 2 to 3 seconds (range: 0.001 to 12 seconds; Fraisse, 1963; Cohen, 1966; Efron, 1967).

primary process   The form of thinking of the unconscious, typified by the fluid symbolism and timelessness of dreams.

psychedelic   Refers to nonordinary experiences of mental events; literally, "mind-manifestation."

psychological time   The inner time of the mind, consisting of the rate and sequence of mental events as well as temporal perspective into the past and future.

psychotic   Refers to defective reality testing, usually accompanied by alterations in the sense of reality.

reinforcement   In this book, the matching of plans of action with goals so that rewards are maximized and punishments are minimized.

script   A person's unwitting life plan, derived largely from parental programming via identification and reinforcements.

secondary process   Rational goal-directed thinking that normally accompanies the waking state.

sequence   The occurrence of events in succession.

sequential processing   The comprehension and analysis of events in terms of linear sequences ordered according to the timeline of past, present, and future. Thought to occur primarily in the left (dominant) cerebral hemisphere.

simultaneous processing   The intuition of patterned wholes as visual-spatial displays. Thought to occur primarily in the right (nondominant) cerebral hemisphere.

spiral   The amplification of deviations from a goal; a snowball effect; a progressive escalation of changes where one change augments other changes.

A "downward spiral" is a vicious cycle that progressively alienates a person from his goals; an "upward spiral" is a virtuous cycle that not only accomplishes initial goals but also creates positive and unforeseen ripple effects.

synchronicity   A notion developed by Jung (1955) to refer to the temporal concurrence of an external event with an inward experience so that the person feels that there is an unusual connection that has meaning beyond that which can be inferred in terms of cause and effect.

synchronization   The proper timing of rates and sequences so that two or more systems are in phase with one another.

temporal disintegration   The breakdown of sequential thinking; more precisely, the incoordination of sequences in the process of attempting to make adjustments in order to reach a goal.

temporal indistinction   The interpenetration and confusion of past, present, and future so that these categories are indistinguishable; an extreme form of temporal disintegration characterized by the time telescoping of sequences.

temporal organization   The sequencing and rearrangement of plans of action toward general life goals within future time perspective; the planning of plans of action to meet evolving images of the future.

temporal perspective   The span of awareness extending into the past or future. Compare *future time perspective.*

tertiary process   A form of thinking proposed to be involved in creativity; probably entails the integration of simultaneous and sequential processing of information in conjunction with primary process.

time   A general dimension of human existence derived largely from the perception or imputation of changes against a background taken to be relatively stable and permanent.

time binding   The capacity of the human brain to store, retrieve, and rearrange events that previously have occurred together in time, that is, as temporally contiguous events.

time diffusion   The feeling that the march of time is chaotic and disorganized; frequently seen as a mistrust of time in identity diffusion.

time disorientation   The inability to locate one's self according to clock or calendar time, such as the inability to tell the date or year.

time estimation   The judgment of the amount of clock time that either has elapsed or is elapsing.

time sense   The subjective feeling of time passing by compared to the amount of clock time.

time telescoping   The collapse of the past and future into the present.

timing   The arrangement and adjustment of rates and sequences so that a goal is reached at an opportune moment.

tracking difficulties   The inability to keep track of sequences over time; a mild to moderate form of temporal disintegration.

transaction   A social exchange between two or more people, usually involving both verbal and nonverbal communications.

unconscious processes   Mental processes that ordinarily take place out of a person's awareness, often involving the influence of past identifications and reinforcements on current expectations and anticipations.

vicious cycle   A snowball effect in which one change augments other changes leading to a downward spiral that progressively alienates a person from his goals.

APPENDIX A

Research Materials

The purpose of this appendix is twofold: (1) to acquaint the interested reader with some of the instruments used to measure psychological time, future outlook, and related constructs and (2) to give an overview of the reliability and construct validity of the instruments. Since details of the previous research can be found in the original scientific reports, this will be a general overview.

TESTS OF TIME ESTIMATION

There are a variety of methods to test a person's estimation of clock time (for review, see Doob, 1971). We have predominantly used the production method in which the subject is asked to produce an interval of clock time such as 30 seconds. We have preferred the production method because it is straightforward and can be used clinically with just the aid of a second hand on a watch or stopwatch. Also, the production method, compared to other time estimation methods (such as verbal estimation of time already elapsed, comparison of durations, and reproduction of an interval just witnessed) is generally more accurate and reliable (Clausen, 1950). It should be noted that these different methods may give opposite results if the terms *overestimation* or *underestimation* are used (Bindra and Waksberg, 1956). For example, if a subject gives 15 seconds when asked to produce 30 seconds, his internal tempo can be interpreted to be going twice as fast as clock time, but if he gives 15 seconds when asked to verbally estimate a 30-second interval that has already elapsed, this implies that his internal tempo is twice as slow as clock time. Unfortunately, some investigators have not taken into account these different implications of the various methods and, as a result, have reported confusing findings.

The 30-Second Production Test

This simple test has been useful for studying changes in time sense during acute mental illness (Melges and Fougerousse, 1966) and is remarkably sensitive for detecting differences between the effects of various psychoactive drugs (Tinklenberg et al., 1972, also personal communication).

The instructions are as follows: "When I say 'go,' I want you to tell me when 30 seconds—one-half of a minute—are up. Do you understand? Please repeat back the instructions to me. . . . Fine. Now go. . . ." The subject is asked to do this task twice in consecutive fashion in order to evaluate the consistency of his time production.

Normal subjects have been found to give a mean production of 25.92 seconds (s.d. 11.85) for the 30-second standard. Patients with acute mental illness (excluding organic brain disease) at the time of admission to a psychiatric hospital gave a mean production of 14.80 seconds (s.d. 8.73), and after an average of nine days of hospitalization gave a mean production of 19.60 seconds (s.d. 11.15). At a particular time of testing, repeat testing of the same individual generally shows high consistency; for example, even with the highly disturbed mental patients, the correlation of the repeat testing at the time of admission was .86 (Melges and Fougerousse, 1966).

Because of the variability between individuals, as reflected in the standard deviations cited above, this test is most useful for studying changes over time, using each subject as his own control. Normal subjects retested approximately one week later show only 1–2 seconds difference, whereas there can be marked changes within an individual recovering from mental illness or after withdrawing from a psychoactive drug. In studying changes over time, the 30-second production test can be scored for the magnitude of change in the produced number of seconds (for example, early testing = 14 seconds; later testing = 26 seconds; thus, magnitude of change = 12 seconds) or for change in degree of inaccuracy (for example, in above example, early testing inaccuracy $[30 - 14] = 16$ seconds; later testing inaccuracy $[30 - 26] = 4$ seconds; percent change in inaccuracy $(16/4) = 400\%$ improvement). Scoring for magnitude is indicated when one is interested in inferring changes in internal rate; scoring for inaccuracy is indicated when one is interested in how well the subject is in tune with standards of clock time.

Other Time Production Tests

Of course, there are many variants of time production tasks. Longer or shorter intervals can be used. Ordinarily, the subject or patient is not given feedback in order to minimize the effect of learning on later retesting. However, feedback about the degree of inaccuracy can be used as a special test to see how well the subject temporally integrates feedback about time itself. For example: "You were 9 seconds short of 30 seconds; now let's try it again to see if you can come closer to 30 seconds." With acutely psychotic patients, it is remarkable how little they correct their time estimations even when given feedback.

A continuous type of production task is the operant schedule called the "differential reinforcement of low rates" (Sidman, 1956; Melges and Poppen, 1976). Essentially, this means that when subjects wait long enough for a prescribed period, they are reinforced each time they wait long enough. If their responses are premature, the clock resets and they again have to wait for the prescribed period until reinforcement is again available. This requires a timing apparatus with some means of signaling reinforcement, such as a light flashing, a token, or a piece of candy. This procedure has been shown to be sensitive for demonstrating improvement in schizophrenics (Angle, 1973).

TESTS OF TEMPORAL DISORGANIZATION

Temporal disorganization is a general construct referring to disturbances in the rate, sequential ordering, and goal-directedness of mental processes (Melges et al., 1974). There are a number of psychological tests relevant to this construct, such as various tests of memory, the Porteus maze, and different ways to analyze the temporal organization of spontaneous speech. Since we were interested in brief tests that could be used repeatedly to show changes in acutely disturbed psychiatric patients or subjects undergoing a psychotomimetic experience, we developed some special cognitive and subjective report tests for this purpose.

Goal-Directed Serial Alternation Test (GDSA)

The GDSA tests a person's capacity to organize sequences serially in order to meet a goal. That is, the person has to keep in mind the goal as he makes sequential adjustments to reach the goal. It requires simple arithmetic operations that involve a process similar to arranging words in linear fashion while composing a sentence in order to make a point. It has the advantage over analysis of sentence structure in that it can be scored numerically (Melges et al., 1970).

The instructions are as follows: "I want you to try to reach a goal, a number I will give you, by going through some steps. The goal you are to reach is the number 50, exactly. Starting at 110, you are to try to reach the number 50 by going back and forth between two steps. First you subtract 7, then you add 1, 2, *or* 3. Keep repeating these alternate steps of subtracting 7, then adding 1, 2, or 3 until you reach the goal of 50. You can subtract past the goal of 50 and then add on, if you wish. Work as fast as you can but also be accurate. Do you understand?   . . . Repeat back the instructions to me. Fine. . . . Start now.'' The tester times the performance and records each operation, which the patient states aloud. For repeat testing, in order to avoid practice effects, the starting number can be varied between 114 and 106, and the goal number can be varied between 54 and 46.

This test is scored for time taken and the number of mistakes. The types of mistakes include loss of place, no alternation, blocking, forgetting what to subtract (7), forgetting what to add (1, 2, or 3), miscalculations, forgetting the goal number, failure to adjust to goal, and disregarding the goal number (as when the person just keeps subtracting and adding but goes way past the goal number). As detailed in a previous report (Melges et al., 1970a), overall performance on the GDSA is measured as the time (seconds) $+ C$ (1 + number of mistakes), with C equal to 39, which was the average number of seconds associated with errorless performance for a group of normal, bright graduate students. (C may have to be modified accordingly for different samples.) Since the GDSA is a goal-directed task, failure to reach the goal exactly is weighted as three mistakes for the overall GDSA performance score.

The GDSA is particularly useful as a cognitive test of tracking difficulties (Melges et al., 1970a). Although it is somewhat dependent on intact immediate memory functions and the ability to concentrate on simple arithmetic operations, these factors are not the whole story. For example, in one study the regular serial subtraction of 7s from 100 was not significantly impaired, but the GDSA was markedly impaired in the same subjects during THC intoxication (Melges et al., 1970a). This indicates that the subjects could concentrate adequately, but they had difficulty in temporally integrating information at the right time in order to make serial adjustments to reach a goal. To quote one subject on THC: ''I'd pick out a number now and then go ahead. . . . Coming back, I'd forget which number I just did or what I was supposed to do next.'' Only during THC intoxication did subjects completely disregard the goal, going right past it and not bringing it into awareness at the right time, even though when prompted they remembered the goal accurately. This is a classic example of lack of temporal integration. It did not occur during baseline of placebo control periods.

The usefulness of the GDSA in demonstrating tracking difficulties during THC intoxication has been replicated by Casswell and Marks (1973). Other cognitive and EEG tests also have demonstrated impairment of tracking information over time during THC intoxication and in schizophrenia (Braff et al., 1977; Saccuzzo and Braff, 1981).

The application of the GDSA to randomly selected psychiatric patients who are acutely disturbed is sometimes difficult. One problem is that some acute patients have such severe tracking difficulties that they cannot repeat back the instructions of the GDSA. Another problem is that at least average intelligence is necessary to perform the task, and we have found that the GDSA works best for showing changes over time in reasonably intelligent psychiatric patients. Attempts are now being made to simplify the test so that it has wider applicability for giving an objective measurement of tracking difficulties in all types of psychiatric patients.

Temporal Integration Inventory (TII)

This subjective report instrument measures a person's appraisal of how well he can integrate, yet keep distinct, past, present, and future during the process of pursuing goals. As outlined below, it is scored for temporal *dis*integration. As predicted, changes in the TII were highly correlated with changes in overall GDSA performance ($r = .72; P < .0001$). This finding lends validity to using each of these measures as tests of the construct of temporal disintegration (Melges et al., 1970a, 1970b).

The TII consists of 14 statements.

TII

1   Sometimes I feel absent from the present, swept into the past and future as if I were really there.
2   My past, present, and future seem quite integrated with each other.
3   My past, present, and future seem like separate islands of experience with little relation to each other.
4   Things seem to be happening in the proper sequence, and it is easy for me to tell what comes before or after.
5   My past and future seem to have collapsed into the present, and it is difficult for me to tell them apart.
6   I can keep in mind memories, perceptions, and expectations all at once without confusing which is which.
7   My past, present, and future seem all muddled up and mixed together.
8   When I am remembering my past or imagining my future, I still realize that I am here in the present.

9 Things seem to be happening to me rather than my making things happen.

10 My short-term goals seem to fit my long-term goals.

11 My sense of self-direction seems to be impaired.

12 My thoughts and actions are organized toward what I want to do or say next.

13 I feel I have little control over what happens to me in the immediate future.

14 I am confident that my plans will accomplish my goals.

Although the items were intermixed during actual testing of subjects, the TII statements are listed above according to its two components: temporal distinction and goal-directedness. The first eight statements relate to temporal distinction—that is, orderly indexing memories as past, perceptions as present, and expectations as future, without confusion of these temporal categories. In addition, items 1 and 8 refer to what Minkowski (1933) termed the "I–here–now" position, meaning that the present is used as a reference point for experience, and the person does not get lost in fantasies of the past and future as though he were "really there." Statements 9 through 14 relate to goal-directedness—that is, adjusting plans of action to reach goals and control outcomes. Previous theoretical and review papers have detailed those concepts: Plans of actions are hierarchies of sequential acts; goals are the desired outcomes of these acts (Miller, Galanter, and Pribram, 1960; Melges and Bowlby, 1969).

Subjects respond to each statement on a six-point scale, ranging from "not at all" to "extremely." The TII items labeled above with odd numbers reflect temporal disintegration, and thus are scored positively; even-numbered items are scored negatively. Thus scoring of the TII in this way gives a total score which reflects temporal disintegration so that higher scores indicate greater psychopathological disturbance.

When 30 normal subjects were tested two weeks apart, the test–retest correlation of the TII was .83 ($P < .001$). Care was taken to make sure that these subjects were normal to begin with (for example, no psychiatric history, stable interpersonal relationships, actively working, and so forth) and, during the two-week interval, had no unusual emotional and mental disturbance. The 95% confidence intervals for the mean change in the TII in these normal subjects over the two-week period were -0.98 to $+2.58$. This indicates that the TII scores change very little during stable conditions. On the other hand, the TII is sensitive to measuring changes over time, as in the THC experiments and clinical investigations.

Tracking Difficulties

In previous studies, temporal disintegration was related to difficulties in immediate or "working" memory, such that there were disturbances in retaining, coordinating, and serially indexing those memories, perceptions, and expectations that were relevant to a goal being pursued (Melges et al., 1970a, 1970b). The tracking difficulties inventory consists of items reporting subjective difficulties in immediate memory and in maintaining attention over time. The items were culled from tape recordings of previous experiments with tetrahydrocannabinol and from reports of acutely ill schizophrenics (Bleuler, 1950; Chapman, 1966). The items are as follows:

1 Thoughts slip away before I can quite grasp them.
2 My attention shifts rapidly from one thing to another.
3 Many different thoughts are racing through my mind.
4 I can recall and select the appropriate thought at the right time.*
5 I tend to lose my train of thought.
6 I forget what I have just said or what I intend to say.
7 I tune out such that my attention to the outside world wavers.
8 My mind goes blank at times, as if my memory is blocked.
9 It seems that my mind is racing and I cannot sort out the thoughts that I want.
10 I forget the first part of a sentence by the time I've gotten to the second part.
11 I can keep track of what I'm saying and what others are saying.*

The items above labeled with an asterisk are phrased in the direction of normality and therefore are scored in the opposite direction than the other items. Subjects respond to each item on a four- to seven-spaced scale ranging from "not at all" to "frequently." They are to answer the statements in terms of the last few minutes or, for some clinical situations, of the last hour. Specifying a recent time period like this increases the accuracy of the reports. It also helps compare changes over time, as when subjects are tested several hours later in a drug experiment or days later when evaluating changes in psychiatric patients. It should be emphasized that all these measures of temporal disorganization can show marked changes just one day later after a psychotic patient has been hospitalized. In this regard, I feel strongly that a psychosis should be studied *while* it is occurring, and that retrospective accounts of a psychosis are frequently invalid since patients usually view the experience like a dream for which recall is imprecise and vague.

Temporal Disorganization

This inventory consists of a composite of items taken from previous inventories of temporal disintegration, tracking difficulties, and other statements used in our research. The inventory was made brief and to the point during pilot studies with acutely disturbed patients. Because of its brevity, it lacks some of the precision of the previous inventories. Nevertheless, it has been useful in detecting overall changes in temporal disorganization during acute mental illness (Melges and Freeman, 1977).

This general inventory of temporal disorganization consists of 20 statements, with four statements comprising each of its five subcomponents. In the lists below, the statements with an asterisk are phrased in the direction of normality so as to avoid response sets. In actual practice, the inventory statements are usually intermixed and presented in random order. Patients are carefully instructed and reminded to reply in terms of their experiences on the day of testing, and the statements are read aloud by the research assistant with the patient looking on and also reading. Patients reply in terms of "not at all," "occasionally" (1–2 times per hour), "often" (5–10 times per hour), "frequently" (more than 20 times per hour).

The statements reflecting overall temporal disorganization in terms of its subcomponents are as follows:

1   *Rate-duration changes.*   My mind seems to be racing. My mind seems to be going slowly. I'm unsure how much clock time has gone by (unless I look at a clock). My mind seems to be going at its usual rate.*

2   *Tracking difficulties.*   I tend to lose my train of thought. I forget what I've just said or intend to say. My mind goes blank at times. I can keep track of what I'm thinking about.*

3   *Temporal indistinction.*   My past and future seem to have collapsed into the present, and it is difficult for me to tell them apart. My past, present, and future seem all muddled up and mixed together. Sometimes I feel absent from the present, swept into the past or future as if I were really there. It's easy for me to tell whether something is a memory, a perception, or an expectation.*

4   *Impaired goal-directedness.*   My sense of self-direction seems to be impaired. I lose control over my thinking. It's hard for me to direct my thoughts to what I intend to think or say. My thoughts and actions are organized toward what I want to do or say next.*

5   *Desynchronization.*   My mind switches between speeding up and slowing down. I am having two or more trains of thought at the same time.

Some of my experiences seem to have happened before in the exact same way. My mind swings back and forth in opposite directions.

TESTS OF PSYCHOTIC SYMPTOMS

The format of these inventories is the same as those described above, such as the TII. That is, subjects responded to each statement in terms of a four- to six-point scale, ranging from "not at all" to "extremely" or "frequently." The statements are intermixed when administered, but will be reported here in terms of the appropriate category.

Depersonalization

Depersonalization is measured by 12 statements (hereafter abbreviated as the DP inventory) that Dixon (1963) found to have a factor loading of greater than 0.50 on depersonalization. Statements of the DP inventory refer to feelings of estrangement and unreality about the self. For example: "My body seems detached, as if my body and self are separate," and "I feel like a stranger to myself."

The statements listed below are those used in my initial studies of depersonalization. Most of the items reflect feelings of self-estrangement, but in a later study I also added some statements reflecting body image diffusion, such as, "My body boundaries feel fluid and changing" (Freeman and Melges, 1977). The statements reflecting self-estrangement are as follows:

1   I feel like a stranger to myself.
2   My body seems detached, as if my body and self are separate.
3   I have the feeling that I am two people. One is "going through the motions" while the other "me" is observing me.
4   My ordinary feelings of self-awareness seem different: There seems to be a greater difference between self and not-self.
5   My body feels it is not part of me.
6   My ordinary feelings of self-awareness seem different: There seems to be less difference between self and not-self.
7   There is little distinction between "me" and "not me"—There is feeling, but it is not me feeling.
8   Things I have been used to in the past now begin to seem strange.
9   Other people seem strange and unfamiliar.

10   It is as if there is a wall or veil between me and other people.

11   Things around me seem to behave in an odd way.

12   It is as if I am about to receive some great revelation or mystical awareness.

Delusional Ideation

This inventory was designed after a thorough review of the literature on delusions. Pilot studies with delusional psychiatric patients and hashish-intoxicated normal subjects helped to refine the statements and make the inventory brief. Not all types or aspects of delusions (for example, delusions of worthlessness) are reflected in its three categories: feelings of persecution, influence, and grandiosity. (Statements below marked with an asterisk are phrased in the direction of normality so as to avoid response sets; accordingly, they are scored in the reverse direction of the other statements phrased in the direction of psychopathology.)

Persecutory items include the following: I have the feeling that I might be being tricked or manipulated; I feel that it is safe to trust other people right now;* I am suspicious that other people have motives that are unclear to me; something strange is going on in the world around me.

Influence items include the following: Somebody seems to be controlling my mind; my thoughts and feelings seem imposed upon my by some outside force; I myself am in control of what I do or say;* some persons seem to be able to read my mind without my speaking.

Grandiosity items are as follows: Things that happen around me seem to have special hidden messages for me; I feel that my ''psychic'' powers are the same as anyone else;* I am having profound relevations and insights; I feel compelled to transmit my original insights to mankind.

The above items indicate delusionallike or bizarre ideation and do not, of course, reflect fixed delusional ideas of an idiosyncratic nature, often impervious to contradiction, as seen at later stages of some types of psychiatric illness (see Chapter 8). Our focus was not on the maintenance of fixed delusional ideas; rather, it was on the emergence of delusionallike ideation during different experimental conditions, using each subject as his own control. That is, if a person responded ''extremely'' to the above statements during one condition and ''not at all'' during another condition, I was interested in the processes involved in such a difference.

The total delusionallike inventory score consists of the sum of all statement scores combined, that is, the sum of the persecutory, influence, and grandiosity categories.

Symptoms of Inner–Outer Confusion

The symptoms of inner–outer confusion were derived from Schneider's first-rank symptoms of schizophrenia and refined from other studies (Schneider, 1959; Carpenter, Strauss, and Muleh, 1973; Mellor, 1972), with four statements in each of the subcomponents below. (The last statement, marked with an asterisk, in each of the below subcomponents is phrased in the direction of normality.)

1 *Auditory hallucinations.* I hear my inner thoughts spoken aloud. I hear voices outside my head arguing or talking about me. Voices comment on my actions at the time that I do them. All the voices that I hear come from myself or persons I can see talking.*

2 *Experiences of influence.* I am made to feel emotions that are not my own. Outside forces put impulses into me. Forces other than myself make me do or say things that I don't intend. I myself am in control of what I do, think, and feel.*

3 *Thought diffusion.* Thoughts that are not my own are put into my mind. My inner thoughts are broadcast to other people even when I don't speak aloud. Some outside force or person takes my thoughts away. My inner thoughts are contained within my head and nobody can read my mind.*

4 *Delusional perception.* Something strange is going on in the world around me. Unusual coincidences are happening to me that seem to have special meanings for me and my future. Something I see or hear suddenly takes on a profound significance for me and my future. The coincidences that happen to me are just ordinary chance happenings, with no special meaning for me or my future.*

5 *Somatic passivity experiences.* Somebody or something touches me even when nobody is around. Unusual sensations are put into my body. My body is controlled by outside forces. My bodily movements seem normally under my control.*

Although most of the Schneiderian symptoms listed above can be conceptualized as inner–outer confusion, some of Schneider's symptom descriptions (for example, thought-echo and delusional perception) may not be readily interpreted in this way. For the purposes of our research, compared to such constructs as diffusion of ego or body boundaries, these Schneiderian symptoms investigated questions relevant to inner–outer confusion that were specific enough to be measured by scaled subjective report methods.

TESTS RELEVANT TO FUTURE-ORIENTED RECONSTRUCTION (FOR) THERAPY

The tests outlined below have been used in systematic research as well as for clinical evaluation during therapy and follow-up (see Chapter 12). For ease of repeated administration and to keep the format similar and brief, we largely have used semantic differential tests. Semantic differential tests consist of opposite words separated by seven-point scales upon which a subject rates a specified concept (Osgood, Suci, and Tannenbaum, 1957). For example, the concept of "My View of My Own Future Three Months Ahead" can be rated in terms of the bipolar scale of optimism versus pessimism as follows:

OPTIMISM   __: __: __: __: __: __: __: PESSIMISM

If the subject feels very optimistic, he checks the space on the far left; if he feels very pessimistic, he checks the space on the far right; if his feeling is somewhere between these extremes, he may so indicate on the intervening spaces.

Eriksonian Semantic Differential of the Self-Image (ESD)

This scale was generated through correlating and testing a number of antonyms related to the bipolar constructs of Erikson's (1959) epigenetic life-cycle stages of personality development. In order to make the test brief and understandable, we chose one antonym pair that was rated by a group of graduate students familiar with Erikson's writings as being both representative and readily comprehendible. In the scales below, the first eight antonyms are related to the eight identity stages outlined by Erikson. The bottom four scales are commonly used in semantic differential tests. It can be seen that the positively keyed word of each antonym is varied from right to left so as to avoid response sets; scoring of the test has to take this into account.

My Own View of Myself Now

TRUSTING   __: __: __: __: __: __: __: DISTRUSTING

SELF-   __: __: __: __: __: __: __: SELF-
  CONSCIOUS   ASSURED

ASSERTIVE   __: __: __: __: __: __: __: DEFENSIVE

INADEQUATE   __: __: __: __: __: __: __: COMPETENT

REAL	__: __: __: __: __: __: __:	UNREAL
DISTANT	__: __: __: __: __: __: __:	WARM
CARING FOR OTHERS	__: __: __: __: __: __: __:	SELF-ABSORBED
PHONY	__: __: __: __: __: __: __:	SINCERE
STRONG	__: __: __: __: __: __: __:	WEAK
PASSIVE	__: __: __: __: __: __: __:	ACTIVE
GOOD	__: __: __: __: __: __: __:	BAD
MASCULINE	__: __: __: __: __: __: __:	FEMININE

Of course, if the subject is a man, masculine is the positive pole; if a woman, feminine is the positive pole. Various temporal views of the self-image can be rated by the ESD. That is, besides "My Own View of Myself Now," subjects can rate "How I Would Like to View Myself Three Months in the Future" or "My View of Myself Five Years Ago When My Husband Left Me" (see Chapter 12).

When 30 normal subjects were tested two weeks apart, the test–retest reliability of the ESD was .83 ($P < .001$; Melges et al., 1971). Thus this test is stable during stable conditions, but also is sensitive to changes over time in psychiatric patients.

Future Outlook Inventory (FOI)

This is also a semantic differential test with a format similar to that of the ESD. The concepts that can be rated on the FOI scales refer to the person's outlook on the future, such as "My Feelings about My Own Future Right Now," "My Feelings about My Own Future Three Months from Now," "My Feelings about My Own Future Five Years from Now," and so forth. The antonyms presented below were selected on the basis of ratings from normal subjects of a number of similar polar-opposite words. This was done to make the inventory brief and understandable for repeated use (Melges et al., 1971).

The format of the FOI is presented below with the positive pole of the bipolar scales varied from left to right.

My Feelings about My Own Future Three Months from Now

OPTIMISM	__:	__:	__:	__:	__:	__:	__:	PESSIMISM
CHALLENGE	__:	__:	__:	__:	__:	__:	__:	FAMILIARITY
CONFIDENCE	__:	__:	__:	__:	__:	__:	__:	UNCERTAINTY
INDIFFERENCE	__:	__:	__:	__:	__:	__:	__:	COMMITMENT
PURPOSE	__:	__:	__:	__:	__:	__:	__:	AIMLESSNESS
URGENCY	__:	__:	__:	__:	__:	__:	__:	CALMNESS
CONFUSION	__:	__:	__:	__:	__:	__:	__:	MEANING
PROGRESSION	__:	__:	__:	__:	__:	__:	__:	REGRESSION
RESTRICTION	__:	__:	__:	__:	__:	__:	__:	CHOICE
HOPE	__:	__:	__:	__:	__:	__:	__:	DESPAIR

When 30 normal subjects were tested two weeks apart, the test–retest reliability of the FOI was .83 $(P < .001)$. As with all the semantic differential tests presented in this section, each scale is scored from one to seven, with seven representing the score given to the positive pole. The scales are then summed for the total FOI score. In the normal subjects, the 95% confidence intervals for mean change over two weeks were -1.92, $+0.92$, whereas psychiatric patients undergoing therapy showed a mean change of $+17.67$.

Another useful test of future outlook is the Hopelessness Scale (Beck et al., 1974).

Tests of Emotion

In systematic research, I have generally used the Nowlis-Green Mood Adjective Check List (Melges and Fougerousse, 1966). However, since that test takes fairly long to complete, recently I have preferred a semantic differential test of emotions, especially for clinical assessment. The concept rated is "My Feelings at Present" in terms of the following bipolar scales:

ANGRY	__:	__:	__:	__:	__:	__:	__:	PEACEFUL
CALM	__:	__:	__:	__:	__:	__:	__:	ANXIOUS

DEPRESSED	__: __: __: __: __: __: __:	ELATED
PLEASANT	__: __: __: __: __: __: __:	UNPLEASANT
GUILTY	__: __: __: __: __: __: __:	FREE (FOR-GIVING OF MYSELF)
LOVING	__: __: __: __: __: __: __:	HATEFUL (TOWARD OTHERS)
SAD	__: __: __: __: __: __: __:	GLAD
RELAXED	__: __: __: __: __: __: __:	UPTIGHT
ASHAMED	__: __: __: __: __: __: __:	JOYOUS
HAPPY	__: __: __: __: __: __: __:	UNHAPPY

It can be seen that there are two scales related to common negative emotions seen in psychiatric patients. That is, anger is related to the angry, hateful scales; anxiety to the anxious, uptight scales; depression to the depressed, sad scales; guilt to the guilty, ashamed scales; and overall unpleasantness to the unpleasant, unhappy scales. These separate emotions can be examined, but usually the entire emotion scales are summed for a total score of negative emotions to be used for measuring changes over time during psychotherapy.

Modified Internal–External Control Inventory

This test measures the degree to which a person believes he has control over outcomes. It was developed originally by Rotter (1966) and his co-workers as a measure of enduring beliefs about the role of skill versus chance in determining one's destiny. We modified the statements to refer to current and personal states of mind, rather than enduring traits or beliefs about humanity, and we also made it brief so that it could be used repeatedly with the same subjects (Melges and Weisz, 1971).

The modified internal–external control inventory is a forced-choice test in which the subject must choose between two alternative statements as reflecting his current state of mind. In the statements presented below, those marked with an asterisk indicate internal control. The inventory is scored for the degree of internal control by simply summing the number of internal-control preferences made by the subject.

Instructions: Please choose either *a* or *b* to indicate your current state of mind for each of the numbered paired statements listed below.

1   **(a)**   Many of the unhappy things in my own life right now are partly due to bad luck.

    (b)   My present misfortunes are a result of the mistakes I have made.*

2   **(a)**   Right now I feel I am getting the respect I deserve in this world.*

    (b)   Right now, no matter how hard I try, my personal worth is going unrecognized.

3   **(a)**   At present, no matter how hard I try, some people just don't like me.

    (b)   If some people don't like me at this time, it must be that I don't understand how to get along with them.*

4   **(a)**   At this time, I feel that what is going to happen will happen.

    (b)   At this time, trusting to fate will not turn out as well for me as making a decision to take a definite course of action.*

5   **(a)**   If I am successful in the near future, it will be a matter of hard work; luck has little or nothing to do with it.*

    (b)   If I am successful in the near future, it will depend mainly on being in the right place at the right time.

6   **(a)**   When I am making my present plans, I am almost certain that I can make them work.*

    (b)   Right now I feel it is unwise to plan too far ahead because many things may turn out to be a matter of good or bad fortune anyway.

7   **(a)**   In my present case, getting what I want has little or nothing to do with luck.*

    (b)   Presently, I might just as well decide what to do by flipping a coin.

8   **(a)**   Right now, life seems somewhat controlled by accidental happenings.

    (b)   For the way I feel now, there is really no such thing as "luck."*

9   **(a)**   Right now, I feel that I have little influence over the things that are happening to me.

    (b)   It is impossible for me to believe that chance or luck plays an important role in what is happening to me.*

10   **(a)**   Presently, I am lonely because I don't try to be friendly.*

   (b)   At present, there's not much use in trying too hard to please people; if they like me, they like me.

11 **(a)**   What happens to me is my own doing.*

   (b)   At present, I feel that I don't have enough control over the direction my life is taking.

APPENDIX B

The Change Correlation Method

Throughout this book, we have emphasized the importance of vicious cycles (spirals) in psychopathology. A vicious cycle, or spiral, occurs when one change augments another change. In this appendix, we will outline a method that we have developed for investigating psychopathological spirals.

A key problem in any science is the development of appropriate research designs for conducting crucial experiments about the nature of the phenomena under question. In psychiatry and psychology, the phenomena under study are often changeable, subjective, and unique to an individual's life course and situation (Melges, 1972). For example, it would be difficult to study emotion without asking an individual what he is experiencing at a particular time in a certain situation and how his inner experiences change over time. In similar fashion, an individual's sense of time and his outlook on the personal future are changeable, subjective, and individualistic. Thus in order to study variables related to a person's sense of time and future outlook, we developed a research method that could test hypotheses about changes in subjective phenomena as an individual is studied over time. This method is called the change correlation method (CCM).

The central question of the CCM is, What changes with what? That is, as an individual is studied longitudinally, changes over time in a variable are tested for whether they correlate with contemporaneous changes in other variables (Melges et al., 1971). This focus on relationships between changes within an individual (or a system) over time is different from the traditional cross-sectional comparison of groups, and may produce quite different results (Kraemer, 1978). By analogy, the CCM is like studying a single engine's moving parts over time rather than comparing a group of engines with another group of engines each measured at only one point in time. Thus the CCM attempts to capture concomitant variation within an individual (or system).

This appendix was written in collaboration with Helena C. Kraemer, Ph.D., Associate Professor of Psychiatry and Biostatistics, Stanford University School of Medicine.

ADVANTAGES OF THE CHANGE CORRELATION METHOD

The CCM has the following advantages:

1　The question What changes with what? is highly relevant to a systems approach to psychiatric problems. As noted, in order to discover and test whether a vicious cycle, or spiral, is taking place, it is necessary to study the possible influence of a change in one variable upon other variables as an individual or system is followed over time. In a systems approach to psychiatry, there often is an interaction between biopsychosocial variables (Engel, 1977, 1980). For example, a psychological change may induce concomitant biological and social changes, which, in turn, may affect the degree of psychological change. A cybernetic system cannot be adequately investigated unless changes in its parameters are studied in relation to one another over time (Melges, 1972). This pertains to the study of an individual or a family.

2　Subjective changes can be systematically investigated in terms of their relationship to other concomitant changes. Many of the core phenomena of psychiatry are subjective events that can change rapidly. These include emotions, pain, self-images, delusions, and hallucinations. In order to study such subjective phenomena adequately, the investigator has to be able to test hypotheses about how the subjective changes might be related to other changes. The hypothesized other changes may be psychological in nature, or they may be biological or social variables that can be used for corroborating the subjective changes (Stoyva and Kamiya, 1968).

3　Intermittent disturbances can be systematically investigated. Many psychiatric disorders are essentially intermittent. These include episodes of panic, tracking difficulties (loosening of associations), and hallucinations (see Chapter 7). To study such intermittent phenomena adequately, the investigator needs a research design that enables the study of changes within an individual *when* they arise. For example, a schizophrenic patient may hallucinate intermittently for five minutes out of an hour; the proper study of hallucinations should focus on the relevant five minutes, not the other times (except for comparison). The CCM, by focusing on changes within an individual, allows for the study of such intermittent changes.

4　Each subject is used as his own control for a series of measurements. That is, each subject is compared to himself at other times. This intensive study of an individual through time enhances the likelihood of finding factors that are influencing the changes (Chassan, 1979; Dukes, 1965; Barlow and Hersen, 1973; Warnock, Mintz, and Tremlow, 1979). Moreover, by comparing the individual to himself, many pertinent variables in psychiatry (for example, differences in heredity, development, and belief) are readily controlled. On such variables, it is almost impossible to find another individual who can serve as an exact "matched" control.

5   Individual and aggregate data can be compared. The CCM not only is a single-case research design but also enables a series of individuals to be tested for concomitant variation, using the same statistic. As illustrated later, each individual studied over time constitutes a test of the hypothesized related changes. Important individual differences may be discovered in this way.

6   Longitudinal clinical studies of covarying changes can be further studied by manipulation experiments in order to replicate, as well as rule out, alternative hypotheses about mutual interaction between variables. That is, if changes in two or more variables are found to rise and fall concomitantly as psychiatric patients are studied longitudinally, and this concomitant variation holds up for a number of individuals, then the investigator can attempt to deliberately increase one of the variables in normal subjects in order to test whether related changes in the other variables are thereby induced (see Chapter 7). Or the investigator can treat or correct one variable to see if this influences the other variables.

ILLUSTRATION: TEMPORAL DISINTEGRATION AND DEPERSONALIZATION

To illustrate the use of the CCM, we will summarize how we used this method to test an hypothesis about related changes in both clinical and experimental investigations. The hypothesis was that changes in the temporal disintegration of sequences are related to changes in depersonalization. As noted in Chapter 7, temporal disintegration refers to impaired sequential thinking with lack of goal-directedness. Depersonalization refers to strangeness and unfamiliarity about the self. The rationale for the hypothesis was that as temporal disintegration became worse, such that there would be discontinuity between the sequences of past, present, and future, the individual would then lose the customary time frames through which he becomes familiar with himself and would then feel strange and unfamiliar—that is, depersonalized (see Chapter 7). Essentially we were hypothesizing a spiral: as temporal disintegration became worse, depersonalization would also become worse as the individual was studied over time.

The instruments used to measure these changes were the Temporal Integration Inventory and the Depersonalization Inventory (see Appendix A).

Using the CCM, we tested this hypothesis by going back and forth between longitudinal studies of psychiatric patients and experimental manipulation studies in which temporal disintegration was induced in normal subjects by tetrahydrocannabinol, or THC, (see Chapter 7). Details of the research can be found in previously published works (Melges et al., 1970b; Melges et al., 1974; Melges and Freeman, 1977; Freeman and Melges, 1977). The results of each of these studies, which are summarized in Table 8, confirmed the hypothesis.

For the top three studies listed in Table 8, the correlation coefficients are "average intrasubject r's," which represent summary statements, across the individuals studied, of the within-subject correlated changes over time within an individual. The procedures for computing the average intrasubject r will be presented later. From Table 8, it can be seen that the dynamic interrelationship between changes in temporal disintegration and depersonalization, originally found in longitudinal studies of psychiatric patients, was further confirmed by the THC studies. That is, rather than there just being a relationship between concomitant changes during the course of psychiatric illness, the induction of temporal disintegration in normal subjects was accompanied by changes in depersonalization.

After the manipulation studies, we then returned to larger samples of psychiatric patients. Again, as indicated on the bottom two lines of Table 8, the hypothesis was confirmed. These latter two studies, however, differ from the CCM. One involved the study of a group of psychiatric patients studied on

Table 8   Summary of Studies of Temporal Disintegration and Depersonalization

Study	Method	Correlation Coefficient	Significance[a]
Psychiatric patients	Correlated changes, within subjects	.83	.01
Oral THC	Correlated changes, within subjects	.87	.0001
Smoked THC	Correlated changes, within subjects	.92	.0001
Psychiatric patients	Correlated changes, pre–post	.52	.001
Psychiatric patients	Single-time correlation	.66	.001

[a]Significance for studies using within-subject correlated changes was determined by the z-transformation as well as the T transformation. For THC studies, significance was at about 1 in 1 million.

admission and then shortly before discharge from a hospital. This represents a study of pre–post changes over a number of patients. The substantial correlation indicates that the changes are related, but unlike the CCM the findings do not indicate that, within the same individual, the worsening of temporal disintegration is related to the worsening of depersonalization, while improvement of temporal disintegration is related to improvement of depersonalization. Since the CCM captures these directional changes within the same individual, we believe that "stronger inferences" about dynamically related changes can be made from the finding of substantial correlations using the CCM as compared to pre–post correlations (Melges et al., 1971). In particular, the covariance of changes toward worsening and improvement within the same individual is important for the delineation of a psycho-pathological spiral.

In this regard, the single-time correlation at the bottom of Table 8, although significant, does not provide grounds for inferring a spiral. These psychiatric patients were tested only once, shortly after admission to a hospital. Although such a single-time correlation is commonly employed in psychiatric research, it does not tell whether changes are dynamically related. By contrast, the correlations listed on the top three lines of the table do show that changes in temporal disintegration and depersonalization are dynamically related in terms of intensity and time.

However, these dynamic interrelationships do not necessarily imply a cause–effect relationship between the variables. Nevertheless, since the induction of temporal disintegration in normal subjects was found to slightly precede the appearance of depersonalization and greater degrees of temporal disintegration produced greater degrees of depersonalization (see Chapter 7), the dynamic relationship between the changes may be approximating the notion of causality.

The main point of this illustration is to show how the CCM can be used for systematic replication in testing and comparing the strength of a hypothesized relationship between changes in different samples and conditions.

LIMITATIONS OF THE CHANGE CORRELATION METHOD

The limitations of the CCM stem largely from what kind of question is being asked.

1 If the question or hypothesis pertains to a comparison of groups such as diagnostic categories, the CCM is not applicable. However, if the hypothesis pertains to a comparison of intrapatient changes in variables, the average intrasubject r of one group can be compared to that of another group.

2   If the question or hypothesis pertains to testing the overall or average effect of a type of treatment for a defined group of patients, the CCM is not applicable. Nevertheless, as emphasized by Barlow and Hersen (1973) and Chassan (1979), single-case designs are often more effective than group comparisons for determining specific treatment effects. The rationale is much like that of a good clinician who systematically observes concomitant variation between variables as he follows a patient or family longitudinally. The CCM can be used for such a purpose in clinical settings.

3   The CCM is limited to questions that pertain to contemporaneous relationships from one test session to the next. It correlates *changes* over time, not states at a given time nor the effect of an earlier state on a later state. Serial changes are not necessarily stochastically dependent upon one another, whereas serial states are (Melges et al., 1974). This assumption particularly holds if the researcher makes sure that intrinsic change, rather than just random variation, has occurred over time. The independent judgment of an outside observer (who does not know the hypothesis) can serve to make sure that a significant clinical change has occurred. Nevertheless, if one is interested in the effect of an earlier change on later changes, time-series analysis and trend analysis are more appropriate methods (Chassan, 1979; Box and Jenkins, 1970). In this regard, the CCM can be modified to study the effect of earlier changes on later changes, rather than just concomitant changes, by using sets of time-lag correlations. This is a possible way of extending the CCM to get closer to testing cause–effect relationships, rather than mutual causality as with concomitant changes.

4   Another possible limitation of the CCM as here presented is that it is a bivariate technique. Yet the study of two variables through time has the advantage of carefully defining and measuring the variables, thereby avoiding diffuse "fishing expeditions" of multiple variables. It is our bias that salient hypotheses about clinical disorders are more likely to arise from astute clinical observations than huge correlation matrices. Obviously, a hypothesis often involves more than two variables, and a number of variables can be studied pairwise using the CCM, if necessary. For those hypotheses requiring multivariate study of concomitant variation within individuals over time, the methods developed by Cattell (1952) and Mefford (1967) are useful. These methods employ similar logic to that of the CCM.

STATISTICAL PROCEDURES OF THE CCM

Since the CCM can be used for systematically testing hypotheses about interrelated changes in clinical practice, its basic steps will be outlined here so as to encourage clinical research in psychiatric practice (Melges, 1972). The initial steps can be carried out by a secretary or other staff assistant. The final steps of computing the within-subject correlations and finding the average intrasubject r ordinarily require the help of a statistician who has access to a computer, but they can be done by a psychiatrist or psychologist who has a reasonable knowledge of statistics.

The steps of the CCM are as follows:

1 Set up the design to ensure that, at the time of subsequent testing, the individual is definitely in a different state than at the time of the preceding test session. An outside observer can be used to report either a definite improvement or worsening of the symptom under study.

2 For each individual studied, compute changes from one test session to the next for each variable under study, ending with k changes per individual.

3 For each individual studied, compute either the Pearson correlation coefficient or the Spearman rank correlation coefficient between contemporaneous changes in two variables. The first form is used when data are approximately normally distributed; the second form is appropriate for any quantitative data. Do the same pairwise procedure if other variables were hypothesized to be relevant to the proposed covarying processes.

4 Find the average intrasubject correlation coefficient for all individuals studied by:

    (a) For each intrasubject correlation coefficient, obtain the corresponding Fisher's z-transformation (for example, by using Table 14, "The z-transformation of the correlation coefficient, $z = \tanh^{-1} r$," on page 139 in *Biometrika Tables for Statisticians*, volume I, edited by E. S. Pearson and H. O. Hartley, Cambridge University Press, 1962.

    (b) Sum the z-transformation values, and compute the average z for the number of subjects. Using the same table as above, convert this average z-transformation back into a correlation coefficient r. The latter is the average of the correlated changes of the variables under consideration across the number of subjects studied.

5 Obtain significance of the average intrasubject r as follows:

    (a) Having already found the corresponding average z-transformation, compute X by

$$X = [n \, (k - 3)]^{1/2} \bar{z}$$

where $\bar{z}$ = average z-transformation; n = number of subjects used; and k = number of changes per subject.

    (b) X is a standard normal deviate. One might determine the significance of X by looking up the corresponding P value (for example, in

Table 1, page 104, in *Biometrika Tables for Statisticians,* referenced above). This P value will be the significance level of the average intrasubject r.

6 Test for the homogeneity of the intrasubject correlations in order to find whether there are significant individual differences. This is done by finding the significance of X^2_{n-1}, where n is the number of subjects used (see Kraemer, 1979). If X^2_{n-1} is significant, this means that the correlations are not homogeneous; that is, some individual differences exist in the sample. In this case, further hypotheses about individual differences or subgroups should be formulated and tested.

SUMMARY AND CONCLUSIONS

The change correlation method is designed to study concomitant variation between changes as an individual or system is studied longitudinally over time. It is useful for testing possible interactions between variables that may be contributing to a psychopathological spiral.

Bibliography

Aaronson, B. S. Behavior and the place names of time. *American Journal of Hypnosis: Clinical, Experimental, Theoretical* 9:1–17, 1966.

Aaronson, B. S. Hypnotic alterations of space and time. *International Journal of Parapsychology* 10:5–36, 1968.

Adams-Webber, J. R. *Personal Construct Theory*. New York: John Wiley & Sons, 1979.

Adey, W. R., Bell, F. R., and Dennis, B. J. Effects of LSD–25, psilocybin and psilocin on temporal lobe EEG patterns and learned behavior in the cat. *Neurology* 12:591–602, 1962.

Adler, A. *The Science of Living*. New York: Greenberg, 1929.

Akiskal, H. S., and McKinney, W. T. Overview of recent research in depression. *Archives of General Psychiatry* 32:285–305, 1975.

Alexander, F., and French, T. M. *Psychoanalytic Therapy*. New York: Ronald Press, 1946.

Allport, G. W. *Becoming*. New Haven: Yale University Press, 1955.

Ames, F. A. A clinical and metabolic study of acute intoxication with cannabis sativa and its role in the model psychoses. *Journal of Mental Science* 104:972–999, 1958.

Ames, L. The development of the sense of time in the young child. *The Journal of Genetic Psychology* 68:97–125, 1946.

Anderson, C. M. Family intervention with severely disturbed inpatients. *Archives of General Psychiatry* 34:697–702, 1977.

Angle, H. V. The role of chlorpromazine in maintaining timing behavior in chronic schizophrenics. *Psychopharmacologia* 28:185–194, 1973.

Arieti, S. The processes of expectation and anticipation. *Journal of Nervous and Mental Disease* 106:478–481, 1947.

Arieti, S. Hallucinations, delusions, and ideas of reference treated with psychotherapy. *American Journal of Psychotherapy* 16:52–60, 1962.

Arieti, S. *Interpretation of Schizophrenia*. New York: Basic Books, 1974.

Arieti, S. *Creativity: The Magic Synthesis*. New York: Basic Books, 1976.

Arieti, S. A psychotherapeutic approach to severely depressed patients. *American Journal of Psychotherapy* 32:33–47, 1978.

Arieti, S., and Bemporad, J. *Severe and Mild Depression*. New York: Basic Books, 1978.

Arkin, A. M., and Battin, D. A. technical device for the psychotherapy of pathological bereavement, in *Bereavement: Its Psychosocial Aspects*. Edited by B. Schoenberg et al. New York: Columbia University Press, 1975, pp. 351–356.

Arnold, M. B. *Emotion and Personality, I*. New York: Columbia University Press, 1960.

Aronson, H, Silverstein, A. B., and Klee, G. D. The influence of lysergic acid diethylamide (LSD-25) on subjective time sense. *Archives of General Psychiatry* 1:469–472, 1959.

Arthur, A. Z. Theories and explanations of delusions: a review. *American Journal of Psychiatry* 121:105–115, 1964.

Artiss, K. L., and Bullard, D. M. Paranoid thinking in everyday life: The function of secrets and disillusionment. *Archives of General Psychiatry* 14:89–93, 1966.

Baddeley, A. D. *The Psychology of Memory*. New York: Basic Books, 1976.

Balken, E. R. A delineation of schizophrenic language and thought in a test of imagination. *Journal of Psychology* 16:239–271, 1943.

Bandler, R., Grinder, J., and Satir, V. *Changing with Families*. Palo Alto, Calif.: Science and Behavior Books, 1976.

Bandura, A. Behavior theory and the models of man. *American Psychologist* 29:859–869, 1974.

Bandura, A. Self-efficacy: Toward a unifying theory of behavioral change. *Psychological Review* 84:191–215, 1977.

Bannister, D., and Fransella, F. A grid test of schizophrenic thought disorder. *British Journal of Social and Clinical Psychology* 5:95–102, 1966.

Bannister, D., and Mair, J. M. M. *The Evaluation of Personal Constructs*. London: Academic Press, 1968.

Barlow, D. H., and Hersen, M. Single-case experimental designs. *Archives of General Psychiatry* 29:319–325, 1973.

Bartlett, F. C. *Remembering*. Cambridge, England: Cambridge University Press, 1932.

Bateson, G. *Navan*. Palo Alto, Calif.: Stanford University Press, 1958.

Bear, D. M., and Fedio, P. Quantitative analysis of interictal behavior in temporal lobe epilepsy. *Archives of Neurology* 34:454–467, 1977.

Beck, A. T. *Depression*. New York: Hoeber Medical Division, Harper & Row, 1967.

Beck, A. T. Cognition, affect, the psychopathology. *Archives of General Psychology* 24:495–500, 1971.

Beck, A. T. *Cognitive Therapy and Emotional Disorders*. New York: International Universities Press, 1976.

Beck, A. T., Laude, R., and Bohnert, M. Ideational components of anxiety neurosis. *Archives of General Psychiatry* 31:319–325, 1974.

Beck, A. T., Rush, A. J., Shaw, B. F., and Emery, G. *Cognitive Therapy of Depression*. New York: The Guilford Press, 1979.

Beck, A. T., Weissman, A., Lester D., and Trexler, L. The measurement of pessimism: The hopelessness scale. *Journal of Consulting and Clinical Psychology* 42:861–865, 1974.

Bender, L. Psychopathic disorders in children, in *Handbook of Correctional Psychology*. Edited by R. M. Lindner and R. B. Seliger. New York: Philosophical Library, 1947.

Ben-Dov, G., and Carmon, A. On time space and the cerebral hemispheres: A theoretical note. *International Journal of Neuroscience* 7:29–33, 1976.

Benton, A. L., van Allen, M. W., and Fogel, N. L. Temporal orientation in cerebral disease. *Journal of Nervous and Mental Disease* 139:110–119, 1964.

Bergson, H. The evolution of life, in *Man and the Universe: The Philosophers of Science*. Edited by S. Commins and R. N. Lindscott. New York: Random House, 1947, pp. 274–293.

Berkowitz, L. The judgmental process in personality functioning. *Psychological Review* 67:130–142, 1960.

Berne, E. *Transactional Analysis in Psychotherapy*. New York: Grove Press, 1961.

Berne, E. *What Do You Say After You Say Hello? The Psychology of Human Destiny*. New York: Grove Press, 1972.

Bernstein, L., and Dana, R. H. *Interviewing and the Help Professions*. New York: Appleton-Century-Crofts, 1970.

Bibring, E. The mechanism of depression, in *Affective Disorders*. Edited by P. Greenacre. New York: International Universities Press, 1953.

Bindra, D., and Waksberg, H. Methods and terminology in studies of time estimation. *Psychological Bulletin* 53:155–159, 1956.

Blanck, G., and Blanck, R. *Ego Psychology: Theory and Practice*. New York: Columbia University Press, 1974.

Bleuler, E. (1911) *Dementia Praecox or the Group of Schizophrenias*. Translated by J. Zinkin. New York: International Universities Press, 1950, pp. 14–15.

Bogen, J. E. The other side of the brain: An appositional mind, in *The Nature of Human Consciousness: A Book of Readings*. Edited by R. E. Ornstein. New York: Viking, 1974, pp. 101–125.

Bogen, J. E., and Bogen, G. M. The other side of the brain: III. The corpus callosum and creativity. *Bulletin of the Los Angeles Neurological Society* 34:191–220, 1969.

Bonaparte, M. Time and the unconscious. *International Journal of Psychoanalysis* 21:427–468, 1941.

Boulding, K. E. General systems theory—the skeleton of science. *Management Science* 2:197–208, 1956.

Bowen, M. Theory in the practice of psychotherapy, in *Family Therapy*. Edited by P. J. Guerin. New York: Gardener Press, Division of John Wiley & Sons, 1976, pp. 42–90.

Bowers, M. B. *Retreat from Sanity: The Structure of Emerging Psychosis*. New York: Human Sciences Press, 1974.

Bowers, M. B., and Freedman, D. X. "Psychedelic" experiences in acute psychoses. *Archives of General Psychiatry* 15:240–248, 1966.

Bowlby, J. Processes of mourning. *International Journal of Psychoanalysis* 42:317–340, 1961.

Bowlby, J. Pathological mourning and childhood mourning. *Journal of the American Psychoanalytic Association* 11:500–541, 1963.

Bowlby, J. *Attachment and Loss, Volume I: Attachment*. London: Hogarth Press, 1969.

Bowlby, J. *Attachment and Loss, Volume II: Separation*. New York: Basic Books, 1973.

Bowlby, J. *Attachment and Loss, Volume III: Loss*. New York: Basic Books, 1980.

Box, G. E. P., and Jenkins, C. M. *Time Series Analysis: Forecasting and Control*. San Francisco: Holden-Day, 1970.

Brady, J. P. Studies on the metronome effect on stuttering. *Behavioral Research and Therapy* 7:197–204, 1969.

Braff, D. L., and Beck, A. T. Thinking disorder in depression. *Archives of General Psychiatry* 31:456–459, 1974.

Braff, D. L., Callaway, E., and Naylor, H. Very short-term memory dysfunction in schizophrenia. *Archives of General Psychiatry* 34:25–30, 1977.

Braff, D. L., Silverton, L., Saccuzzo, D. P., and Janowsky, D. S. Impaired speed of visual information processing in marihuana intoxication. *American Journal of Psychiatry* 138:613–617, 1981.

Brain, Lord. Some reflections on brain and mind. *Brain* 86:381–402, 1963.

Broadbent, D. E. *Perception and Communication*. New York: Pergamon Press, 1958.

Bromberg, W. Marijuana intoxication. *American Journal of Psychiatry* 91:303–330, 1934.

Bronowski, J. *The Identity of Man*. New York: American Museum of Science Books, 1966.

Buckley, W. (Ed.) *Modern Systems Research for the Behavioral Scientist*. Chicago: Aldine Publishing Company, 1968.

Buhler, C., and Massarik, F. (Eds.) *The Course of Human Life: A Study of Goals in the Humanistic Perspective*. New York: Springer Publishing Company, 1968.

Burns, N. M., and Gifford E. C. Time estimation and anxiety. *Journal of Psychological Studies* 12:19–27, 1961.

Callaway, E. Schizophrenia and interference. *Archives of General Psychiatry* 22:193–208, 1970.

Callaway, E., and Naghdi, S. An information processing model for schizophrenia. *Archives of General Psychiatry* 39:339–347, 1982.

Cameron, N. Paranoid reactions, in *Personality Development and Psychopathology*. Boston: Houghton Mifflin Company, 1963, pp. 470–515.

Campos, L. P. The relationship between some factors of parental deprivation and delay of need gratification (unpublished doctoral thesis). Lansing: Michigan State University, 1963.

Campos, L. P. Relationship between time estimation and retentive personality traits. *Perceptual and Motor Skills* 23:59–62, 1966.

Cannon, W. B. *The Wisdom of the Body.* New York: W. W. Norton Company, 1932.

Carpenter, W. T., Strauss, J. S., and Muleh, S. Are there pathognomonic symptoms of schizophrenia? *Archives of General Psychiatry* 28:847–852, 1973.

Casswell, S., and Marks, D. F. Cannabis and temporal disintegration in experienced and naive subjects. *Science* 179:803–805, 1973.

Cattell, R. B. The three basic factor-analytic research designs—their interrelations and derivatives. *Psychological Bulletin* 49:499–520, 1952.

Cautela, J. R. Covert reinforcement. *Behavior Therapy* 1:33–50, 1970.

Chambers, J. Maternal deprivation and the concept of time in children. *American Journal Orthopsychiatry* 31:406–419, 1961.

Chapman, J. The early symptoms of schizophrenia. *British Journal of Psychiatry* 112:225–251, 1966.

Chassan, J. B. *Research Design in Clinical Psychology and Psychiatry.* New York: Irvington Publishers, 1979.

Chisholm, R. M., and Taylor, R. Making things to have happened. *Analysis* 20:73–78, 1960.

Clausen, J. An evaluation of experimental methods of time judgment. *Journal of Experimental Psychology* 40:756–761, 1950.

Cloward, R. A., and Ohlin, I. E. *Delinquency and Opportunity: A Theory of Delinquent Gangs.* New York: The Free Press of Glencoe, 1960.

Coelho, G. V., Hamburg, D. A., and Adams, J. E. *Coping and Adaptation.* New York: Basic Books, 1974.

Cohen, B. D. Self-editing deficits in schizophrenia, in *The Nature of Schizophrenia: New Approaches to Research and Treatment.* Edited by L. C. Wynne, R. L. Cromwell, and S. Matthysse. New York: John Wiley & Sons, 1978, pp. 313–319.

Cohen, J. Subjective time. In *The Voices of Time.* Edited by J. T. Fraser. New York: George Braziller, 1966, pp. 257–278.

Cohen, J. *Psychological Time in Health and Disease.* Springfield, Ill.: Charles C. Thomas, 1967.

Collins, P. J., Kietzman, M. L., Sutton, S., and Shapiro, E. Visual temporal integration in psychiatric patients, in *The Nature of Schizophrenia: New Approaches to Research and Treatment.* Edited by L. C. Wynne, R. L. Cromwell, and S. Matthysse. New York: John Wiley & Sons, 1978, pp. 244–253.

Conrad, K. Die Beginnende Schizophrenie: Versuch einer Gestaltanalyse des Wahns [*Commencing Schizophrenia: An Attempt at a Gestalt Analysis of Delusion*]. Stuttgart: Thieme, 1968.

Cooper, L. F., and Erickson, M. H. *Time Distortion in Hypnosis* (2nd ed.). Baltimore: Williams and Wilkins, 1959.

Cottle, T. J., and Klineberg, S. L. *The Present of Things Future: Explorations of Time in Human Experience.* New York: Macmillan Publishing Company, 1974.

Cousins, N. Anatomy of an illness. *New England Journal of Medicine* 295:1458–1463, 1976.

Davanloo, H. *Basic Principles and Techniques in Short-Term Dynamic Psychotherapy.* New York: Spectrum Publications, 1978.

Dean, S. R. (Ed.) *Psychiatry and Mysticism.* Chicago: Nelson-Hall, 1975.

Deardorff, C. M., Melges, F. T., Hout, C. N., and Savage, D. J., Situations related to drinking of alcohol: A factor analysis of questionnaire responses. *Journal of Studies on Alcohol* 36:1184–1195, 1975.

Delgado, J. M. R. *Physical Control of the Mind.* New York: Harper Colophon Books, Harper & Row, 1969.

Delgado, J. M. R. "Future Research in the Brain." Special lecture given at the American Psychiatric Association Annual Meeting, Chicago, Ill., May, 1979.

Detre, T. P., and Jarecki, H. G. *Modern Psychiatric Treatment.* Philadelphia and Toronto: J. B. Lippincott Co., 1971.

DeWied, D. Hormonal influences on motivation, learning, and memory processes. *Hospital Practice* (Jan):125–131, 1976.

Diagnostic and Statistical Manual of Mental Disorders (DSM-III). 3rd ed. Washington, D.C.: American Psychiatric Association, 1980.

Dilling, C. A., and Rabin, A. I. Temporal experience in depressive states and schizophrenia. *Journal of Consulting Psychology* 31:604–608, 1967.

Dimond, S. J. The structural basis of timing. *Psychological Bulletin* 62:348–350, 1964.

Dixon, J. C. Depersonalization phenomena in a sample population of college students. *British Journal of Psychiatry* 109:371–375, 1963.

Docherty, J. P., Van Kammen, D. P., Siris, S. G., and Marder, S. R. Stages of onset of schizophrenic psychosis. *American Journal of Psychiatry* 135:420–426, 1978.

Dollard, J., and Miller, N. E. *Personality and Psychotherapy.* New York: McGraw-Hill, 1950.

Doob, L. W. *Patterning of Time.* New Haven, Conn.: Yale University Press, 1971.

Douglas, R. J. The hippocampus and behavior. *Psychological Bulletin* 67:416–442, 1967.

Douglas, R. J., and Pribram, K. H. Learning and limbic lesions. *Neuropsychologia* (Oxford) 4:197–220, 1966.

Dukes, W. F. "N = 1." *Psychological Bulletin* 64:74–79, 1965.

Ebbinghaus, H. *Memory.* Translated by H. Ruyer and C. E. Bussenius. New York: Teachers College Press, 1913.

Edelstein, E. Changing time perception with antidepressant drug therapy. *Psychiatrica Clinica* 7:375–382, 1974.

Efron, R. The effect of handedness on the perception of simultaneity and temporal order. *Brain* 86:261–284, 1963a.

Efron, R. Temporal perception, aphasia, and deja vu. *Brain* 86:403–424, 1963b.

Efron, R. The duration of the present, in *Interdisciplinary Perspectives of Time, Annals of the New York Academy of Sciences* 138:713–729, 1967.

Eisenbud, J. Research in precognition, in *Psychiatry and Mysticism.* Edited by S. R. Dean. Chicago: Nelson-Hall, 1975, pp. 101–110.

Eisler, F. *Psycholinguistics: Experiments in Spontaneous Speech.* London: Academic Press, 1968.

Ellinwood, E. H., Jr. Amphetamine psychoses: II. Theoretical implications. *International Journal of Neuropsychiatry* 4:45–54, 1968.

Ellis, A. *Reason and Emotion in Psychotherapy.* New York: Lyle Stuart, 1962.

Engel, G. L. Is grief a disease? *Psychosomatic Medicine* 23:18–22, 1961.

Engel, G. L. Anxiety and depression–withdrawal: The primary affects of unpleasure. *International Journal of Psychoanalysis* 43:89–97, 1962.

Engel, G. L. The need for a new medical model: a challenge for biomedicine. *Science* 196:129–136, 1977.

Engel, G. L. The clinical application of the biopsychosocial model. *The American Journal of Psychiatry* 137:535–544, 1980.

Engel, G. L., and Morgan, W. L. *Interviewing the Patient.* London: W. B. Saunders Company, 1973.

Engel, G. L., and Romano, J. Delirium: A syndrome of cerebral insufficiency. *Journal of Chronic Diseases* 9:260–277, 1959.

Engelmann, W. A slowing down of circadian rhythms by lithium ions. *Z Naturforsch* 28:733–736, 1973.

Epley, D., and Ricks, D. R. Foresight and hindsight on the TAT. *Journal of Projective Techniques and Personality Assessment* 27:51–59, 1963.

Erickson, M. H. Pseudo-orientation as a hypnotherapeutic procedure. *Journal of Clinical and Experimental Hypnosis* 2:261–283, 1954.

Erickson, M. H., and Rossi, E. L. *Hypnotherapy: An Exploratory Casebook.* New York: Irvington Publishers, 1979.

Erikson, E. H. Identity and the life cycle. *Psychological Issues* 1:1–171, 1959.

Erikson, E. H. *Identity, Youth and Crisis*. New York: W. W. Norton & Co., Inc., 1968.

Ezekiel, R. S. The personal future and Peace Corps competence. *Journal of Personality and Social Psychology*, Monograph Supplement, 8:1–26, 1968.

Ezriel, H. H. Notes on psychoanalytic group therapy: II. Interpretation and research. *Psychiatry* 15:119–126, 1952.

Faschingbauer, T. R., Devaul, R. A., and Zisook, S. Development of the Texas inventory of grief. *American Journal of Psychiatry* 134:696–698, 1977.

Fenichel, O. *The Psychoanalytic Theory of Neurosis*. New York: Norton, 1945.

Fischer, R. The biological fabric of time, in *Interdisciplinary Perspectives of Time, Annals of the New York Academy of Science* 138:440–488, 1967.

Fleck, S. Family Functioning and Family Pathology. *Psychiatric Annals* 10:17–36, 1980.

Flynn, J. P., MacLean, P. D., and Kim, C. Effects of hippocampal after-discharges on conditioned responses, in *Electrical Stimulation of the Brain: An Interdisciplinary Survey of Neuro-behavioral Systems*. Edited by D. E. Sheer, Austin, Tex.: University of Texas Press, 1961.

Fogel, S., and Hoffer, A. Perceptual changes induced by hypnotic suggestion for the posthypnotic state: I. General account of the effect on personality. *Journal of Clinical and Experimental Psychopathology* 23:24–35, 1962.

Fowler, D. R., and Longabaugh, R. The problem-oriented record. *Archives of General Psychiatry* 32:831–836, 1975.

Fraisse, P. *The Psychology of Time*. New York: Harper & Row, 1963.

Frank, J. D. The role of hope in psychotherapy. *International Journal of Psychiatry* 5:383–395, 1968.

Frank, J. D. Psychotherapy: The restoration of morale. *American Journal of Psychiatry* 131:271–274, 1974.

Frank, J. D. *Psychotherapy and the Human Predicament*. Edited by P. E. Dietz. New York: Schocken Books, 1978.

Frankenhauser, M. *Estimation of Time: An Experimental Study*. Stockholm, Sweden: Almquist and Wiksell, 1959.

Frankl, V. E. *The Unheard Cry for Meaning*. New York: Simon and Schuster, 1978.

Fraser, J. T. (Ed.) *The Voices of Time*. New York: George Braziller, 1966.

Fraser, J. T. *Of Time, Passion, and Knowledge*. New York: George Braziller, 1975.

Fraser, J. T. Temporal levels: sociobiological aspects of a fundamental synthesis. *Journal of Social and Biological Structure* 1:339–355, 1978.

Fraser, J. T. Temporal levels and reality testing. *International Journal of Psychoanalysis* 62:3–26, 1981.

Freeman, A. M., and Melges, F. T. Depersonalization and temporal disintegration in acute mental illness. *American Journal of Psychiatry* 134:679–681, 1977.

Freeman, A. M., and Melges, F. T. Temporal disorganization, depersonalization, and persecutory ideation in acute mental illness. *American Journal of Psychiatry* 135:123–124, 1978.

French, T. M. *The Integration of Behavior* (Vol. I: Basic Postulates). Chicago: University of Chicago Press, 1952.

French, T. M. *Psychoanalytic Interpretations*. Chicago: Quadrangle Books, 1970.

Freud, S. (1901) *The Interpretation of Dreams*. New York: Basic Books, 1960.

Freud, S. (1908) On creative writers and daydreaming. *Standard Edition*, 9. Translated by J. Strachey. Frome, Great Britain: Butler & Tanner, 1959, pp. 141–154.

Freud, S. (1911) Formulations regarding the two principles in mental functioning, in *Collected Papers, Vol. IV*. Translated by J. Riviere. New York: Basic Books, 1959, pp. 13–21.

Freud, S. (1911) Psycho-analytic notes upon an autobiographical account of a case of paranoia (dementia paranoides), in *Collected Papers, Vol. III*. Translated by A. Strachey and J. Strachey. New York: Basic Books, 1959, pp. 387–470.

Freud, S. (1915) The unconscious, in *Complete Psychological Works*, Standard Edition, vol. 14. Translated and edited by J. Strachey. London: Hogarth Press, 1964, pp. 159–215.

Freud, S. (1917) Mourning and melancholia, in *Standard Edition*, vol. 14. London: Hogarth Press, 1957, pp. 243–360.

Freud, S. (1920) Beyond the pleasure principle, in *Standard Edition*, vol. 18. London: Hogarth Press, 1957, pp. 7–64.

Freud, S. (1927) *The Problem of Anxiety*. Translated by H. A. Bunker. New York: W. W. Norton, 1936.

Freud, S. (1933) New introductory lectures on psychoanalysis: Dissection of the cyclical personality (Lecture 31), in *The Complete Psychological Works of Sigmund Freud* (vol. 22). London: Hogarth Press, 1964.

Friedman, M., and Rosenman, R. H. *Type A Behavior and Your Heart*. New York: Alfred A. Knopf, 1974.

Furlong, W. B. The flow experience: The fun in fun. *Psychology Today* June 1976, pp. 35–38.

Galin, D. Implications for psychiatry of left and right cerebral specialization. *Archives of General Psychiatry* 31:572–583, 1974.

Gascon, G. G., and Gilles, F. Limbic dementia. *Journal of Neurology and Neurosurgery and Psychiatry* 36:420–430, 1973.

Gergen, K. J. Self theory and the process of self-observation. *Journal of Nervous and Mental Disease* 148:437–448, 1969.

Geschwind, N. Specialization of the human brain. *Scientific American* 241:180–201, 1979.

Gjessing, R., Gjessing, L. R. Some main trends in the clinical aspects of periodic catatonia. *Acta Psychiatrica Scandinavica* 37:1–13, 1961.

Goldberger, L., and Holt, R. R. Experimental interference with reality contact (perceptual isolation): Method and group results. *Journal of Nervous and Mental Disease* 127:99–112, 1958.

Goldrich, J. M. A study of time orientation: The relation between memory for past experience and orientation to the future. *Journal of Personality and Social Psychology* 6:216–221, 1967.

Goldstein, K. *The Organism*. New York: American Book Company, 1939.

Goldstein, K., and Scheerer, M. Abstract and concrete behavior: An experimental study with special tests. *Psychological Monographs*, Vol. 53, No. 239, 1941.

Goldstone, S., Nurnberg, H. G., and Lhamon, W. T. Effects of trifluoperazine, chlorpromazine, and haloperidol upon temporal information processing by schizophrenic patients. *Psychopharmacology* 65:119–124, 1979.

Goleman, D. *The Varieties of the Meditative Experience*. New York: Irvington Publishers, 1977.

Goodwin, B. C. *Analytical Physiology of Cells and Developing Organisms*. New York: Academic Press, 1976.

Gordon, W. J. J. *The Metaphorical Way of Learning and Knowing*. Cambridge, Mass.: Porpoise Books, 1971.

Goulding, M. M., and Goulding, R. L. *Changing Lives through Redecision Therapy*. New York: Brunner/Mazel Publishers, 1979.

Goulding, R. L., and Goulding, M. M. *The Power Is in the Patient: A TA/Gestalt Approach to Psychotherapy*. San Francisco: TA Press, 1978.

Gray, W., Duhl, E. J., and Rizzo, N. D. (Eds.) *General Systems Theory and Psychiatry*. Boston: Little, Brown & Co., 1969.

Greenblatt, M. The grieving spouse. *American Journal of Psychiatry* 135:43–47, 1978.

Greenblatt, M., and Solomon, H. C. Studies of lobotomy, in *The Brain and Human Behavior*, Proceedings of the Association for Research in Mental Disease, Vol. 26. Edited by H. C. Solomon, S. Cobb, and W. Penfield, Baltimore: The Williams & Wilkins Co., 1958, pp. 19–34.

Grinker, R. R. Miller, J. Sabshin, M., Nunn, R., and Nunnally, J. C. *The Phenomena of Depressions*. New York: Paul B. Hoeber, 1961.

Gross, A. Sense of time in dreams. *Psychoanalytic Quarterly* 18:466–495, 1949.

Gur, R. E. Cognitive concomitants of hemispheric dysfunction in schizophrenia. *Archives of General Psychiatry* 36:269–278, 1979.

Halberg, F. Physiologic considerations: rhythmometry with special reference to emotional illness, in *Cycles Biologiques et Psychiatrie,* edited by D. E. Ajuriaguerra. Paris: Masson et Cie, 1968, pp. 73–126.

Halberg, F. Chronobiology. *Annual Review of Physiology* 31:675–725, 1969.

Haley, J. *Problem–Solving Therapy: New Strategies for Effective Family Therapy.* San Francisco: Jossey-Bass Publishers, 1977.

Halleck, S. L. *Psychiatry and the Dilemmas of Crime.* New York: Hoeber Medical Division, Harper & Son, Publishers Inc., 1967.

Hamburg, D. A., and Adams, J. E. A perspective on coping behavior. *Archives of General Psychiatry* 17:277–284, 1967.

Harper, R. G., Wiens, A. N., and Matarazzo, J. D. *Nonverbal Communication: The State of the Art.* New York: John Wiley and Sons, 1978.

Hartocollis, P. Time as a dimension of affects: *Journal of the American Psychoanalytic Association* 20:92–108, 1972.

Hartocollis, P. Origins of time: A reconstruction of the ontogenetic development of the sense of time based on object relations theory. *Psychoanalytical Quarterly* 43:243–261, 1974.

Hartocollis, P. Time and affects in borderline disorders. *International Journal of Psychoanalysis* 59:157–163, 1978.

Havens, L. L. The existential use of the self. *American Journal of Psychiatry* 131:1–10, 1974.

Heath, R. G. Marijuana: Effects on deep and surface electroencephalograms of man. *Archives of General Psychiatry* 26:577–584, 1972.

Heath, R. G., Fitzjarrel, A. T., Fontana, C. J., and Garey, R. E. Cannabis sativa: Effects on brain function and ultrastructure in Rhesus monkeys. *Biological Psychiatry* 15:657–690, 1980.

Hering, D. W. The time concept and time sense among cultured and uncultured peoples, in *Time and its Mysteries.* Eight lectures given at the James Arthur Foundation, New York University. New York: Collier Books, 1962, pp. 83–111.

Hearnshaw, L. S. Temporal integration and behavior. *Bulletin of the British Psychological Society* 30:1–20, 1956.

Hilgard, E. R. *Hypnotic Susceptibility.* New York: Harcourt, Brace & World, 1965.

Hilgard, J. R. *Personality and Hypnosis: A Study of Imaginative Involvement.* Chicago: University of Chicago Press, 1970.

Hilgard, J. R., and Newman, M. F. Anniversaries in mental illness. *Psychiatry* 22:113–121, 1959.

Hilgard, J. R., and Newman, M. F. Parental loss by death in childhood as an etiological factor among schizophrenic and alcoholic patients compared with a non-patient community sample. *Journal of Nervous and Mental Disease* 137:14–28, 1963.

Hine, F. R., Pfeiffer, E., Maddox, G. L., Hein, P. L., and Friedel, R. O. *Behavioral Science: A Selective View.* Boston: Little, Brown and Company, 1972.

Hoagland, H. *Consciousness and the Chemistry of Time.* New York: Josiah Macy Foundation, 1950.

Holden, C. Cancer and the mind: How are they connected? *Science* 200:1363–1369, 1978.

Holubar, J., and Machek, J. Time sense and epileptic EEG activity. *Epilepsia* 3:323–328, 1962.

Horney, K. *New Ways in Psychoanalysis.* New York: W. W. Norton, 1939.

Horney, K. *Neurosis and Human Growth: The Struggle Toward Self-Realization.* New York: W. W. Norton, 1950.

Horowitz, M. J. *Image Formation and Cognition.* New York: Appleton-Century-Crofts, 1970.

Horowitz, M. J. A cognitive model of hallucinations. *American Journal of Psychiatry* 132:789–795, 1975.

Horowitz, M. J. *Stress Response Syndromes.* New York: Jason Aronson, 1976.

Horowitz, M. J., Wilner, N., Marmar, C., and Krupnick, J. Pathological grief and the activation of latent self-images. *American Journal of Psychiatry* 137:1157–1162, 1980.

Huxley, A. *The Doors of Perception.* New York: Harper & Row, 1963.

Isbell, H., Gorodestky, C. W., Jasinski, D., Claussen, U., Spulak, F., and Kort, F. Effects of (-)delta-9-tetrahydrocannabinol in man. *Psychopharmacologia* 14:115–123, 1967.

Izard, C. E. *Human Emotions.* New York: Plenum Press, 1977.

Jackson, D. D. A suggestion for the technical handling of paranoid patients. *Psychiatry* 26:306–307, 1963.

Jacobsen, C. F. Functions of frontal association areas in primates. *Archives of Neurology and Psychiatry* 33:558–569, 1935.

James, W. (1890) The stream of consciousness, in *The Principles of Psychology.* New York: Dover Press, 1950, pp. 224–290.

James, W. *Psychology: The Briefer Course.* New York: Henry Holt & Company, 1892.

James, W. H., and Rotter, J. B. Partial and 100% reinforcement under chance and skill conditions. *Journal of Experimental Psychology* 55:397–403, 1958.

Janis, I. L., and Mann, L. *Decision Making: A Psychological Analysis of Conflict, Choice, and Commitment.* New York: The Free Press, a division of Macmillan Publishing Company, 1977.

Jaques, E. *A General Theory of Bureaucracy.* New York: John Wiley & Sons, 1976.

Jaspers, K. *General Psychopathology.* Translated by J. Hoenig and M. W. Hamilton. Manchester and Chicago: Manchester University Press and Chicago University Press, 1963.

Jaspers, K. Delusion and awareness of reality. *International Journal of Psychiatry* 6:25–38, 1968.

Jaynes, J. *The Origin of Consciousness in the Breakdown of the Bicameral Mind.* New York: Houghton Mifflin Co., 1976.

Jenkins, H. M. Sequential organization in schedules of reinforcement, in *Theory of Reinforcement Schedules.* Edited by W. N. Schoenfeld and J. Farmer. New York: Appleton-Century-Crofts, 1970.

Jenner, E. A. The effects of an altered time regime on biological rhythms in a 48-hour periodic psychosis. *British Journal of Psychiatry* 114(507):215–224, 1968.

John, E. R. A model of consciousness, in *Consciousness and Self-Regulation,* (vol. 1). Edited by G. E. Schwartz and D. Shapiro. New York: Plenum Press, 1976, pp. 1–50.

John, E. R. How the brain works—a new theory. *Psychology Today* (May):48–52, 1976.

Johnson, D. T., and Speilberger, C. D. The effects of relaxation training and the passage of time on measures of state- and trait-anxiety. *Journal of Clinical Psychology* 24:20–23, 1968.

Johnsson, A., Pflug, B., Engelmann, W., and Klemke, W. Effect of lithium carbonate on circadian periodicity in humans. *Pharmako Psychiat.* 12:423–425, 1979.

Jones, M. R. Time, our lost dimension: Toward a new theory of perception, attention and memory. *Psychological Review* 83:323–355, 1976.

Joslyn, D., and Hutzell, R. R. Temporal disorientation in schizophrenic and brain-damaged patients. *American Journal of Psychiatry* 136:1220–1222, 1979.

Jung, C. G. *The Structure and Dynamics of the Psyche, Collected Works.* New York: Pantheon, 1960.

Jung, C. G. (1955) Synchronicity: An acausal connecting principle, in *The Nature of Human Consciousness.* Edited by R. E. Ornstein. New York: Viking Press, 1973, pp. 445–457.

Kafka, M. S., Naber, D., and Wehr, T. A. Imipramine and circadian rhythms. Reported in *Psychiatric News,* December 21, 1979, p. 3.

Kagan, J. Perspectives: the form of early development. *Archives of General Psychiatry* 36:1047–1054, 1979.

Kahn, P. Time orientation in perceptual and cognitive organization. *Perceptual and Motor Skills* 23:1059–1066, 1966.

Kanfer, F. H., and Karoly, P. Self-control: A behavioristic excursion into the lion's den. *Behavior Therapy* 3:398–416, 1972.

Kanfer, F. H., and Marston, A. R. Determinants of self reinforcement in human learning. *Journal of Experimental Psychology* 66:245–254, 1963.

Kantor, D., and Lehr, W. *Inside the Family: Toward a Theory of Family Process.* San Francisco: Jossey-Bass Publishers, 1975.

Kappers, C. U. *The Evolution of the Nervous System in Convertebratae, Vertebratae and Man*. Haarlam: Bohn, 1930.

Karagulla, S., and Robertson, E. E. Psychical phenomena in temporal lobe epilepsy and the psychoses. *British Medical Journal* 26:748–752, 1955.

Karpman, S. Fairy tales and script drama analysis. *Transactional Analysis Bulletin* 7:39–43, 1968.

Kasdin, A. E., and Wilson, G. T. Criteria for evaluating psychotherapy. *Archives of General Psychiatry* 35:407–418, 1978.

Kelley, C. R. *Manual and Automatic Control*. New York: John Wiley & Sons, 1968.

Kelly, G. A. *The Psychology of Personal Constructs* (vols. I and II). New York: W. W. Norton & Co., 1955.

Kenna, J. C., and Sedman, G. The subjective experience of time during lysergic acid diethylamide (LSD-25) intoxication. *Psychopharmacologia* 5:280–288, 1964.

Kierkegaard, S. *The Concept of Dread*. Translated by W. Lowrie. Princeton, N.J.: Princeton University Press, 1944.

King, A. E. *Psychomotor Aspects of Mental Disease*. Cambridge, Mass.: Harvard University Press, 1954.

Kinsbourne, M. (Ed.) *Asymmetrical Function of the Brain*. New York: Cambridge University Press, 1978.

Kipling, R. "If-" in *The Works of Rudyard Kipling* (vol. XXI). New York: Charles Scribner, 1925.

Kirstein, L., and Bukberg, J. Temporal disorganization and primary affective disorder. *American Journal of Psychiatry* 136:1313–1316, 1979.

Klaf, F. S. Evidence of paranoid ideation in overt homosexuals. *Journal of Social Therapy* 7:48–51, 1961.

Kline, P. *Fact and Fantasy in Freudian Theory*. London: Methuen & Co., 1972.

Klineberg, S. L. Future time perspective and the preference for dealyed reward. *Journal of Personality and Social Psychology* 8:253–257, 1968.

Kluckhohn, F. R., and Strodtbeck, F. B. *Variations in Value Orientations*. Evanston, Ill.: Row, Peterson & Company, 1961.

Korzybski, A. (1926) *Time-Binding: The General Theory*. New York: E. P. Dutton & Co., 1949.

Kosbab, F. P. Imagery techniques in psychiatry. *Archives of General Psychiatry* 31:283–291, 1974.

Kovacs, M., and Beck, A. T. Maladaptive cognitive structures in depression. *American Journal of Psychiatry* 135:525–533, 1978.

Kraemer, H. C. Individual and ecological correlation in a general context. *Behavioral Science* 23:67–72, 1978.

Kraemer, H. C. Test of homogeneity of independent correlation coefficients. *Psychometrika* 44:329–335, 1979.

Krauss, H. H. Anxiety: The dread of a future event. *Journal of Individual Psychology* 23:88–93, 1967.

Kripke, D. F., Mullaney, D. J., Atkinson, M., and Wolf. S. Circadian rhythm disorders in manic depressives. *Biological Psychiatry* 13:335–351, 1978.

Kris, E. *Psychoanalytic Explorations of Art*. New York: International Universities Press, 1952.

Kümmel, F. Time as succession and the problem of duration, in *The Voices of Time*. Edited by J. T. Fraser. New York: George Braziller, 1966, pp. 31–55.

Lager, E. N., and Zwerling, I. Time orientation and psychotherapy in the ghetto. *American Journal of Psychiatry* 137:306–309, 1980.

Laing, R. D., Phillipson, H., and Lee, A. R. *Interpersonal Perception*. New York: Springer Publishing Company; and London: Tavistock Publications, 1966.

Lakein, A. *How to Get Control of Your Time and Your Life*. New York: The New American Library, 1974.

Lang, P. J., and Buss, A. H. Psychological deficit in schizophrenia. II: Interference and activation. *Journal of Abnormal Psychology* 70:77–106, 1965.

Lashley, K. S. *Brain Mechanisms and Intelligence*. Chicago: Chicago University Press, 1929.

Lashley, K. S. The problem of serial order in behavior, in *Cerebral Mechanisms in Behavior*. Edited by L. A. Jeffress. New York: John Wiley & Sons, 1951, pp. 112–136.

Lashley, K. S. Cerebral organization and behavior, in *The Brain and Human Behavior* (vol. XXXVI). Edited by H. C. Solomon, S. Cobb, and W. Penfield. Baltimore: Williams & Wilkins Co., 1958, pp. 1–18.

Lawson, J. S. McGhie, A., and Chapman, J. Perception of speech in schizophrenia. *British Journal of Psychiatry* 110:375–380, 1964.

Lazarus, A. A. Learning theory in the treatment of depression. *Behavioral Research and Therapy* 6:83–89, 1968.

Lazarus, A. A. *Behavior Therapy and Beyond*. New York: McGraw-Hill Book Company, 1971.

Lazarus, A. *In the Mind's Eye*. New York: Rawson Associates Publishers: Associates Publishers, 1977.

Lazarus, A. Styles not systems. *Psychotherapy Theory, Research, Practice* 15:359–361, 1978.

Lazarus, R. S. *Psychological Stress and the Coping Process*. New York: McGraw-Hill Book Company, 1966.

Lazowick, L. On the nature of identification. *Journal of Abnormal Social Psychology* 51:175–183, 1955.

Lee, D. Codifications of reality: lineal and nonlineal. *Psychosomatic Medicine* 12:89–97, 1950.

Leuner, H. Guided affective imagery (GAI). *American Journal of Psychotherapy* 23:4–22, 1969.

Levine, M., and Spivack, G. Incentive, time conception, and self-control in a group of emotionally disturbed boys. *Journal of Clinical Psychology* 15:110–113, 1959.

Levinson, D. J., Darrow, C. N., Klein, E. B., Levinson, M. H., and McKee, B. *The Seasons of a Man's Life*. New York: Alfred A. Knopf, 1978.

Levy, D. L., Holzman, P. S., and Proctor, L. R. Vestibular responses in schizophrenia. *Archives of General Psychiatry* 35:972–981, 1978.

Levy, L. H. *Psychological Interpretation*. New York: Holt, Rinehart and Winston, 1963.

Lewin, K. Time perspective and morale, in *Civilian Morale*. Edited by W. Goodwin. Boston: Houghton Mifflin Co., 1942, pp. 48–70.

Lewis, A. The experience of time in mental disorder. *Proceedings of the Royal Society of Medicine* 25:611–620, 1931.

Lewis, W. C. *Why People Change: The Psychology of Influence*. New York: Holt, Rinehart & Winston, 1972.

Lhamon, W. T., and Goldstone, S. Temporal information processing in schizophrenia. *Archives of General Psychiatry* 28:44–51, 1973.

Lindemann, E. Symptomatology and management of acute grief. *American Journal of Psychiatry* 101:141–148, 1944.

Linnoila, M., Seppala, T., Mattila, M. J., Vihko, R., Pakarinen, A., and Skinner, T., III. Cloripramine and doxepin in depressive neuroses. *Archives of General Psychiatry* 37:1295–1302, 1980.

Litchfield, P. M., and Sattler, J. M. An hypothesis: The existential notion of intentional time as a dimension of psychological health. *Journal of General Psychology* 79:257–270, 1968.

Luce, G. G. *Biological Rhythms in Medicine and Psychiatry*. Washington, D.C.: United States Government Printing Office, 1970.

Luce, G. G. *Body Time: Physiological Rhythms and Social Stress*. New York: Pantheon Books, 1971.

Ludwig, A. M. Altered states of consciousness. *Archives of General Psychiatry* 15:225–234, 1966.

MacAndrew, C., and Edgerton, R. B. *Drunken Comportment: A Social Explanation*. Chicago: Aldine Publishing Company, 1969.

MacKay, D. M. Self-organization in the time domain, in *Self-Organizing Systems*. Edited by M. C. Yovits, D. T. Jacobs, and G. D. Goldstein. Washington, D.C.: Spartan Books, 1962, pp. 37–48.

MacKay, D. M. Cerebral organization and the conscious control of action, in *Brain and Conscious Experience*. Edited by J. C. Eccles. New York: Springer-Verlag, 1966, pp. 422–445.

MacKay, D. M. *Information, Mechanism and Meaning*. Cambridge, Mass.: M.I.T. Press, 1969.

MacKenzie, R. A. *The Time Trap*. New York: Amacom, a division of American Management Association, 1972.

MacKinnon, R. A., and Michels, R. *The Psychiatric Interview in Clinical Practice*. Philadelphia: W. B. Saunders Company, 1971.

MacLean, P. D. Psychosomatic disease and the "visceral brain"—Recent developments bearing on the Papez theory of emotion. *Psychosomatic Medicine* 11:338–353, 1949.

Maddison, D. C., and Viola, A. The health of widows in the year following breavement. *Journal Psychosomatic Research* 12:297–306, 1968.

Magoun, H. W. *The Waking Brain*. Springfield, Ill.: Charles C. Thomas Publisher, 1963.

Mann, J. *Time-Limited Psychotherapy*. Cambridge, Mass.: Harvard University Press, 1973.

Manschreck, T. C., and Petri, M. The paranoid syndrome. *Lancet* II (July): 251–253, 1978.

Margulies, A., and Havens, L. L. The initial encounter: What to do first? *The American Journal of Psychiatry* 138:421–428, 1981.

Marks, I. M. *Living with Fear*. New York: McGraw-Hill, 1978.

Marmor, J. Short-term dynamic psychotherapy. *American Journal of Psychiatry* 136:149–155, 1979.

Maruyama, M. The second cybernetics: Deviation amplifying mutual causal processes. *American Scientist* 51:164–179, 1963.

Maslow, A. H. Peak-experiences as acute identity experiences. *American Journal of Psychoanalysis* 21:254–260, 1961.

Maslow, A. H. *Toward a Psychology of Being* (2nd ed.). Princeton, N.J.: Van Nostrand Company, 1968.

Masserman, J. H. Psychotherapy as the mitigation of uncertainties. *Archives of General Psychiatry* 26:186–188, 1972.

May, R. Contributions of existential psychiatry, in *Existence*. Edited by R. May, E. Angel, and H. Ellenberger. New York: Basic Books, 1958.

McDonald, N. Living with schizophrenia. *Canadian Medical Association Journal* 82:218–221, 1960.

McGaugh, J. L. Time-dependent processes in memory storage. *Science* 153:1351–1358, 1956.

McGhie, A., and Chapman, J. Disorders of attention and perception in early schizophrenia. *British Journal of Medical Psychology* 34:103–116, 1961.

McGhie, A., Chapman, J., and Lawson, J.S. Effect of distraction on schizophrenic performance: I. Perception and immediate memory. *British Journal of Psychiatry* III:383–390, 1965.

McIsac, W. M., Fritchie, G. E., Idanpann-Heikkila, J. E., Ho, B. T., and Englert, L. F., Distribution of marijuana in monkey brain and concomitant behavioral effects. *Nature* 230:593–594, 1971.

McPherson, F. M. Thought-process disorder, delusions of persecution and 'non-integration' in schizo-phrenia. *British Journal of Medical Psychology* 42:55–57, 1969.

Mednick, S. A. Birth defects in schizophrenia. *Psychology Today* (April):49–81, 1971.

Meehl, P. E. Schizotaxia, schizotypy, schizophrenia. *American Psychologist* 17:827–828, 1962.

Meerloo, J. A. The time sense in psychiatry, in *The Voices of Time*. Edited by J. T. Fraser. New York: George Braziller, 1966, pp. 235–252.

Meerloo, J. A. *Along the Fourth Dimension*. New York: The John Day Company, 1970.

Mefford, R. B., Jr.: Structuring physiological correlates of mental processes and states: The study of biological correlates of mental processes, in *Handbook of Multivariate Experimental Psychology*. Edited by R. B. Cattell. Chicago: Rand McNally and Company, 1967.

Meichenbaum, D. *Cognitive-Behavior Modification: An Integrative Approach*. New York: Plenum Press, 1977.

Melges, F. T. Postpartum psychiatric syndromes. *Psychosomatic Medicine* 30:95–108, 1968.

Melges, F. T. Integrating psychiatric research with clinical training: N = 1. *Journal of Nervous and Mental Disease* 154:206–212, 1972.

Melges, F. T. Future oriented psychotherapy. *American Journal of Psychotherapy* 26:22–33, 1972.

Melges, F. T. The mental status examination, in *Psychiatric Treatment: Crisis, Clinic and Consultation.* Edited by C. P. Rosenbaum and J. E. Beebe. New York: Mc-Graw-Hill Book Company, 1975, pp. 529–538.

Melges, F. T. Tracking difficulties and paranoid ideation during hashish and alcohol intoxication. *American Journal of Psychiatry* 133:1024–1028, 1976.

Melges, F. T. Psychiatric interview and approach to the patient, in *Psychiatry and Behavioral Sciences.* Edited by D. A. Hamburg, J. D. Barchas, P. A. Berger, and G. R. Elliott. Cambridge: Oxford University Press (in press).

Melges, F. T., Anderson, R. E., Kraemer, H. C., Tinklenberg, J. R., and Weisz, A. E. The personal future and self-esteem. *Archives of General Psychiatry* 25:494–497, 1971.

Melges, F. T., and Bowlby, J. Types of hopelessness in psychopathological process. *Archives of General Psychiatry* 20:690–699, 1969.

Melges, F. T., and DeMaso, D. R. Grief resolution therapy: Reliving, revising, and revisiting. *American Journal of Psychotherapy* 34:51–61, 1980.

Melges, F. T., and Fougerousse, C. E. Time sense, emotions and acute mental illness. *Journal of Psychiatric Research* 4:127–140, 1966.

Melges, F. T., and Freeman, A. M. Persecutory delusions: A cybernetic model. *American Journal of Psychiatry* 132:1038–1044, 1975.

Melges, F. T., and Freeman, A. M. Temporal disorganization and inner-outer confusion in acute mental illness. *American Journal of Psychiatry* 134:874–877, 1977.

Melges, F. T., and Hamburg, D. A. Psychological effects of hormonal influences in women, in *Human Sexuality in Four Perspectives.* Edited by F. A. Beach. Baltimore: The Johns Hopkins University Press, 1976, pp. 269–295.

Melges, F. T., and Harris, R. F. Anger and attack: a cybernetic model of violence, in *Violence and the Struggle for Existence.* Edited by D. N. Daniels, M. D. Gilula, and F. M. Ochberg. Boston: Little, Brown and Co., 1970, pp. 97–127.

Melges, F. T., and Poppen, R. Expectation of rewards and emotional behavior in monkeys. *Journal of Psychiatric Research* 13:11–21, 1976.

Melges, F. T., Tinklenberg, J. R., Deardorff, C. M., Davies, N. H., Anderson, R. E., and Owen, C. A. Temporal disorganization and delusional-like ideation: Processes induced by hashish and alcohol. *Archives of General Psychiatry* 30:855–861, 1974.

Melges, F. T., Tinklenberg, J. R., Hollister, L. E., and Gillespie, H. K. Marihuana and temporal disintegration. *Science* 168:1118–1120, 1970a.

Melges, F. T., Tinklenberg, J. R., Hollister, L. E., and Gillespie, H. K. Temporal disintegration and depersonalization during marihuana intoxication. *Archives of General Psychiatry* 23:204–210, 1970b.

Melges, F. T., Tinklenberg, J. R., Hollister, L. E., and Gillespie, H. K. Marihuana and the temporal span of awareness. *Archives of General Psychiatry* 24:564–567, 1971.

Melges, F. T., and Weisz, A. E. The personal future and suicidal ideation. *Journal of Nervous and Mental Disease* 153:244–250, 1971.

Mellor, C. S. First rank symptoms of schizophrenia. I. The frequency in schizophrenics on admission to a hospital. II. Differences between individual first rank symptoms, in *Annual Review of the Schizophrenic Syndrome.* Edited by R. Cancro. New York: Brunner-Mazel, 1972, pp. 13–29.

Meltzoff, J., and Kornreich, M. *Research in Psychotherapy.* New York: Atherton Press, 1970.

Menninger, K. *Man Against Himself.* New York: Harcourt, 1938.

Mezey, A. G., and Cohen, S. L. The effect of depressive illness on time judgment and time experience. *Journal of Neurology, Neurosurgery, and Psychiatry* 24:269–270, 1961.

Mezey, A. G., and Knight, R. J. Time sense in hypomanic illness. *Archives of General Psychiatry* 12:184–186, 1965.

Michotte, A. Causality and activity, in *Readings in Perception*. Edited by D. C. Beardslee and M. Wertheimer. Princeton, N.J.: Van Nostrand, 1958, pp. 382–389.

Miller, G. A. The magical number 7, plus or minus 2: Some limits on our capacity for processing information. *Psychological Review* 63:81–97, 1956.

Miller, G. A., Galanter, E., and Pribram, K. H. *Plans and the Structure of Behavior*. New York: Holt, Rinehart and Winston, 1960.

Miller, J. G. *Living Systems*. New York: McGraw-Hill Book Company, 1976.

Miller, L. L. Cannabis and the brain with special reference to the limbic system, in *Marihuana*. Edited by N. G. Nahas and W. D. M. Patton. New York: Pergamon Press, 1979.

Miller, M. H. Time and the character disorder. *Journal of Nervous and Mental Disease* 138:535–540, 1964.

Mills, L., and Rollman, G. B. Hemispheric asymmetry for auditory perception of temporal order. *Neuropsychologia* 18:41–47, 1980.

Milner, B. Psychological defects produced by temporal lobe excision. *Research Publication of the Association for Research in Nervous and Mental Disease* 36:244–257, 1958.

Milner, B. Some effects of frontal lobectomy in man, in *The Frontal Granular Cortex and Behavior*. Edited by J. M. Warren and K. Akert. New York: McGraw-Hill Book Company, 1964, pp. 313–334.

Minkowski, E. (1927) *La Schizophrenie: Psychopathologie des Schizoides et des Schizophrenes*. Paris: Desclee de Brouwer, 1953.

Minkowski, E. Das Zeit und das Raumproblem in der Psychopathologie. *Wien, Klin. Woch.* 44:346–350, 380–384, 1931.

Minkowski, E. (1933) *Lived Time*. Translated by Nancy Metzel. Evanston, Ill.: Northwestern University Press, 1970.

Mintz, I. The anniversary reaction: A response to the unconscious sense of time. *Journal of the American Psychoanalytic Association* 19:720–735, 1971.

Minuchin, S. *Families and Family Therapy*. Cambridge, Mass.: Harvard University Press, 1974.

Mischel, W. Preference for delayed reinforcement and social responsibility. *Journal of Abnormal and Social Psychology* 62:1–7, 1961.

Mischel, W. Toward a cognitive social learning reconceptionalization of personality. *Psychological Review* 80:252–283, 1973.

Mo, S. S., Kersey, R., and Huang, D. D. Weakness and instability of time expectancy in schizophrenia. *Journal of Clinical Psychology* 34:37–44, 1978.

Monat, A. Temporal uncertainty, anticipation time, and cognitive coping under threat. *Journal of Human Stress* 2:32–43, 1976.

Monroe, R. R. The episodic psychoses of Vincent Van Gogh. *Journal of Nervous and Mental Disease* 166:480–488, 1978.

Moos, R. H., Kopell, B. S., Melges, F. T., Yalom, I. D., Lunde, D. T., Clayton, R. B., and Hamburg, D. A. Fluctuations in symptoms and moods during the menstrual cycle. *Journal of Psychosomatic Research* 13:37–44, 1969.

Moreau (de Tours), J. *Du Hachisch et de l'alienation mentale, etudes psychologiques*. Paris: Libraria de Fortin, Masson, 1845.

Mowrer, O. H., and Ullman, A. D. Time as a determinant in integrative learning. *Psychological Review* 52:61–90, 1945.

Mowrer, O. H. *Learning Theory and Personality Dynamics*. New York: The Ronald Press Co., 1950.

Mowrer, O. H. *Learning Theory and Behavior*. New York: John Wiley & Sons, 1960.

Mullan, S., and Penfield, W. Illusions of comparative interpretation and emotion. *Archives of Neurology and Psychiatry* 81:269–284, 1959.

Nannum, A. Time in psychoanalytic technique. *Journal of the American Psychoanalytic Association* 20:736–750, 1972.

Naranjo, C. Present-centeredness in Gestalt therapy, in *Gestalt Therapy New*. Edited by J. Fagan and I. L. Shepherd. New York: Science and Behavior Books, 1977, pp. 47–69.

Needham, J. Time and knowledge in China and the West, in *The Voices of Time*. Edited by J. T. Frazer. New York: George Braziller, 1966, pp. 92–135.

Neff, W. D. Temporal pattern discrimination in lower animals and its relation to language perception in man, in *Disorders of Language*. Edited by A. V. S. DeReuck and M. O'Connor. London: Churchill, 1964, pp. 183–199.

Neisser, U., *Cognitive Psychology*. New York: Appleton-Century-Crofts, 1967.

Neugarten, B. L. Time, age, and the life cycle. *The American Journal of Psychiatry* 136:887–894, 1979.

Newell, S. Chemical modifiers of time perception, in *The Future of Time*. Edited by H. Yaker, H. Niederland, W. G. *The Schreber Case: Psychoanalytic Profile of a Paranoid Personality*. New York: Quadrangle/New York Times Book Company, 1974.

Osmond, and F. Cheek, Garden City, N.Y.: Anchor Books, Doubleday and Company, 1972, pp. 351–388.

Norman, D. A. Comments on the information structure of memory, in *Attention and Performance* III. Edited by A. F. Sanders. Amsterdam: North Holland Publishing Company, 1970, pp. 293–303.

Nowlis, V. Research with the mood adjective check list, in *Affect, Cognition, and Personality*. Edited by S. Tomkins and C. Izard. New York: Springer, 1965, pp. 352–389.

Noyes, R., and Kletti, R. Depersonalization in the face of life-threatening danger: A description. *Psychiatry* 39:19–27, 1976.

Olds, J. Pleasure centers in the brain. *Scientific American* 195:105–116, 1965.

Olds, J., Mink, W. D., and Best, P. J., Single unit patterns during anticipatory behavior. *Electroencephalography and Clinical Neurophysiology* 26:144–158, 1969.

Orme, J. E. Knowledge of the year: Brain damage and memory for designs. *Diseases of the Nervous System* 27:202–203, 1966.

Orme, J. E. *Time, Experience and Behavior*. London: Iliffe Books, 1969.

Ornstein, R. E. *On the Experience of Time*. New York: Penguin Books, 1969.

Ornstein, R. E. *The Psychology of Consciousness*. San Francisco: W. H. Freeman, 1972.

Osgood, C. E., Suci, G. J., and Tannenbaum, P. H. *The Measurement of Meaning*. Urbana, Ill.: University of Illinois Press, 1957.

Paivio, A. *Imagery and Verbal Processes*. New York: Holt, Rinehart and Winston, 1971.

Papez, J. W. A proposed mechanism of emotion. *Archives of Neurology and Psychiatry* 38:725–743, 1937.

Papp, P., Silverstein, O., and Carter, E. Family sculpting in preventive work with well families. *Family Process* 12:197–212, 1973.

Parkes, C. M. *Bereavement: A Study of Grief in Adult Life*. London: Tavistock, 1972.

Pattison, E. M., Llamas, R., and Hurd, T. Social network mediation of anxiety. *Psychiatric Annals* 9:56–67, 1979.

Pavlov, I. P. *Conditioned Reflexes*. New York: Dover, 1927.

Pearl, D., and Berg, P. S. Time perception and conflict arousal in schizophrenia. *Journal of Abnormal and Social Psychology* 66:332–338, 1963.

Penfield, W. The role of the temporal cortex in certain psychical phenomena. 29th Maudsley Lecture. *Journal of Mental Science* 101:451–465, 1955.

Penfield, W. Functional localization in temporal and deep Sylvian areas, in *The Brain and Human Behavior*. (Vol. 26.) Edited by H. C. Solomon, S. Cobb, and W. Penfield. Baltimore: Williams and Wilkins Company, 1958, pp. 210–226.

Perls, F. S. *Ego, Hunger, and Aggression*. New York: Vintage Books, 1969.

Perls, F. *The Gestalt Approach and Eye Witness to Therapy*. Palo Alto, Calif.: Science and Behavior Books, 1973.

Pervin, L. A. The need to predict and control under conditions of threat. *Journal of Personality* 31:570–587, 1963.

Peterfreund, E. *Information, Systems, and Psychoanalysis*. New York: International Universities Press, 1971.

Petrie, A. *Personality and the Frontal Lobes*. London: Routledge & Kegan Paul, Ltd., 1952.

Petrie, A. Effects of chlorpromazine and of brain lesions on personality, in *Psychopharmacology*. Edited by H. D. Pennes. New York: Harper and Row, 1958.

Pettitt, T. F. Anality and time. *Journal of Consulting and Clinical Psychology* 33:170–174, 1969.

Piaget, J. *The Psychology of Intelligence*. London: Routledge & Paul, 1950.

Piaget, J. Time perception in children, in *The Voices of Time*. Edited by J. T. Fraser. New York: George Braziller, 1966, pp. 202–216.

Piaget, J., and Inhelder, B. *The Early Growth of Logic in the Child*. New York: Harper & Row, 1964.

Pittendrigh, C. S. On temporal organization in living systems. *Harvey Lectures* 56:93–125, 1961.

Platt, J. J., and Eisenman, R. Internal–external control of reinforcement, time perspective, adjustment, and anxiety. *The Journal of General Psychology* 79:121–128, 1968.

Plutchik, R. *The Emotions: Facts, Theories, and New Models*. New York: Random House, 1962.

Polya, G. *How to Solve It*. Princeton, N.J.: Princeton University Press, 1945.

Popper, K. R. *Conjectures and Refutations*. New York: Basic Books, 1965.

Portmann, A. Preface to a science of man. *Diogenes* 40 (Winter), 1962, p. 3.

Powers, W. T. *Behavior: The Control of Perception*. Chicago: Aldine Publishing Company, 1973.

Premack, D. Toward empirical behavior laws. I. Positive reinforcement. *Psychological Review* 66:219–233, 1959.

Prescott, J. W. Neural timing mechanisms, conditioning, and the CS–UCS interval. *Psychophysiology* 2:125–131, 1966.

Pribram, K. H. Reinforcement revisited: A structural view, in *Nebraska Symposium on Motivation*. Edited by M. Jones. Lincoln, Nebr.: University of Nebraska Press, 1963, pp. 113–159.

Pribram, K. H. *Languages of the Brain*. Englewood Cliffs, N.J.: Prentice-Hall, 1971.

Pribram, K. H. Problems concerning the structure of consciousness, in *Consciousness and the Brain*. Edited by G. G. Globus, G. Maxwell, and I. Savodnic, New York: Plenum Press, 1976.

Pribram, K. H. Holonomy and structure in the organization of perception, in *Proceedings of the Conference of Images, Perception and Knowledge*. University of Western Ontario, 1976.

Pribram, K. H., and Melges, F. T. Psychophysiological basis of emotion, in *Handbook of Clinical Neurology* (vol. III). Edited by P. J. Vinken and G. W. Bruyn. Amsterdam: North Holland Publishing Company, 1969, pp. 316–342.

Pribram, K. H., and Tubbs, W. E. Short-term memory parsing and the primate frontal cortex. *Science* 156:1765–1767, 1967.

Rabin, A. I. Future time perspective and ego strength, in *The Study of Time III*. Edited by J. T. Fraser, N. Lawrence, and D. Park, New York: Springer-Verlag, 1978, pp. 294–306.

Raimy, V. *Misunderstandings of the Self*. San Francisco: Jossey-Bass Publishers, 1975.

Rapaport, D. The structure of psychoanalytic theory: A systematizing attempt. *Psychological Issues* 2:1–158, 1960.

Rees, W. D. The bereaved and their hallucinations, in *Bereavement: Its Psychosocial Aspects*. Edited by B. Schoenberg. New York: Columbia University Press, 1975, pp. 66–71.

Renner, M. Ein transozeanversuch zum zeitsinn der honigbiene. *Naturwiss* 42:540–541, 1955.

Rescher, N., and Urquhart, A. *Temporal Logic*. New York: Springer-Verlag, 1971.

Restak, R. M. *The Brain: The Last Frontier*. New York: Doubleday, 1979.

Richter, C. P. *Biological Clocks in Medicine and Psychiatry*. Springfield, Ill.: Thomas, 1965.

Riddle, M., and Roberts, A. H. Psychosurgery and the porteus maze tests. *Archives of General Psychiatry* 35:493–497, 1978.

Riesman, D. On autonomy, in *The Self in Social Interaction*. Edited by C. Gordon and K. J. Gergen. New York: John Wiley & Sons, 1968, pp. 445–461.

Rochester, S. R. Are language disorders in acute schizophrenia actually information-processing problems?, in *The Nature of Schizophrenia: New Approaches to Research and Treatment*. Edited by L. C. Wynne, R. L. Cromwell, and S. Matthysse. New York: John Wiley & Sons, 1978, pp. 329–336.

Rokeach, M. *The Open and Closed Mind*. New York: Basic Books, 1960.

Rosenberg, M. *Conceiving the Self*. New York: Basic Books, 1979.

Rothenberg, A. The process of Janusian thinking and creativity. *Archives of General Psychiatry* 24:194–205, 1971.

Rothenberg, A. Homospatial thinking in creativity. *Archives of General Psychiatry* 33:17–26, 1976.

Rothenberg, A. Einstein's creative thinking and the general theory of relativity: A documented report. *American Journal of Psychiatry* 136:38–43, 1979.

Rotter, J. B. Generalized expectancies for internal vs. external control of reinforcement. *Psychological Monographs* 80:1–28, 1966.

Rush, A. J., and Beck, A. T. Cognitive therapy of depression and suicide. *American Journal of Psychotherapy* 32:201–219, 1978.

Russell, J. L. Time in Christian thought, in *The Voices of Time*. Edited by J. T. Fraser. New York: George Braziller, 1966, pp. 59–76.

Saccuzzo, D. P., and Braff, D. L. Early information processing deficit in schizophrenia. *Archives of General Psychiatry* 38:175–182, 1981.

Sackeim, H. A., Gur, R. C., Saucy, M. C. Emotions are expressed more intensely on the left side of the face. *Science* 202:434–436, 1978.

Sagan, C. *The Dragons of Eden: Speculations of the Evolution of Human Intelligence*. New York: Ballantine Books, 1977.

Salzinger, K. The immediacy hypothesis of schizophrenia, in *The Future of Time*. Edited by H. Yaker, H. Osmond, and F. Cheek. Garden City. N.Y.: Doubleday and Company, 1972, pp. 272–292.

Salzman, L. Psychotherapy of the obsessional. *American Journal of Psychotherapy* 33:32–40, 1979.

Satir, V. *Conjoint Family Therapy*. Palo Alto, Calif.: Science and Behavior Books, 1967.

Scheflen, A. E. The significance of posture in communication systems. *Psychiatry* 27:316–331, 1964.

Scheflen, A. E. Human communication: Behavioral programs and their integration. *Behavioral Science* 13:44–55, 1968.

Scher, J. M. The depressions and structure: An existential approach to their understanding and treatment. *American Journal of Psychotherapy* 25:369–384, 1971.

Schilder, P. Psychopathology of time. *Journal of Nervous and Mental Diseases* 83:530–546, 1936.

Schmale, A. H. Relationship of separation and depression to disease: A report on a hospitalized medical population. *Psychosomatic Medicine* 20:259–277, 1958.

Schneider, K. *Clinical Psychopathology*. Translated by M. W. Hamilton. New York: Grune & Stratton, 1959.

Schoenberg, B., Gerber, I., Wiener, A., Kutscher, A. H., Peretz, D., and Carr, A. C. *Bereavement: Its Psychosocial Aspects*. New York: Columbia University Press, 1975.

Schonbach, P. Cognition, motivation, and time perception. *Journal of Abnormal Social Psychology* 58:195–202, 1959.

Schreber, D. P. *Memoirs of My Nervous Illness*. Translated and edited by I. MacAlpine and R. A. Hunter. London: Wm. Dawson & Sons, 1955.

Schwab, J. J., Chalmers, J. M. Conroy, S. J., et al. Studies in grief: A preliminary report, in

Bereavement: Its Psychosocial Aspects. Edited by B. Schoenberg et al. New York: Columbia University Press, 1975, pp. 78–90.

Schwartz, D. A. A re-view of the "paranoid" concept. *Archives of General Psychiatry* 8:349–361, 1963.

Scoville, W. B., and Milner, B. Loss of recent memory after bilateral hippocampal lesions. *Journal of Neurology, Neurosurgery and Psychiatry* 20:11–21, 1957.

Sedman, G. Theories of depersonalization: A re-appraisal. *British Journal of Psychiatry* 117:1–14, 1970.

Seeman, M. V. Time and schizophrenia. *Psychiatry* 36:189–195, 1976.

Segraves, R. T. Conjoint marital therapy: A cognitive behavior model. *Archives of General Psychiatry* 35:450–455, 1978.

Serban, G. The process of neurotic thinking. *American Journal of Psychotherapy* 28:418–429, 1974.

Shakow, D. Psychological deficit in schizophrenia. *Behavioral Science* 8:275–305, 1963.

Shapiro, D. *Neurotic Styles*. New York: Basic Books, 1965, pp. 54–107.

Sheehy, G. *Passages: Predictable Crises in Adult Life*. New York: E. P. Dutton & Company, 1974.

Shorr, J. E. *Psycho-Imagination Therapy*. New York: Intercontinental Book Corporation, 1972.

Shostrum, E. L. Time as an integrating factor, in *The Course of Human Life*. Edited by C. Buhler and F. Massarik. New York: Springer Publishing Company, 1968, pp. 351–358.

Sidman, M. Time discrimination and behavioral interaction in a free operant situation. *Journal of Comprehensive Physiology and Psychology* 49:469–473, 1956.

Siegman, A. W., and Feldstein, S. (Eds.) *Of Speech and Time*. New York: John Wiley & Sons, 1979.

Silber, J. R. The pollution of time, in *Bostonia*, Boston University Alumni Magazine, September, 1971.

Silverman, P. R. The widow as caregiver in a program of preventive intervention with other widows, in *Support Systems and Mutual Help*. Edited by C. G. Killeli. New York: Grune and Stratton, 1976, pp. 233–243.

Simon, T. W. Control systems and teleological systems. *Behavioral Science* 20:325–330, 1975.

Singer, J. L. Delayed gratification and ego development: Implications for clinical and experimental research. *Journal of Consulting Psychology* 19:259–266, 1955.

Singer, J. L. *Imagery and Daydream Methods in Psychotherapy and Behavior Modification*. New York: Academic Press, 1974.

Singer, J. L., Wilinsky, H., and McCraven, V. G. Delaying capacity, fantasy, and planning ability: A factorial study of some basic ego functions. *Journal of Consulting Psychology* 20:375–383, 1956.

Skinner, B. F. *Science and Human Behavior*. New York: Macmillan, 1953.

Smeltzer, W. E. Time orientation and time perspective in psychotherapy. *Dissertation Abstracts* 29, 1969, 3922-B.

Sollberger, A. *Biological Rhythm Research*. London: Elsevier Publishing Company, 1965.

Sommerhoff, G. *Logic of the Living Brain*. New York: John Wiley & Sons, 1974.

Speer, D. C. Family systems: Morphostasis and morphogenesis, or is homeostasis enough? *Family Process* 9:259–278, 1970.

Sperry, R. W., Gazzaniga, M. S., and Bogen, J. E. Role of neocortical commissures, in *Handbook of Clinical Neurology*. Edited by P. J. Vinken and C. W. Bruyn. Amsterdam: North Holland Publishers, 1969.

Spiegel, D. Man as timekeeper. *The American Journal of Psychoanalysis* 41:5–12, 1981.

Spiegel, H., Fishman, S., and Shor, J. A hypnotic ablation technique for the study of personality development: a preliminary report. *Psychosomatic Medicine* 7:273–278, 1945.

Spiegel, H., and Spiegel, D. *Trance and Treatment: Clinical Uses of Hypnosis*. New York: Basic Books, 1978.

Spitz, R. A. On anticipation, duration, and meaning. *Journal of the American Psychoanalytic Association* 20:721–735, 1972.

Spohn, H. E., Lacoursiere, R. B., Thompson, K., and Coyne, L. Phenothiazine effects on psychophysiological dysfunction in chronic schizophrenics. *Archives of General Psychiatry* 34:633–644, 1977.

Squires, K. C., Wickens, C., Squires, N. K., and Donchin, E. The effect of stimulus sequence on the wave-form of the cortical event-related potential. *Science* 193:1142–46, 1976.

Steffy, R. A. An early cue sometimes impairs process schizophrenic performance, in *The Nature of Schizophrenia: New Approaches to Research and Treatment.* Edited by L. C. Wynne, R. L. Cromwell, and S. Matthysse. New York: John Wiley & Sons, 1978, pp. 225–232.

Stein, M. I. *Stimulating Creativity, Vols. I & II.* New York: Academic Press, 1974, 1975.

Stein, M. I. Methods to stimulate creative thinking. *Psychiatric Annals* 8:65–75, 1978.

Stenbeck, A. Object loss and depression. *Archives of General Psychiatry* 12:144–151, 1965.

Stevens, J. R., Mark, V. H., Erwin, F., Pacheco, P., and Suematsu, A. Deep temporal stimulation in man. *Archives of Neurology* 21:157–169, 1969.

Stevenson, I., and Greyson, B. Near-death experiences. *Journal of American Medical Association* 242:265–267, 1979.

Stone, G., Callaway, E., Jones, R. T., et al. Chlorpormazine slows delay of visual short-term memory. *Psychonomic Science* 16:229–230, 1969.

Storrow, H. A. *Introduction to Scientific Psychiatry.* New York: Meredith Publishing Company, 1967.

Stotland, E. *The Psychology of Hope.* San Francisco: Jossey-Bass, 1969.

Stoyva, J., and Kamiya, J. Electrophysiological studies of dreaming as the prototype of a new strategy in the study of consciousness. *Psychological Review* 75:192–205, 1968.

Stransky, E. Zur lehre von der dementia praecox. *Zbl. Nervenheilk* 27:1, 1904.

Straus, E. W. Disorders of personal time in depressive states. *Southern Medical Journal* 40:254–259, 1947.

Stroebel, C. F. Biological rhythms in psychiatry, in *Comprehensive Textbook of Psychiatry II.* Edited by A. N. Freedman, H. I. Kaplan, and D. J. Sadock. Baltimore: Williams & Wilkins Company, 1980, pp. 211–228.

Strupp, H. H. Specific vs. non-specific factors in psychotherapy and the problem of control. *Archives of General Psychiatry* 23:393–401, 1970.

Strupp, H. H. The therapist's theoretical orientation: an overrated variable. *Psychotherapy: Theory, Research, and Practice* 15:314–317, 1978.

Sullivan, H. S. *The Interpersonal Theory of Psychiatry.* Edited by H. S. Perry and M. L. Gawel, New York: W. W. Norton & Company, 1953.

Susskind, D. J. The idealized self-image (ISI): A new technique in confidence training. *Behavior Therapy* 1:538–541, 1970.

Swanson, D. W., Bohnert, P. J., and Smith, J. A. *The Paranoid.* Boston: Little, Brown & Co., 1970.

Talland, G. A. Psychological studies of Korsakoff's Psychosis. VI. Memory and learning. *Journal of Nervous and Mental Disease* 130:366–385, 1960.

Talland, G. A. *Deranged Memory.* New York: Academic Press, 1965.

Talland, G. A. *Disorders of Memory and Learning.* Baltimore: Penguin Books, 1968.

Tart, C. T. (Ed.) *Altered States of Consciousness.* New York: John Wiley & Sons, 1969.

Teahan, J. E. Future time perspective, optimism, and academic achievement. *Journal of Abnormal Social Psychology* 57:379–380, 1958.

Tennant, F. S., and Groesbeck, C. S. Psychiatric effects of hashish. *Archives of General Psychiatry* 27:133–136, 1972.

Thacore, V. R., and Shukla, S. P. R. Cannabis psychosis and paranoid schizophrenia. *Archives of General Psychiatry* 33:383–386, 1976.

Tiger, L. *Optimism: The Biology of Hope*. New York: Simon & Schuster, 1979.

Tillich, P. *The Courage to Be*. New Haven, Conn.: Yale University Press, 1952.

Tinklenberg, J. R., Kopell, B. S., Melges, F. T., and Hollister, L. E. Marihuana and alcohol: Time production and memory functions. *Archives of General Psychiatry* 27:812–815, 1972.

Tinklenberg, J. R., Roth, W. T., and Kopell, B. S. Marihuana and ethanol: Differential effects on time perception, heart rate, and subjective response. *Psychopharmacology* 49:274–279, 1976.

Tomkins, S. S. *Affect, Imagery, Consciousness* (Vols. I and II). New York: Springer, 1962, 1963.

Trommsdorff, G., and Lamm, H. An analysis of future orientation and some of its social determinants, in *The Study of Time, II*. Edited by J. T. Fraser and N. Lawrence. New York: Springer-Verlag, 1973.

Turner, E. Hippocampus and memory. *Lancet* 2:1123–1126, 1969.

Usdansky, G., and Chapman, L. J. Schizophrenic-like responses in normal subjects under time pressure. *Journal of Abnormal and Social Psychology* 60:143–146, 1960.

Valenstein, E. S. *Brain Control: A Critical Examination of Brain Stimulation and Psychosurgery*. New York: John Wiley & Sons, 1973.

Vauhkonen, K. On the pathogenesis of morbid jealousy. *Acta Psychiatr. Scand.* 44 (suppl. 202):5–261, 1968.

Vernon, J. A., and McGill, T. E. Time estimations during sensory deprivation. *Journal of General Psychology* 69:11–18, 1963.

Volkan, V. D. "Re-grief" therapy, in *Bereavement: Its Psychosocial Aspects*. Edited by B. Schoenberg. New York: Columbia University Press, 1975, pp. 344–350.

Von Bertolanffy, L. *General Systems Theory*. New York: George Braziller, 1968.

Von Forster, H. Memory without record, in *The Anatomy of Memory*. Edited by D. P. Kimble. Palo Alto, Calif.: Science and Behavior Books, 1965, pp. 388–433.

Von Franz, M. L. Time and synchronicity in analytic psychology, in *The Voices of Time*. Edited by J. T. Fraser. New York: George Braziller, 1966, pp. 218–232.

Von Monakow, C., and Mourgue, A. *Biologische Einfuehrung in das Studium der Neurologie und Psychopathologie*. Stuttgart: Enke Verlag, 1930.

Wachtel, P. L. Psychodynamics, behavior therapy, and the implacable experimenter: An inquiry into the consistency of personality. *Journal of Abnormal Psychology* 82:324–334, 1973.

Wallace, M. Future time perspective in schizophrenia. *Journal of Abnormal Social Psychology* 52:240–245, 1956.

Wallace, M., and Rabin, A. I. Temporal experience. *Psychological Bulletin* 57:213–236, 1960.

Wallis, R. *Time: Fourth Dimension of the Mind*. New York: Harcourt Brace and World, 1966.

Walter, W. G., Cooper, R., Aldridge, V. J., McCallum, W. C., and Winter, A. L. Contingent negative variation: An electrical sign of sensory motor association and expectancy in the human brain. *Nature* 203:380–384, 1964.

Warnock, J. A., Mintz, S. I., and Tremlow, S. W. Single-case documentation of psychiatric treatment effectiveness. *Bulletin of the Menninger Clinic* 43:137–144, 1979.

Watzlawick, P. *How Real Is Real?* New York: Random House, 1976.

Watzlawick, P. *The Language of Change: Elements of Therapeutic Communication*. New York: Basic Books, 1978.

Watzlawick, P., Weakland, J. H., and Fisch, R. *Change*. New York: W. W. Norton, 1974.

Wehr, T. A., and Goodwin, F. K. Rapid cycling in manic-depressives induced by tricyclic antidepressants. *Archives of General Psychiatry* 36:555–559, 1979.

Wehr, T. A., and Goodwin, F. K. Biological rhythms in psychiatry, in *American Handbook of Psychiatry. Volume VII. Advances and New Directions*. Edited by A. Arieti and H. K. H. Brodie. New York: Basic Books, 1981, pp. 46–74.

Wehr, T. A., Muscettola, G., and Goodwin, F. K. Urinary three-methoxy-four-hydroxyphenylglycol circadian rhythm. *Archives of General Psychiatry* 37:257–263, 1980.

Weil, A. T., and Zinberg, N. E. Acute effects of marihuana on speech. *Nature* 222:434–437, 1969.

Weil, A. T., Zinberg, N. E., and Nelson, J. M. Clinical and psychological effects of marihuana in man. *Science* 162:1234–1242, 1968.

Weinberger, D. R., Torrey, E. F., Neophytides, A. N., and Wyatt, R. J. Lateral cerebral ventricular enlargement in chronic schizophrenia. *Archives of General Psychiatry* 36:735–739, 1979.

Weinstein, A. D., Goldstone, S., and Boardman, W. K. The effect of recent and remote frames of reference on temporal judgments of schizophrenic patients. *Journal of Abnormal Social Psychology* 57:241–244, 1958.

Weitzenhoffer, A. M. Explorations in hypnotic time distortions. I: Acquisition of temporal reference frames under conditions of time distortion. *Journal of Nervous and Mental Disorders* 138:354–366, 1964.

Wender, P. Vicious and virtuous circles: The role of deviation amplifying feedback in the origin and perpetuation of behavior. *Psychiatry* 31:309–324, 1968.

Wetzel, R. D. Hopelessness, depression and suicide intent. *Archives of General Psychiatry* 33:1069–1073, 1976.

Wexler, B. E. Cerebral laterality in psychiatry: A review of the literature. *American Journal of Psychiatry* 137:279–291, 1980.

Wexler, B. E., and Heninger, G. R. Alterations in cerebral laterality during acute psychotic illness. *Archives of General Psychiatry* 36:278–288, 1979.

White, R. W. Ego and reality in psychoanalytic theory. *Psychological Issues* 3:1–210, 1963.

Whorf, B. L. *Language, Thought and Reality.* Cambridge, Mass.: M.I.T. Press, 1956, pp. 57–58.

Wiener, N. *Cybernetics.* Cambridge, Mass.: M.I.T. Press, 1948.

Williams, N., and Zangwill, O.L. Disorders of temporal judgment associated with amnesiac states. *Journal of Mental Science* 96:484–493, 1950.

Wohlford, P. F. Determinants of extension of personal time. Unpublished doctoral thesis, Duke University, 1964. Ann Arbor, Michigan: University Microfilms, Inc.

Wohlford, P. F. Extension of personal time, affective states, and expectation of personal death. *Journal of Personality and Social Psychology* 3:559–566, 1966.

Wolfe, T. *Look Homeward Angel.* New York: Charles Scribner, 1952.

Woolf, L. S. *The Journey, Not the Arrival Matters—An Autobiography of the Years 1939–1969.* New York: Harcourt, Brace & World. 1970.

Wyrick, R., and Wyrick, L. Time experience during depression. *Archives of General Psychiatry* 34:1441–1443, 1977.

Yalom, I. D. *The Theory and Practice of Group Psychotherapy.* New York: Basic Books, 1970.

Yalom, I. D. *Existential Psychotherapy.* New York: Basic Books, 1980.

Yufit, R. I., Benzies, B., Fonte, M. E., and Fawcett, J. A. Suicide potential and time perspective. *Archives General Psychiatry* 23:158–163, 1970.

Zahn, T. P., Carpenter, W. T., and McGlashan, T. H. Short-term outcome, clinical improvement, and reaction time performance in acute schizophrenia, in *The Nature of Schizophrenia: New Approaches to Research and Treatment.* Edited by L. C. Wynne, R. L. Cromwell, and S. Matthysse. New York: John Wiley & Sons, 1978, pp. 273–279.

Zangwill, O. L. Some qualitative observations on verbal memory in cases of cerebral lesion. *British Journal of Psychology* 37:8–19, 1946.

Zimbardo, P. G., Marshall, G., and Maslach, C. Liberating behavior from time-bound control: Expanding the present through hypnosis. *Journal of Applied Social Psychology* 1:305–323, 1971.

Zimbardo, P. G., Marshall, G., White, C., and Maslach, C. Objective assessment of hypnotically induced time distortion. *Science* 181:282–284, 1973.

Zitrin, C. M., Klein, D. F., and Woerner, M. G. Treatment of agorophobia with group exposure in vivo and imipramine. *Archives of General Psychiatry* 37:63–72, 1980.

Author Index

Subject Index

Adjustment disorders, 51, 70–71, 287–288
Alcohol, 54–55
Altered states of consciousness, 3, 23, 24, 136, 293
Ambivalence, 71, 105, 199
  and desynchronized transactions, 91–93, 231–235
  family therapy, 276–277
  in grief, 199
Amnestic syndrome, 25, 57, 76–78
Anger, 19, 159, 222, 224–225, 230–231
Anniversary reactions, 69, 87–89, 207
Anticipation, 17, 20–24
  anticipatory alternativism, 264–265
  brain functions, 24–28
  vs. expectation, 20–21, 293
  and psychological organization, 12, 29, 32–33, 38, 45, 219, 240–241
  simultaneous processing of sequences, 23, 27–28
  and thinking, 20–24
Anticipatory control, xviii, 29, 40–42, 293
  abnormal, 42, 285–286
  central proposal about, 40–42
  normal, 284
  in psychosis, loss of, 134–135
  and time problems, impaired by, 43, 46, 72–74, 284
Anti-depressant drugs, 67, 85, 191, 204, 213
Anti-psychotic drugs, 61, 79–80, 109–110, 148, 168
Anti-social personality
  case example, 89–91
  present-orientation, 51, 70, 87, 187–190
Anxiety:
  as dread of future, 47, 215–217

  normal vs. neurotic, 222, 224–225, 227
  spirals of, 227–228, 236
  time urgency, 5
  and uncertainty, 11, 111, 215
  see also Anxiety disorders
Anxiety disorders:
  case example, 91–93
  free-floating anxiety, 221–222
  past, over-focus on, 51
  spirals in, 69, 227–228
  see also Neurosis
Aphasia, 26–27
Assessment, clinical:
  family interviews, 103–106
  of future, 106
  goals of, 75
  of rate and rhythm problems, 81–86
  of sequence problems, 76–81
  of spirals, 106
  of temporal perspective problems, 86–93
  of time problems, 74–107

Behavior modification, 119, 223, 236
Belief, 33
Biological rhythms, 9–10
  and anti-depressant drugs, 67, 112
  brain functions, 24
  definition of, 293
  lithium, slowing of, 67, 82–83, 111–112
  in psychiatric disorders, 66–67
Biopsychosocial approach, 47, 55, 75, 293
Brain, 11–12, 24–28
  and anticipation, 24–28
  brain-mind relationship, 11–13
  cerebral cortex, 25–28
  expectancy, measures of, 28
  frontal cortex, 25